The Secret

The Secret
Love, Marriage, and HIV

Jennifer S. Hirsch, Holly Wardlow,
Daniel Jordan Smith, Harriet M. Phinney,
Shanti Parikh, and Constance A. Nathanson

Vanderbilt University Press • Nashville

© 2009 by Vanderbilt University Press
Nashville, Tennessee 37235
All rights reserved
First Printing 2009

This book is printed on acid-free paper.
Manufactured in the United States of America

Library of Congress Cataloging-in-Publication Data
The secret: love, marriage, and HIV / Jennifer S. Hirsch . . . [et al.].
p. cm.
Includes bibliographical references and index.
ISBN 978-0-8265-1682-4 (cloth : alk. paper)
ISBN 978-0-8265-1683-1 (pbk. : alk. paper)
1. Marriage—Cross-cultural studies. 2. Adultery—Cross-cultural studies.
3. Marital conflict—Cross-cultural studies. 4. Husbands—Sexual behavior—
Cross-cultural studies. 5. HIV infections—Cross-cultural studies.
I. Hirsch, Jennifer S.
GN480.S43 2009
306.73'6—dc22
2009015190

Contents

Acknowledgments

Both collectively and as individuals, we've accumulated quite a list of people without whom the "Love, Marriage, and HIV" project and this book would not have been possible. The project had its genesis in Carlos del Rio's off-the-cuff remark to Jennifer in the spring of 1999 that for most women in the world, their biggest risk of HIV infection comes from having sex with their husbands. For that provocation, and for his encouragement during the sometimes daunting process of submitting an R01 grant application to the National Institutes of Health (NIH), we will be forever grateful. If Carlos was our godfather, Susan Newcomer was certainly our fairy godmother, and we were fortunate indeed to have had such a loyal and enthusiastic project officer. Although he joined us late in our journey, Michael Ames has earned our deepest gratitude for his unflagging enthusiasm for our project and for his willingness to risk taking on such an unconventionally organized approach to scholarship. We thank also our anonymous reviewers, the staff at Vanderbilt University Press (particularly Jessie Hunnicutt), and Lavina Anderson, who prepared the index.

During the initial years of this project, Bruce Knauft and Marjorie Muecke provided critical intellectual support and mentorship as its senior advisors, and we feel lucky to have counted them as part of our intellectual community as we developed the research instruments and conceptual framework, while we were in the field, and during the early processes of data analysis.

The dry phrase "administrative infrastructure" does not begin to capture the critical nature of the logistical and grants management support that made the fun part of this collaboration possible. Enormous thanks are due to Laurie Ferrell and Maria Sullivan at Emory; to Kathryn Valdes and Mayra Pabon at Columbia; to Tom Alarie at Brown; to Elaine Beffa and Gloria Lucy at Washington University in St. Louis; to Deanna Pong at the University of Toronto; and to the Department of Anthropology (and especially John Cady) at the University of Washington. Since mid-2004, the logistical complexity of our collaboration has been somewhat simplified by the fact that the Department of Sociomedical Sciences at Columbia's Mailman School of Public Health, under Richard Parker's visionary leadership, has provided such a congenial home to two of the six of us. We are grateful as well to the students who were such able note-takers at our project meetings: Jenny Higgins, Ellen Stiefvater, and Harris Solomon provided us with very detailed records of our conversations, to which we referred repeatedly during the process of carrying out the research and writing up our findings, and Sonia Alam was patient and meticulous as she compiled the final manuscript.

Each of us has also accrued our own individual set of debts over the years.

Jennifer S. Hirsch:

I thank my husband, John Santelli, for his wry humor (manifest in his frequent reminders to friends and colleagues that everything he knows about infidelity, he learned from his wife); for supporting my work by giving me "permission" to be away from home to do research, as I repeatedly had to reassure my informants in the field; and for driving with the boys and me there and back to show his support. Most of all, I thank him for his willingness to move our family to New York, where on Riverside Drive and in Sociomedical Sciences both my family and this book have found, I think, the best homes imaginable. My parents, David and Ellen Hirsch, have done so much to facilitate what frequently felt to me like an impossible task—raising semi-civilized children while working full-time—as have Araceli Rosas, Jorge Gonzalez, and Brittany Brogdon (my children's wonderful caregivers). They all deserve more thanks than I could ever begin to express.

I also thank Isaac and Jacob, who were never asked their opinion about spending six months in Mexico, where I shamelessly used them as research instruments, toting their cute little gringo selves around town in a quest to ingratiate myself with prospective informants. I learned deep lessons about embodiment and social hierarchy as I watched them shamed, little by little, into kissing the cheeks of adults they did not know by way of greeting, as proper children do. During that time, Isaac (as he never fails to remind me) suffered more than Jacob: dear little easygoing two-year-old Jacob spent the time happily eating tacos in the plaza, playing in the courtyard with our flea-bitten cats, and being taught to curse in Spanish, while already headstrong Isaac was forced to attend one of the town's public schools, where his first sentence in Spanish was "¿Tiene chile el dulce?" (Is that candy spicy?) and he suffered through The Dreaded Scissors Incident. Nonetheless, *lo que no mata endurece* (that which does not kill you makes you stronger), and I thank them both for their forbearance. To my host and dear friend in Degollado, Evangelina Garcia de Lujambio, my deepest gratitude for her friendship and for tolerating our gringo invasion, which so disrupted the calm of her lovely home.

The fieldwork itself would not have been possible without Sergio Meneses Navarro, who was a congenial and thoughtful companion during our time in Degollado—which, despite his Mexican citizenship, I think I can safely say he frequently found as unfamiliar as I did. I am grateful as well to Brenda Thompson, who both helped care for Isaac and Jacob and did the research for her own very fine MPH thesis during those six months (not to mention developing quite an ability at indoor soccer); to Estela Mata Rivera, for her warmth, sense of humor, and colorful commentary; and to Alan and Pati Lujambio, and Pepe and Blanca Lujambio, for their friendship and for opening many doors that would otherwise have remained closed. My colleagues Blanca Pelcastre and Mirka Negroni, both at Mexico's National Institute of Public Health in Cuernavaca, generously provided intellectual support throughout the course of the fieldwork.

Holly Wardlow:

I thank my parents, Lawrence and Diane Wardlow, who have never flagged in being supportive and enthusiastic about my research in Papua New Guinea despite the fact that they really wish I'd manage to dream up a project that would require many months in Venice or Aix. All my love to my partner, Ken, who put up with me being away for six months straight with almost no access to e-mail or telephone. It was very hard, and I plan on never doing that again.

Most of my thanks go to the many, many people in Papua New Guinea who enabled this research to take place. First and foremost, I am grateful that I had such wonderful research assistants: Luke Magala, Michael Parali, Ken Angobe, and Thomas Mindibi. They had very different temperaments and sometimes argued vociferously (with me and with each other) about the best approaches to AIDS prevention, but all were gifted interviewers and all brought a spirit of engaged inquiry to the project. They all were surprised by some of the things they learned from and about their peers, and their moments of surprise and confusion were educational for me as well.

Jacinta Hayabe not only provided a room at the Tari Women's Guest House for doing interviews, but also opened up her family to me, with all its warmth and complications. Joseph Warai and his staff at Community Based Health Care were invaluable: they helped me find my wonderful field assistants, provided interview rooms, and were extremely supportive of the project. Simon Thomas and Geoff Hiatt, employees of Porgera Joint Venture in Tari, were helpful and generous in myriad ways, from inviting me to dinner to providing staff, truck, generator, TV, and VCR so that I could set up an AIDS education project and then train some of their employees to take it over. I also thank Jacinta, Joseph, Simon, and Geoff for making it known that to mess with me would be to mess with them and their respective organizations and clans. They all helped to keep me safe when Tari was going through a difficult and dangerous period.

Pauline Agilo, a nurse at Tari Hospital, generously made time to talk about the HIV-positive cases she had encountered. John Reeder, director of the Papua New Guinea Institute of Medical Research (IMR) at the time, helped push through my research visa more expeditiously than would otherwise have been the case and provided me with a place to stay when I came through Goroka. Many thanks to all the friendly and helpful staff at IMR, Tari District Hospital, and the National AIDS Council.

Thanks especially to June, who visited me almost every day, brought me food she couldn't always spare, and decided to get attached to me even though she had to put up with teasing from "friends" who told her it would all just lead to grief and loss when I had to go home. Finally, "sweet electrical greetings" and all my love to Mary M. Tamia, who can never be thanked enough for being such a devoted, funny, and affectionate friend to me for all these years.

Daniel Jordan Smith:

I would like to thank my many colleagues, friends, and in-laws in Nigeria, who not only made the fieldwork for this project possible, productive, and enjoyable, but also have provided me with a second home in Nigeria during all the years I have been working there. I always have a sense of going home when I return to Ubakala, Umuahia, and Owerri.

For this study, I am especially grateful to my four research assistants: Jane Ibeaja, Frank Ehuru, Chinkata Nwachukwu, and Elizabeth Oduwai Uhuegbu. Their dedicated work made an ambitious agenda possible. In early 2009, I received an e-mail from one of them asking whether we had finally finished our book; given how hard I had pushed them, they are rightfully curious about why this part of the scholarly process is so slow. The fact that more than five years have passed since our fieldwork reinforces their regular reminders to me not to be in too much of a hurry in Nigeria. Da Chinkata, the most senior person among us, often admonished me with the observation that getting people to tell the truth takes time. My research assistants taught me much about the things we were studying by offering insights, posing challenging questions to me, and sharing many of their own life experiences. I owe them each a great debt. In May 2009, I learned that Da Chinkata had passed away. She will be missed, and I dedicate the chapter on Nigeria to her memory.

I would also like to thank my close friend and collaborator, Benjamin Mbakwem, who put me up when I stayed in Owerri, and who continually shared his wisdom about Nigeria, about AIDS, and about the ways his fellow citizens have understood and responded to the epidemic. I am likewise grateful to Dr. Benjamin Nwammadu and Dr. Eugenia Ofundu for allowing me to observe the work they do to prevent HIV and treat AIDS, and for introducing me to many remarkable men and women who willingly shared their life stories.

I must express my deep gratitude to my family in Nigeria—to Christian and Ulumna, to Moses, to Mama, and to Adanna, Ozichi, Chimezie, and Chidibere for making me so welcome and taking such good care of me. And, of course, to my wife, Ada, for providing so much encouragement for my work despite her apprehension about how my anthropology might misrepresent her people. Her fear of that reminds me of my many responsibilities as a scholar.

Finally, I want to thank Jennifer, Harriet, Holly, Shanti, and Connie for the privilege of working with such a dedicated, smart, and productive bunch of scholars. Being part of such a collegial, generous, and fun team has been the most rewarding experience of my professional life.

Harriet M. Phinney:

I would like to dedicate this research to the men and women who were willing to discuss intimate aspects of their marriages and lives in order to help us better understand marital transmission of HIV in Hanoi. I would like to thank Trinh Duy Luan, director of the Institute of Sociology at the Vietnamese Academy of Social Sciences in Hanoi, for agreeing to provide institutional support to the project.

This research would not have been possible without the enthusiasm, dedication, and assistance of Nguyen Huu Minh, vice director of the Institute of Sociology at the time. Nor would it have been nearly as much fun. Minh and I had become friends in graduate school at the University of Washington during the early 1990s, when Minh helped me pass a class in quantitative demographic methodology and I helped him with his English (assistance he really didn't need). At the time, he had spoken of wanting to conduct qualitative ethnographic research. The NIH grant for this project provided us with the opportunity to work together on a research topic both of us have long been interested in: marriage in Vietnam. As co-principal investigator, Minh managed project logistics and accompanied me to nightclubs, bars, and *cafés om*—places into which he himself would not otherwise have ventured. It was instructive to witness his reactions and to see Hanoi through his eyes.

I would like to thank our research assistants—Do Minh Khue, Duong Chi Thien, Nguyen Nga My, Dang Tanh Truc, and Pham Quynh Huong—for their kindness and humor, their interest in the research, and their creativity in locating research informants on their own initiative. Their decision to locate research subjects on their own rather than through official channels proved critical for ensuring our informants' privacy and for eliciting relatively frank responses, which my conducting research in the presence of government officials would not have achieved. Their most valuable contribution, however, did not lie simply in the ability to elicit information. Instead, by virtue of sharing a common history as northern Vietnamese who had lived through an incredibly tumultuous period, they were able to connect intimate aspects of the informants' lives to specific events of the past few decades. As a result, their interviews are rich with historical references and evoke the circumstances that informed personal desires, motivations, and decisions—insights that I as a foreigner could not have drawn. I thank them for this. I would also like to thank Tran Quy Long for transcribing all of the interview tapes.

A number of friends whom I had not seen in over eight years welcomed me back into their lives and provided spaces of kindness and warmth to me and my two children, Eli and Alana: Nguyen Huu Minh and Le Thi Hong Nga; Vu Manh

Loi; Nguyen Thi Linh, Vu Manh Cuong, and their family; Nguyen Hang Nga; David Trees and his family; Phan Thanh Hao; and Tran Thi Ngoi and Tran Van Thu. I also made a number of new friends and acquaintances who were critical in helping me understand the HIV situation and the contemporary context of sexual liaisons in Hanoi: Khuat Thu Hong, Margaret Sheehan, Tran Thi Van Anh, Pham Thi Hanh Van, Anh Anh (my *xe om* driver), and Pauline Oosterhoff. I could not have managed research with two children without Nguyen Thi Kim Thanh, who helped me take care of them and cooked delicious Vietnamese food for us. She became an invaluable source of support and a delightful friend with whom I could discuss my research findings.

Most of all, I want to thank Adam, my husband, for his willingness to let me take our two-year-old daughter and five-year-old son to Hanoi, depriving him of them for six months. It was a difficult time: MSN Messenger just didn't satisfy our desire to be all together in one place. Nonetheless, Eli and Alana have developed into intrepid travelers and keen observers of human behavior, as they demonstrated during their triumphant return to Vietnam for the December 2007 conference on "Modernities and Dynamics of Traditions in Vietnam: Anthropological Approaches" in Binh Chau. While I presented the findings from this research project, Alana networked with anthropologists from Israel, Hanoi, Australia, and New York, and Eli transcended all language barriers by schmoozing with Vietnamese scholars at conference meals.

Shanti Parikh:

My greatest debt is to the residents of Iganga, Uganda, who have with great humor and grace entertained my often culturally inappropriate questions about their sex lives. In doing research in a country so devastated by HIV, I have learned much from the selfless love people have shown to those suffering from and affected by this illness. I am humbled by their determination to lessen the burden of suffering, and it is to their cause that I dedicate my work.

I am most grateful to my spirited research team. I have been fortunate to work with Janet Kagoda and Gerald Isabirye since 1996. Moses Mwesigwa's keen insight allowed him to identify resources and navigate Iganga's social landscape, and John Daniel Ibembe and Harriet Mugulusi each added unique talents and skills to our team. With deep fondness, I remember our many laughter-filled team meetings, late-night debates, and explorations of Iganga's night scene. I thank them for making research fun. I owe special thanks to Robert Batwaula for ensuring everyone ate and rested, Ruth Nakayima for resourcefully identifying participants, and Mrs. Agaati Ojambo, my dear friend, whose strength continues to touch me. Mr. and Mrs. Isaac Basangwa provided our team with not only a lovely place to live and work but also a family to be part of.

Reverend Jackson Muteeba and Catherine Njuba at IDAAC (Iganga Development and AIDS Concern) provided invaluable assistance by connecting us with community groups. The members of NACWOLA (National Community of Women Living with HIV/AIDS in Uganda) and other HIV-positive groups in Iganga touched many people by courageously sharing their stories of survival during the community workshops we organized at the end of our research. I appreciate the mostly male leaders and members of UTODA-Iganga (Uganda Taxi Operators and Drivers Association) who shared with me their concerns about and strategies for dealing with the effects of men's extramarital liaisons on families, the community, and the spread of HIV.

Many dedicated and overworked healthcare professionals and officials helped with this project. I would like to give special recognition to Dr. David Muwanguzi, Francis Kyakulaga, the nurses at Iganga District Hospital and Mulago Hospital in Kampala, and the staff at the Uganda AIDS Commission. While conducting this research, I was affiliated with Makerere Institute for Social Research (MISR) in Kampala, and the faculty and staff at Makerere School of Public Health were instrumental in organizing my lectures based on this research. I benefited tremendously from intellectual exchanges with the faculty at both of these institutes. I also appreciate the intellectual input from my colleagues at Washington University in St. Louis.

The love of my parents carried me through the research phase of this project. My wise mother, the late Eleanor V. Parikh, called me in Uganda every Saturday morning for our "coffee conversations" and to provide sage advice. My memories of my gentle father, the late Arvind M. Parikh, and his love of intellectual inquiry still inspire me. Janet and Ma and Pa Wilson, I appreciate you being mothers to baby Jason David while I was working on this book.

Finally, to my dear husband, Jason K. Wilson, who bravely married a feminist who was in the middle of analyzing data on male infidelity: thank you for your encouragement.

Constance A. Nathanson:
My greatest debts are to Jennifer Hirsch for including me in this wonderful project from its inception, and to Jennifer, Shanti Parikh, Harriet M. Phinney, Daniel Jordan Smith, and Holly Wardlow for their generosity in so warmly welcoming me, a sociologist, into their anthropological midst. I have profited intellectually from their sharp insights and critical minds and socially from their delightful companionship. I have enjoyed every minute of it and thank all five from the bottom of my heart. As always, I owe enormous thanks to my husband, Armand Schwab, for his willingness to read whatever I write, his editorial acumen in finding every missing comma and grammatical error, and his constant support through the inevitable downs as well as ups in life and work.

Arlie Hochschild has written about the inversion of work and reproduction, whereby family feels like work and work feels like family (2003). While we will not here speak to the former, the latter is certainly true; we have all been struck by the depth of the bonds we have formed. These are intellectual, of course, so that we have come to count on Harriet's sensitivity to the power of discourse and her attention to the State; on Shanti's historically rich framing of adolescent sexuality, and her attention to both pleasure and danger in a field site in which people seemed to talk a great deal about both; on the lyricism of Holly's prose, and her piercing ability to articulate ideas that lay just below the surface of our collective discussions; on Connie's genius for abstraction and her generosity as a reader; on Dan's discipline—he is the only one of us who has never, ever, missed a self-imposed deadline—and his wide-ranging interests, which have stretched our discussions to include governmentality, corruption, and whether men who are unfaithful might still truly love their wives; and on Jennifer's creative intellect, her grantsmanship, her amazing talent for pushing without being pushy, and her firm conviction that good food is an essential ingredient of good research. Without Jennifer, none of this would have come to pass.

So yes, intellectual—but personal as well. Since the start of our collaboration, we have collectively mourned the loss of three parents and one sister; celebrated two promotions to tenure, a wedding, and the births of two sons, a daughter, and a niece; endured three institutional transitions, two of which also included transcontinental moves; shared (largely at Jennifer's urging) many, many fabulous meals; read countless drafts of each other's work; together walked the halls of Congress; enjoyed many collective presentations (including one at the 2005 American Anthropological Association (AAA) meeting during which the fire alarm went off every time Holly uttered the word "vagina"); and we have become, quite unexpectedly, each other's family. Working together has changed forever our understanding of what scholarship can be. We began this project, to be sure, looking for love—in order to study it, not to feel it. But one of the things the men and women we interviewed were looking for was a love that would acknowledge them as individuals, and make them feel seen and treasured for their own particular mix of gifts and talents and quirks, and there is perhaps no other word for the feeling we have all come to feel for one another. Our deepest thanks are to each other.

The Secret

Introduction

> Adultery is the foundation of society, because
> in making marriage tolerable, it assures the
> perpetuation of the family.
> —Henry Gauthier-Villars

Chigozie and Ihunanya married in 1994.[1] They first met in Lagos, Nigeria's huge commercial capital, where each had been a young migrant struggling to find a better life in the city. To hear them tell their story, they married because they fell in love, though they both acknowledged that it had been easier to convince their extended families they were a good match because they hailed originally from neighboring Igbo-speaking communities in southeastern Nigeria. By 2004, they had four children, had moved back to Chigozie's natal community, and had managed to cobble together a modest living through Chigozie's small business of selling medicine in his semi-rural community's urbanizing marketplace and Ihunanya's low-level civil service job in the nearby state capital. In extended interviews conducted separately with husband and wife, each described their marriage as solid and stable. Their individual narratives emphasized the joint project of raising and educating their children, the goal of developing their household economically, and the challenges of meeting their obligations to kin and community. Both described the union as a "modern marriage," drawing many contrasts with their parents' marriages. On the question of love, Ihunanya and Chigozie each said that they had married for love and that they still loved each other.

Most details of their respective accounts of their marriage coincided remarkably, but their stories diverged on the topic of extramarital sex. Their accounts differed on the facts as well as on the significance of those facts—specifically, on whether men's infidelity reflects men's commitment to their marriages. Ihunanya was emphatic: she had never had extramarital sex and said she believed that Chigozie had been faithful during their marriage as well. In contrast, Chigozie admitted to having had more than one extramarital sexual relationship; he also indicated that he knew that in at least one instance Ihunanya had suspected as much. Their accounts deviated even further when Ihunanya said that cheating would be an unacceptable breach in a love marriage, while Chigozie strongly asserted that the fact that he had had extramarital sex did not mean that he did not love his wife and family. His discretion, he said, was itself evidence of his dedication to the marriage. Both husband and wife agreed that men's extramarital sex was common—and much more common for men than for married women. They concurred that a man's infidelity was not necessarily sufficient grounds for divorce, though Chigozie insisted that his wife's infidelity would be. Similar stories turned out to be common in southeastern Nigeria: of couples who characterized their marriages as modern and based on love; of husbands who cheated on their wives but remained committed to their marriages; and of wives who said that their own husbands had not cheated on them, even as they acknowledged that men's infidelity was rampant.

As anthropologists and other scholars have long noted, marriage is a fundamental economic, social, and cultural institution in almost every known society—an institution that most people anticipate, engage in, and evaluate both individually and collectively, no matter their cultural context, social class, country of origin, ethnic group, or religious background. Further, the institution of marriage sits at the nexus of large-scale social processes and intimate life, between the concrete tasks of economic subsistence and the biological and social imperatives of reproduction, and in the unfolding of an individual's life course. As such, marriage is the focus of pragmatic strategies and behavior, and the locus of intense moral scrutiny and social preoccupation.

Across the social sciences, marriage has always been a topic of great interest, both because of what it reveals about universal aspects of the human social condition and because of the tremendous diversity of marriage customs that characterize the world's societies. In this book, we build on anthropology's tradition of engagement with marriage, providing a comparative perspective that draws on long-term research in five countries: Mexico, Nigeria, Papua New Guinea, Uganda, and Vietnam. Beyond examining the common and divergent aspects of marital customs, relationships, and experiences in the societies we have studied, we also explore how marriage has been changing in each of these settings, how these transformations have intertwined with new conceptions of and aspirations for intimacy as well as with enduring forms of gender inequality, and how all of these unfolding processes are deeply implicated in the global HIV epidemic. We are particularly concerned with the troubling fact that for many women around the world, their greatest risk of contracting HIV comes from having sex with their husbands or long-term permanent partners (Pan American Health Organization 2009). As such, we necessarily examine extramarital sexual behavior, and especially men's extramarital sexual behavior, not only because men's infidelity is implicated in the marital transmission of HIV, but also because it is central to the social organization and unequal gender dynamics of contemporary marriage across all five societies.

We break new ground by approaching the social organization of extramarital sex and the changing nature of marriage as mutually constitutive. We are not quite as cynical about the relation between marriage and infidelity as Henry Gauthier-

Villars, the nineteenth-century Parisian rake quoted at this chapter's beginning. We do, however, show that extramarital sex is an officially secret but actually widespread (and widely acknowledged) social practice, rather than something men do because their bodies demand it and women can't stop them. We take the title of this book from that secret, as we explore here the considerable efforts involved in maintaining a shared silence about just how much a part of everyday life extramarital sex is in these five very different contexts. "The secret" is one that men keep from their wives (and sometimes wives from their husbands), but it is also a secret that husbands and wives share together as they keep it from their neighbors. It seemed at times almost a secret that entire communities were trying to keep from themselves, insisting on the ideal of marital fidelity even though the conditions that promote infidelity were so clearly woven into the fabric of everyday life.

Our notion of "the secret" is in some ways parallel to that presented by Michael Taussig as "the public secret": "That which is generally known but cannot be spoken" (1999: 50). The public secret, he argues, is a powerful form of social knowledge, taking shape quite differently from the way that Michel Foucault articulated sex as a topic whose hidden-ness is everywhere revealed and regulated through discourse. This idea of "the secret"—a shared understanding about that which is both known and known to be unspeakable—finds echoes as well in Veena Das's work on national honor and the partition of India. Das calls attention to Bourdieu's distinction between official and practical kinship, and writes:

> The complete truth of marriage, as [Bourdieu] says, resides in its twofold truth—its official image, which is made up of rules and rituals, and the actual alliance, which results from the internal political functions of marriage. He gives several instances of the "self-serving" lies to which a group may give allegiance in order to conceal from itself its failure to find honorable solutions to problem cases. (Das 1995: 218–19)

By pointing to these gaps—both between what is known and can be said and between the way things are and the way they are supposed to be—Taussig, Das, and Bourdieu articulate how power is constituted, and specific interests protected, through the telling and retelling of these "self-serving" lies (Bourdieu 1990: 178). Similarly, our work explores whose interests are served and how inequality is reproduced through the keeping of these secrets. As the following chapters make clear, both men and women go to great lengths and demonstrate a clear sense of agency (albeit constrained) in their efforts to create protective silences around men's extramarital sexual behavior. While they do so to accomplish critical social goals—in particular, to construct marriages that feel privately *and* publicly successful—the collective consequence of these practices is to reproduce forms of social organization that provide men with greater access not just to the pleasures of extramarital sex but also to other valuable resources that are cultivated in socially male spaces. Conversely, do failures to keep "the secret"—either through the direct challenges of aggrieved wives in Huliland in Papua New Guinea or Iganga in Uganda, or through the HIV-prevention billboards that, in urging people to love faithfully, seek to uncover and delegitimize men's extramarital partnerships—open the door to new genres of "honorable solutions"? Framing the collectively preserved silences about extramarital sex as a fundamental part of social organization highlights the processes through which inequality is reproduced or contested.

The chapters in this book lead not just toward a deeper understanding of extramarital relations, but also toward a more comprehensive vision of the social organization of marriage and sexual behavior. The meanings and the logistics of extramarital sex are shaped by what marriage is, and vice versa, through the ways in which intersecting ideas about masculinity and femininity, livelihood possibilities, and social institutions all shape sexual desires and behavior. In other words, if we include both officially sanctioned sexuality and supposedly prohibited but nonetheless practiced sexuality within our focus, and examine the overlaps and connections between licit and illicit sexuality, we can develop a richer understanding of how marriage and sexuality vary within and across societies.

The material we present in this book is the result of a five-year collaborative research project, "Love, Marriage, and HIV: A Multisite Study of Gender and HIV Risk," supported by the US National Institutes of Health (NIH). Our study was funded during a period when recognition of the feminization of the global HIV epidemic was increasing, and this growing attention to women and HIV included a new awareness that marriage itself was a "risk factor" for many women. As medical anthropologists, we are interested in the health implications of our research. As individuals who have lived for many years and developed close personal relationships in the communities where we have worked, we feel not only obliged but in fact highly motivated to use our anthropological skills to support the response to AIDS. We have already published a number of articles that focus on the policy and programmatic lessons of our work (Hirsch et al. 2007; Parikh 2007; Smith 2007; Wardlow 2007; Phinney 2008b), and we will continue to try, as best we can, to collaborate with public health colleagues in the countries we study to make the research we do relevant to their work. We also believe, however, that our research on HIV has taught us a great deal about the connections between economic inequality, sexuality, morality, and marriage, and so in this book we have expanded our focus, moving from looking just at the public health implications of our research toward a broader exploration of these widespread changes in intimacy.

Much of our leverage in addressing these issues comes from the comparative nature of our work. As we will explain in Chapter 1, comparative ethnographic research of the kind we conducted has become relatively rare (although it is perhaps entering a renaissance). Our comparative approach runs against anthropology's predominant tradition of an individual researcher immersed in a single particular setting. Moreover, the assumptions of a comparative project can be uncomfortable in a discipline that has developed important critiques of universalizing theories and generalizations. Nonetheless, we have found the comparative endeavor to be analytically productive and intellectually gratifying. By preparing together for our research, communicating with each other while we were doing fieldwork, and sharing our findings in depth, we learned much more than we would have otherwise. Working comparatively enabled us to see the particularities and similarities in how the men and women we came to know built their sexual lives at the intersection of intense economic pressures, complex obligations to families and kin, rapidly shifting cultural contexts, and widely varying notions about love, intimacy, pleasure, and desire.

Background and Theoretical Context

Throughout this volume, we draw on and speak to many strands of our disciplinary history as anthropologists: an old and largely abandoned tradition of comparative work, the galvanizing efforts of feminist anthropologists dating back to the 1970s, the longstanding tradition of political-economic anthropology, the emerging anthropology of love and the established but still vital anthropology of sexuality, the intellectual ferment of the relatively young field of medical anthropology, and the new turn toward public anthropology, which reminds us not just to attend to power, inequality, and injustice, but also to make our research and writing accessible and useful to audiences beyond the ivory tower. In addition, we look at public health itself as a terrain of cultural contact, where culture-bound assumptions and moralities shape and constrain how theories are imported from the social sciences, so that what we know is profoundly shaped by what it is imaginable to ask. Many of the contexts, meanings, and consequences of the HIV epidemic are obscured or entirely elided when seen through the conventional lenses of public health programs. We suggest that an anthropology of public health and HIV that includes an attention to inequality and power, the insights of gender theory, and the intimate perspectives of ethnography can both provide greater analytical understanding and lay the groundwork for better public health policies and programs.

Gender and HIV

This first background section locates our work historically in relation to one of the literatures on which we will build, and calls attention to the field of public health itself as a culture-bound project. Specifically, we use the example of how gender has been conceptualized and deployed in health initiatives to highlight the fact that the culture of public health is shaped by unexamined assumptions about how societies operate and what people value. This is therefore an anthropology not just *in* public health but *of* public health—studying public health as a social field. Over the HIV pandemic's almost three decades, the way that researchers and policy-makers have thought of the intersection between gender and HIV has undergone three major shifts.

The first major shift involved drawing public attention (and funding) to the fact that women were also being infected with HIV and dying from AIDS.[2] The earliest feminist activism around HIV and AIDS was focused on taking heterosexual transmission more seriously, getting women to count both epidemiologically and in policy, which ultimately translates into funding and attention. The inclusion of women in epidemiological studies and surveillance of HIV has revealed an increasingly grim picture: in 2008, women accounted for more than half of the approximately thirty-three million individuals worldwide living with HIV or AIDS. The proportion of cases of AIDS that occur among women, however, varies significantly around the world: in sub-Saharan Africa, the most intensely affected region, nearly 60 percent of the cases occur among women, whereas in Asia the figure reaches an estimated 35 percent (UNAIDS 2008). Counting how many women are infected with HIV or diagnosed with AIDS has certainly been a necessary step toward understanding the changing shape of the pandemic: it enables us to say that the face of AIDS is, increasingly, a woman's face. However, as others have pointed out (Fullilove et al. 1990; Holland et al. 1990; Farmer 1996), the inclusion of women in epidemiological and clinical research is just a first step toward revealing the social and cultural factors that created these gendered patterns of HIV infection, and toward developing more effective prevention programs for both women and men.

During the early and mid-1990s, the second wave of research on women, HIV, and AIDS began to explore how unequal social relations between women and men shape patterns of morbidity and mortality among women. In that second wave, the emerging quantitative data served as a jumping-off point for qualitative, ethnographic, and conceptual work that explored the specific paths through which gender inequality contributes to women's risk of HIV infection both in the United States and around the world.[3] This research has been complemented by plenary speeches and innumerable reports from advocacy organizations, nongovernmental organizations (NGOs), and government agencies that have detailed the importance of taking a gendered approach to HIV prevention and, more recently, to AIDS treatment and care (Gupta, Whelan, and Allendorf 2003; Interagency Coalition on AIDS and Development 2005; Greene 2006). The "relative dearth of attention to the needs of women in behavioral and prevention research on HIV/AIDS" noted by Amaro in 1995 certainly no longer exists.

In the pandemic's third decade, prevention-oriented HIV research has come to explore how gender inequality shapes both men's and women's risk of exposure to HIV. Most women who have HIV were infected sexually, and any exploration of why those infections have occurred runs quickly into the fact that men's behavior is a critical element of women's risk. The acknowledgment that men have gender too has drawn on academic work, both from the insight from feminist social science that any real understanding of gender as a system of social inequality will involve analysis of how men contribute to and are affected by that system (Connell 1995), and from the evolving field of "men's studies" (e.g., Kimmel 1987) that has been producing a new generation of scholars who specialize in the study of men *as gendered men*. This new attention to masculinity—a socially and historically variable set of notions about the ideal qualities and behaviors a man would embody—has represented an important innovation in both applied and theoretical social science.[4]

The focus on masculinity as a line of scholarly inquiry in HIV research and as an aspect of HIV programming, however, diverges in critical ways from the transformational promise of the original feminist impulses on which it draws. The preponderance of current work on gender conceptualizes masculinity as simply an attitude or a set of beliefs.[5] This emphasis on ideology as the aspect of gender toward which interventions must be directed has both strategic and intellectual limitations. As an intervention strategy, trying to remake masculinity by encouraging men to develop their critical consciousness about gender is an individual-level approach that ignores the structures of constraint in which they operate. It is certainly true that critical consciousness about one's own role in systems of inequality can potentially become a key element in social transformation, and it is also true that the men who are the focus of this genre of gender and HIV work may exercise considerable power over their wives and children. Nevertheless, to prioritize the necessity of transforming the hearts and minds of some of the globe's least powerful individuals—without considering the ways in which these men's own limited life choices relate to global patterns of power and consumption—seems to us just one more example of framing risk as the product of "exotic" or "primitive" cultures rather than social and global inequalities (Parker and Easton 1998; Farmer 2001; Schoepf 2001). The recurring reliance on ideological and educational interventions reflects the culture of public health in the United States over the last few decades, characterized by a politically conservative emphasis on individual responsibility and personal choice (Watney 1999).

The notion that men's ideas about masculinity influence their behavior certainly represents an advance over biologically essentialist modes of explanation. This more ideational or cognitive approach to gender, however, excludes institutions such as labor markets and family law (to name just two) that have played such critical roles in creating different opportunities and access to resources for men and women. Gender is, in part, in people's heads—in shared ideas about what makes a man or a woman admirable and successful—but it is not all in their heads. Further, the categorization of gender ideologies into "traditional" and "modern" implies a linear process of cultural evolution contradicted by even the most cursory observation as well as recent anthropological theorizations of culture. A focus solely on gender roles or ideologies also ignores the contributions of performance theory, which emphasizes the fluid and situational nature of gender and directs our attention to the strategic way in which people create gendered self-presentations that may vary depending on the context. In sum, the ideological or cognitive approach to gender often used in public health prevention research fails to attend to critical questions of social structure and individual agency. Throughout this volume, we work to reintegrate the field of gender and HIV with the theoretical insights generated by the broader social science of gender.

Public Health, Stigma, and Sexual Moralities

Globally funded HIV prevention interventions have themselves become part of the social and ideological terrain upon which people negotiate gender dynamics, intimacy, and sexual meanings. This does not just mean that public health programs can shape behavior by affecting shared norms. Rather, as Vincanne Adams and Stacy Pigg (Pigg 1997; Adams and Pigg 2005) have demonstrated, these seemingly objective, nonjudgmental programs also unintentionally shape ideas about what constitutes "normal" sexual practice, transforming sex into an object of moral management and making public health discourse an intrinsic part of how people's sexualities are constituted. Similarly, the social and cultural landscapes in each of the settings where we have worked, particularly with regard to people's interpretations and behavioral responses to the AIDS epidemic, have been increasingly reshaped by the policies, programs, and interventions of the global public health industry. However generous and good the intention of these public health interventions, they may generate widespread consequences that range significantly beyond the initial stated aims. Indeed, in many instances, public health strategies and activities have heightened gendered tensions, exacerbated stigma, and obscured political and economic issues in favor of overly cognitive and individualistic approaches.

In both reactionary and progressive ways, public health communications such as billboards and radio spots have sought deliberately to shape shared perceptions of acceptable and unacceptable sexual behavior in order to improve population health. However, these campaigns sometimes have unexpected behavioral outcomes. In Uganda and Nigeria, some prevention messages have linked risky behavior with immorality, leading people to hide or conceal their actions instead of changing them. In Vietnam, HIV prevention efforts have been severely hampered by their association with government efforts to root out what it calls "social evils" such as drug use and prostitution, which has led some to believe that sexual partners are free of risk as long as they do not engage in these particular vices.

On a more positive note, a recent national campaign in Mexico spread the message that homophobia is a disease and linked the rights of sexual minorities with the prevention of HIV transmission. Its rollout was followed by gay pride parades in locations where they had not previously occurred (some organized by individuals who had been trained as part of that sexual rights project), underlining the potential progressive social and cultural consequences of public health interventions.

Gender, Love, and Marriage

Over nearly four decades, the anthropology of gender has grown into a vibrant area of study, moving far beyond its original emphases on including women's voices and exploring the historical origins of gender inequality in order to transform it. The field has shifted from a strict binarism to the exploration of a spectrum of gendered possibilities; from a concern with socially structured roles to analyses of culture, performance, and political economy; and from a narrow localism to a concern with gender as a dialectical construction of both local and global forces. Western anthropologists have also grown more aware of the ways in which our own assumptions about what equality and oppression look like have shaped and limited our research. Current empirical work on gender inequality necessarily and simultaneously explores the intersections between gender and other axes of social inequality such as race, ethnicity, and class.

Frequently absent from the social science of gender, however, is an adequate exploration of how intimacy is negotiated in the context of these multiple forms of inequality. Thus, our focus on love, affect, and sexuality represents a major distinguishing feature of our approach to gender and HIV. In investigating the ways in which men's and women's ideas about love—and their efforts to express this love—shape both extramarital sex and HIV risk, we draw on the growing ethnographic literature on love as an element of modern kinship as well as on limited prior work that looks at emotion and sexual risk (e.g., Kline, Kline, and Oken 1992; Sobo 1995a, 1995b; Worth 1989). We draw in particular on the work of Raewyn Connell (1987, 1995), which we have found useful for its theorization of gender regimes as constituted by the intertwining domains of power, work, and emotion/desire.[6]

Our work also intersects with the burgeoning theoretical and empirical social science literature on modernity. In particular, there are important links between the globally echoing ideology of companionate marriage and three key dimensions of modernity: individualism, commoditized social relations, and narratives of progress, particularly the way in which gender is deployed as a trope to represent progress or its lack. Elsewhere, we have written extensively about how men and women strategically build identities and relationships in relation to shared ideas about the moral nature of historical change, and how they use gendered idioms to express their yearning for modernity or their melancholy at the waning of tradition (Smith 2000; Hirsch 2003a; Parikh 2005; Phinney 2005; Hirsch and Wardlow 2006; Wardlow 2006; Padilla et al. 2007; Knauft 2002). To varying degrees, the chapters in this volume address questions about how people self-consciously locate very diverse experiences of intimacy in relation to narratives of historical change and progress.

The History of Love (in Recent Social Science)

Ethnographic research in diverse locations has noted a shift toward a marital ideal characterized by sexual and emotional intimacy and somewhat less hierarchical relations between the sexes.[7] This widespread emergence of companionate marital ideals (Hirsch and Wardlow 2006; Padilla et al. 2007) should not be understood as signaling some sort of global cultural convergence; rather, similar structural conditions (such as increasing urbanization and declining fertility) have combined with ideological influences (such as religious missionizing and media glorification of romantic love) to create comparable social forms around the world. The specific ideas and practices associated with these marital partnerships suggest that there is considerable diversity in interpretations of similar ideals. In Mexico, for example, shared sexual pleasure is understood to be among the critical characteristics of companionate marriage (Hirsch 2001, 2003a) whereas in Nigeria, Papua New Guinea, and Uganda, models of companionate marriage place more stress on sharing household economic decisions and eating and sleeping together (Smith 2001; Wardlow 2006; Parikh 2007). Across the five field sites represented by this project, heterosociality—the idea that spouses should be social companions who share some degree of emotional intimacy—is a key characteristic of these modern marriages.

Our interest in companionate marriages derives from our awareness—based on a wide range of social science research—that there is a growing hegemony of companionate ideologies around the world. Thus, we explore the dynamics of marital HIV risk within this increasingly prominent cultural form. In some circumstances, love seems to exacerbate risk: our research suggests that the companionate ideal may encourage women to ignore evidence of infidelity and to adopt a strategy of unilateral monogamy as a (not very effective) method of HIV prevention. Elisa Sobo provided early evidence of the relevance of monogamous ideals to risk behavior in her seminal 1995 description of how African-American women's investment in the fiction of mutual monogamy contributes to their reluctance to negotiate for condom use in committed relationships.[8] That work, however, neglected to explore men's experiences of these committed relationships and did not extend its analysis to examine the implications of HIV-risk denial for the global pandemic. The potential salience of love as a risk factor also reflects the relatively robust finding that around the world, the individuals with whom sex workers are most likely to want to use condoms are those with whom they share no affective tie (Pilkington, Kern, and Indest 1994; Mgalla and Pool 1997; Warr and Pyett 1999; Wong et al. 2003; Murray et al. 2007). Although this research on sex workers is not generally used as a lens through which to understand gendered experiences of sexual risk more broadly, it is part of the same widely shared cultural element of modernity in which sexual intimacy is a key arena for the construction and demonstration of emotional closeness.

As cultural anthropologists, we seek to compare and contrast the social processes that have contributed to these striking similarities in ideas about love and marriage, and to look at differences in the emerging models of marital love, with a particular focus on the implications of the companionate ideal for the marital balance of power. Women frequently perceive companionate marriage to be inherently more beneficial than older marital forms (Cole 1991; Collier 1997; Rebhun 1999; Hirsch 2003a). Although love may blunt the edge of socially structured inequalities in power, or even give women a moral language through which to make claims about rights (Mahoney 1995; Petchesky and Judd 1998; Solomon, Yount, and Mbizvo 2007), it can also recruit women to subservient roles, encourage them to embrace ideologies of female suffering and forbearance (Rebhun 1999), or weaken their access to key resources such as female kin (Feldman-Savelsburg 1994; Collier 1997). The emphasis on emotional satisfaction may even undermine a woman's bargaining power, as a woman's partner could use it to justify his desire to walk away from marriage and fatherhood.

Some of the ethnographic research on love has explored it as a means of creating and fostering kinship ties, and as part of a broader shift toward individualism (Collier 1997; Ahearn 2001), within which marriage has become a project for satisfying personal desires rather than a means of satisfying family obligations. A mostly separate body of work has looked at the intersections of affect and more explicitly transactional sex (Mann 2000; Brennan 2004; Reddy 2005; Bernstein 2007; Brennan 2007; Chen 2007; Padilla 2007; Padilla et al. 2007).[9] In this latter literature, men and women use emotional closeness strategically in their quest to transform casual relations into more permanent ones. Here, we draw together the work on love as structure and love as strategy to look at love in relation to both marital and extramarital intimacy.

The Social Organization of Extramarital Sex

In this volume, we take up a domain of practice—extramarital sex—that has received little anthropological attention as such, and endeavor to place it in relation to the broader corpus of sexuality studies. During the 1990s, the social science of sexuality moved from examining the social and cultural organization of sexuality to analyzing the sexual organization of society. In the past, researchers had focused on the variation of practices and ideologies among groups whose non-normative behavior had made them visibly in need of explanation; until recently, heterosexuality had been largely ignored, left as the neutral, normative reference category rather than being held up to examination as a social and cultural construct. For example, with nods to Adrienne Rich's foundational work in this area (1980), both Connell and Roger Lancaster have written about heteronormativity as a fundamental aspect of social organization (Lancaster 1992; Connell 1995).

In this volume, we reweave the anthropology of sexuality into the anthropologies of kinship and gender, looking at how people use intimacy strategically in their lives even if they are not having sex to make babies. In particular, we explore across five varied settings how men use sexuality to build relations with each other. The chapters that follow extend previous work on homosociality by showing how men navigate the tensions between participating actively in these semi-public sites for extramarital relations and upholding their reputations in their communities as upstanding citizens and good husbands.[10] This calls attention to how both men and women invest quite deliberately in building sexual reputations for public consumption—and sometimes the public for whom they strive to present a façade of fidelity includes a spouse. Sexuality is conceptualized as a domain in which it is possible to explore the tensions between social structure and agency—in which people can exercise some agency even in very constrained social circumstances. We also take heed—or at least try to—of Connell's critique of the disembodied and overly abstract nature of most theorizing on sexuality (the brain may be a sexual organ, after all, but it is certainly not the only one) and so seek to portray sexuality as not just an act of cognition.

Within anthropology, there is little work about infidelity per se, with the exception of Barbara de Zalduondo and Jean Maxius Bernard's important 1995 essay, which presents a detailed social and economic explication of both conjugal and extramarital relationships in Haiti. Anthropologists have not been silent about infidelity, but rather have tended to see men's and women's extramarital partnerships as an element of the broader social organization of sexuality and thus not a phenomenon particularly deserving of research as a topic in and of itself. To the extent that ethnographic research on sexuality has featured description and analysis of extramarital sex, the emphasis has been on the connection between ideological aspects of gender inequality and gendered differences in the occurrence and meanings of extramarital relations; less attention has been paid to the socially productive nature of these forms of sexual intimacy.

This is in striking contrast to the fairly extensive writings on infidelity and extramarital sex within psychology and demography, where scholars have approached extramarital sex as the result of a breakdown in an expected order, a deviation from the norm, or sometimes the product or evidence of natural and primordial differences between the two sexes. There is a large body of demographic work in English on infidelity, analyzing population-based data to describe the social and demographic correlates of extramarital sexual behavior.[11] Psychological research on infidelity, not surprisingly, approaches it primarily within a framework of intra- and inter-personal determinants, focusing primarily on how it should be "treated" therapeutically, on how it can be prevented through "infidelity-proofing" a relationship, and on the characteristics of the personalities and partnerships most susceptible to it.[12] As we conducted the research on which this volume draws, however, we gradually realized that in many settings, extramarital sex (particularly for men) is the socially determined "default" option—the normal (though not perhaps the normative) behavior—and that the behavior that demanded explanation, in contrast, was marital fidelity.

Instead of conducting research specifically on extramarital sex, cultural anthropologists have written a great deal on kinship systems. This work describes the varied patterns of what constitutes ideal (and actual) families and households around the world; how new families are formed; the flow of rights, resources, and obligations across those lines of kinship; how relatedness is constructed in culturally variable ways not always grounded in biology; and (increasingly) how kinship forms are transformed by the changing political-economic, ideological, and technological terrain of everyday life.[13] In this volume, we approach extramarital sexuality as a phenomenon best understood in its social organizational relationship to marriage, family, and kinship. Indeed, in our interviews and discussions with men and women across all five settings, the local understandings, desires, anxieties, unwritten rules, strategies, and perceived consequences of infidelity were deeply embedded in contexts and discourses that privileged both the idioms and social structural realities of kinship. By approaching extramarital sex as a feature of social life rather than as an aberration, we think we have achieved a more accurate and nuanced understanding.

Analytical Framework

Working comparatively, one of our goals was to develop concepts and theoretical understandings that would usefully enable us to identify and explain commonalities among five very distinct contexts—the urban capital of Vietnam, a rural migrant-exporting village in Mexico, the highlands of Papua New Guinea, interconnected rural and urban communities in southeastern Nigeria, and a small town along the Trans-Africa Highway in east-central Uganda—while at the same time highlighting and understanding the nature of differences across these sites. Central to our analysis is the notion that in each of these cultural contexts, extramarital sex is a fundamental aspect of social organization. To develop this claim, we frame our work using three analytical concepts: (1) extramarital opportunity structures, (2) sexual geographies, and (3) social risk. These concepts are briefly introduced here, and then further explicated in the five ethnographic chapters.

Extramarital Opportunity Structures
Across all five sites, social organization clearly facilitated men's access to extramarital sex. By calling these elements of social organization "extramarital opportu-

nity structures," we emphasize the ways that meso- and macro-level factors enable men's participation in extramarital relations. In doing so, we draw attention away from the choices made by individuals and stress instead the factors that shape and constrain the options from which they may choose. In contrast to a narrowly economic notion of opportunity structures, we use the term to encompass the social, symbolic, and moral aspects of how society's structures shape behavior. Some of these extramarital opportunity structures were common to all the sites, while others were specific to only one or two. Several of the most common and consequential extramarital opportunity structures are introduced here.

THE DIVISION OF MARITAL LABOR

The gendered social organization and interpersonal dynamics of marriage itself are fundamental aspects of these extramarital opportunity structures. Despite increasingly widespread ideals that emphasize marriage as a site of shared pleasure and intimacy, the fact that women continue to bear primary responsibility for both the care of young children and the household creates opportunities for men to seek pleasure and companionship elsewhere.[14] This is important because, as discussed earlier, to the extent that extramarital sex has been theorized at all within social science, it has been approached as a breakdown of social organization rather than as an element of kinship or an unintentional result of social policy—as an individual, antisocial behavior rather than part of the fabric of society.

For instance, Vietnam's rapidly changing economic climate provides a particularly acute example of the ways that a gendered division of labor in marriage has facilitated men's access to extramarital sex. Women are socially rewarded for being good mothers in ways that privilege the maternal over the marital, thus encouraging them to spend time with their children rather than with their husbands. Men, for their part, are faced with the challenge of mastering the intricacies of a newly emerging market-driven economy in order to shepherd their families safely through this period of rapid social change. One of the specific forms this challenge has taken is the idea that a successful Vietnamese man must express his "modernness" by seeking a wide range of sexual experiences—frequently with someone other than his wife. Women's child-oriented and men's market-oriented kinship obligations create spaces for infidelity.

Ideologies of love and marriage have played a central role in maintaining "the secret"—a sexual regime in which the commonness of extramarital partnerships coexists with a shared commitment to deny their existence. Our comparative work has its genesis in our recognition of the striking resonances across these five very diverse settings in how men and women talk about marriage as something that (in theory, if not always in practice) could be a sphere for individual satisfaction and self-realization, and for the construction of bonds of intimacy in addition to those of obligation. We found that a man's and woman's commitment to the appearance of a successful marriage can lead to a sort of collusion where the man demonstrates his love through discretion rather than fidelity, and the woman works hard to ignore the evidence so as not to shatter the illusion.

LABOR MIGRATION AND ECONOMIC INEQUALITY

As people try to address their obligations to their families against a backdrop of economic hardship, they are often compelled to engage in work-related migration—that is, to be professionally "mobile"—which has facilitated access to extramarital sex in diverse ways. In both Mexico and Papua New Guinea, migration policies and practices have specifically limited women's ability to accompany their husbands and thus exacerbated the risk of migration-related infidelities. The relation between mobility and sexual opportunity includes work that is itself mobile, in professions such as taxi and transport work, which creates opportunities for brief liaisons because access to vehicles means access to potential partners. It includes longer-term labor migration as well, which places men in settings where they crave partners to provide some of the comforts of home (not just sex, but also food and company) to ease the separation from family. This finding about labor-related mobility goes beyond the old saying about a sailor with a girl in every port (which draws attention to the sailor's individual practices), and focuses on how (at least in that case) multiple partnerships are facilitated by naval commerce and warfare. By emphasizing how multiple partnerships are enabled by the fact that men and women all over the world must travel to find the work they need to survive, we point out the inextricable links between "private," intimate behavior and "public" patterns of production and consumption that rely on relatively low-paid labor, particularly in the extractive, agricultural, and service sectors.

Wage labor and economic inequality are critical elements of the terrain facilitating extramarital sex, in ways that extend beyond the case of labor migration. For young Igbo women in Nigeria, success has become increasingly defined by one's achievements as a consumer; incessant exposure to advertising, coupled with relatively limited economic opportunities, makes these young women easy marks for men who have their own need for ostentatious display. In Uganda, married men's economically determined inability to provide adequately for their wives and children makes it all the more tempting for them to spend time with women whose expectations are lower and thus more easily satisfied. Examples could be drawn from Papua New Guinea, Vietnam, and Mexico as well; while they would differ in the specifics, they too would demonstrate the complex and overdetermined relationship between capitalist economic development, wage labor, and men's access to multiple sexual partners.

MASCULINITY, HOMOSOCIALITY, AND PEER GROUPS

In each setting, we found that men's extramarital sexual behavior was frequently at least in part a performance of masculinity for other men. In some instances, such as in the all-male outings of businessmen in Hanoi or mine workers in Papua New

Guinea, peer pressure played a major role in men's decisions to have extramarital sex. In other cases, such as in bars, discos, and social clubs in Mexico and Nigeria, men clearly aimed to affirm their masculinity to fellow men by displaying and entertaining their female lovers in these social spaces. In Nigeria, where men shared stories with each other about their extramarital sexual experiences, the honorific nicknames the men gave to each other that sometimes alluded to sexual prowess exemplified the social rewards of infidelity. In small-town Uganda, boasting about extramarital liaisons was dangerous because news spread quickly, but that did not mean there was no talk of sex: men's joking was full of emasculating nicknames for men who did not have additional lovers to take care of their (assumed) multiple needs. In other words, it was less that extramarital sexuality was actively promoted in men's peer groups, and more that men's monogamy was critiqued as being socially unproductive, limiting, and at times almost impossible, given the wider economic and social realities.

Gender and social class intertwine, so that in most cases, the participation of men in extramarital sexual relations could be accurately described both as performances of masculinity and performances of social class. Indeed, in Papua New Guinea, poor rural men often argued that when they paid women for sex, they were only doing what rich men did but with less money—and they supported these assertions by conjuring up images of urban politicians drinking at glamorous poolside bars. In Mexico, men endeavored to buy the most expensive sex they could afford. For some, this meant seeking out a smooth-skinned beauty from Eastern Europe, while for others "luxury" meant a bar that was nice enough to have running water; these were moments of self-fashioning, in which men used consumption practices to create themselves—not just as men but as men of a certain class. Class, gender, sexuality, intimacy, kinship, and morality were bound up and revealed in the social organization of extramarital sex.

Sexual Geographies

Extramarital opportunity structures are manifest spatially through sexual geographies. Many of the social structures shaping risk correspond to actual physical spaces, making it possible to conceptualize a topography of sexual risk. This is not an entirely new idea—earlier scholars have focused on the Trans-Africa Highway, for example, and on condom promotion in gay bathhouses—but here we advance their work by emphasizing not just the idea of a physical place but also a socially meaningful space. These sexual geographies call attention to the ways in which spaces organize or even incite behavior, denaturalizing the idea that men engage in multiple partnerships because of some naturally occurring bottomless well of lust.

The analytical utility of the concept of sexual geographies is derived from the ability to think about sexual behavior within a space—a space that is given meaning by social realities such as gender, generation, social class, and shared moralities, as well as by economic realities such as the commodification of leisure time and men's greater disposable income. Thus, not only are sexual geographies such as the Trans-Africa Highway created by particular economic and material conditions, but they are also constructed and navigated socially and symbolically. The symbolic dimensions of space—in particular, how places are morally defined vis-à-vis kinship and gender—can be powerful factors in shaping behavior. For example, in the Huli-speaking highlands of Papua New Guinea, one of the principal venues where married men can find extramarital partners is the *dawe anda* (literally, "courtship house"), a male-dominated ritual space where stigmatized women are said to "belong to no one" and are thus available to these men. Likewise, there are outdoor drinking areas in Iganga, Uganda, where men freely entertain lovers and socialize intimately with women brewers because men assume they are not likely to encounter their own wives in these locales. In other words, while in these spaces, people are temporarily exempted from specific kinship obligations; they step outside the social and moral system that governs marriage, rendering extramarital liaisons socially safer.

In each of the societies we studied, much of everyday life is gender-segregated. In Mexico, as throughout Latin America, the street is conceptualized as a male space and the house as a female one. Papua New Guinea presents a more extreme case: husbands and wives often live in different houses, and they address the tasks of biological and social reproduction with some trepidation, with the sexual act itself viewed as potentially polluting (particularly for men). At the same time, men's mobility in the context of mining industries and the rise of wage labor has created situations that not only offer new opportunities for infidelity, but have diminished, at least partly, the compelling nature of customary sexual-avoidance taboos and restrictions. Similarly, in southeastern Nigeria, much of social life can be described as sex-segregated. The venues where married men meet, entertain, and show off their younger extramarital lovers are typically male-dominated social spaces such as bars, nightclubs, and social and sports clubs. Even brothels in Nigeria are organized as male-oriented spaces, such that a man will often interact with other men in a semi-public bar as he selects a sex worker whom he will accompany to her room. These male-dominated social spaces facilitate extramarital sex by providing an encouraging audience for these performances of masculinity. Infidelity feels safer, too, in these protected spaces where men's wives (as well as other women connected to men's kinship and community groups) are not likely to appear and create scandals.

The concept of sexual geography highlights the role of economic organization in shaping sexual risk. In Iganga, the small east-central town in Uganda, a distinct, gendered sexual geography emerges each evening as the town gradually transforms from its lively daytime economy as a center for trading and business into a bustling center for quite a different sort of exchange. Once the married (and other "proper") women have returned to their homes for evening chores, the town's dim lighting and twisting alleyways provide men and "racy" women with the perfect labyrinth through which they can wander virtually unseen. Along the Trans-Africa Highway, the region's main artery for trade, a row of outdoor eateries, pool halls, discos, and bars offer entertainment and distraction for truck drivers, local and transitory businessmen, and unmarried young women. The loud music and the consumption of beer, roasted meat, soda, and liquor contribute to an ideal setting for various transactions, including sexual, between men and often younger women. In Hanoi, under Doi Moi, the urban landscape has become inundated with establishments that provide a variety of sexual services for men.[15] Men can choose from a number of places where they will be offered the opportunity for sexualized encounters with women, either as venues at which to purchase sex or as spaces where lovers can go for privacy, including rest houses, nightclubs, and massage parlors (to name just a few), all of which have become increasingly visible as Vietnam embraces the notion of a market economy.

A further element of the social organization of sexual space in both Mexico and Vietnam is the intricate balance between the intense heteronormativity of everyday life and the relatively frequent occurrence of sexual relations between men. In Vietnam and Mexico, compulsory heterosexuality is a critical part of the terrain within which men find sexual pleasure outside of marriage. All five contexts could be characterized as strongly heteronormative, but in Mexico and to some extent Vietnam that heteronormativity coexists with instances in which men express (and act on) their sexual desire for other men. This is not to say that sex between men is absent from the other sites, but rather that its contours and locations did not appear at the time of our study to have become routinely patterned in a way that was easily visible to us in the sexual landscape. The fact that men in all of our research settings are essentially forced to marry in order to achieve adult status—thus making long-term, publicly acknowledged relations between men that would combine social, sexual, and affective elements nearly impossible—means that men's sexual relations with each other are necessarily sub-rosa, and thus confined to clearly articulated spatial contexts within which they are socially safe.

Social Risk

Our third analytical lens calls attention to the importance of social risk in shaping sexual behavior. We use the concept of social risk to make sense of behaviors commonly misunderstood as unhealthy, uneducated, or irrational within the narrow individualistic and biomedical conceptualization of risk which has dominated public health approaches to the prevention of HIV. We are also writing against the notion that practices with detrimental health effects can be facilely attributed to "culture," implying a concept of culture that locates the causes of behavior in some sort of primordial and unchanging tradition. As developed here, the notion of social risk provides a more complex analytical framework that situates behavior in political-economic, social, and cultural contexts and acknowledges these contexts as changing, power-laden, and often contradictory.

The concept of social risk highlights how men and women who put them-selves "at risk" of HIV infection are engaging in behaviors that generally make good sense in a particular social and cultural context. People are navigating op-portunities and constraints that are often economically, socially, and culturally more salient, significant, and obviously consequential than the biomedical risk of HIV infection. In short, they are prioritizing social risks above the biomedical risk of HIV. Rather than seeing people who make these choices as promiscuous, irrational, or uneducated slaves to culture and tradition, it is more accurate to see them as reacting sensibly to the circumstances in which they live.

In many instances, it is the fear of losing access to important social resources rather than the fear of viral infection that seems to be the strongest influence on practices. Concretely, for example, this means that in Mexico, men perceive "dangerous sex" to be infidelity that is public enough to cause humiliation either to themselves or to their wives; safe sex conversely means sex that can be safely hidden rather than sex that carries no viral or bacterial risk. Socially safe sex in Vietnam is that which poses no risk to the economic foundation of the nuclear unit and to family happiness. As a result, it is more socially acceptable for Viet-namese men to visit a sex worker (who is an epidemiological risk) rather than to take a lover (who is a potential financial risk due to the possibility of emotional and economic demands). Similarly, among the Huli in Papua New Guinea, socially safe sex is that which poses no risk to a man's clan. A man who is caught having sex with a married woman can expect his whole clan to be threatened with warfare by the woman's husband's clan, or with the retaliatory rape of female clan members and demands for compensation for the "theft" of a woman who already "belongs" to someone. Not surprisingly, Huli men typically limit their extramarital partners to widows and sex workers. Ugandan and Nigerian conceptualizations of "safe sex" echo those found in Mexico, with one troubling wrinkle: the barrage of com-munication campaigns associating the risk of HIV with illicit, immoral sex have made condoms something to be avoided, and thus "safe sex" has come to mean sex that is presumptively and apparently monogamous rather than sex that is actu-ally monogamous. Rather than using a condom as an element of safe sex, men and women commonly strive to avoid using condoms to demonstrate that the sex they are having is already safe sex.

Plan of This Book

In the following chapter, we locate our project in relation to the broader anthro-pological history and theorization of comparative research. Comparative research grew to prominence early in our disciplinary history, but later fell out of favor. We explore the earlier projects on comparative research and its promises, and then discuss what changed in anthropological thinking and trends that made comparative research come to be seen as problematic. We also explore the ways in which the premises and methods of our comparative ethnography differ from previous approaches. Our approach includes the analysis of relations of inequality, attention to both meaning and structure, an iterative method that enables insights from one field site to inform research directions in other field sites, and an explicitly critical sensibility about the limitations of comparability, given anthropology's commitment to that which is peculiarly local about each specific society. Through a discussion of our methods, we provide a candid and reflexive review of the benefits and challenges of this kind of collaborative and comparative endeavor, arguing in particular for the utility of the critical comparative approach for anthropologists who seek to engage with policy.

Chapters 2 through 6 present some of the key empirical findings from the fieldwork in each location. Set in a rural, migrant-exporting town in western Mexico, Chapter 2 examines reputation as an aspect of sexual identity, using the notion of sexual projects to explore how people's crafting of respectable identities fits into their larger life plans. It develops further the concept of sexual geographies, showing how they reflect the broader social and economic organization of gender inequality, and provides some insight into why it makes sense to men to spend so freely on extramarital sex. Turning to Nigeria, Chapter 3 demonstrates how the concept of social risk can help unravel and address the complex behavioral dynamics driving the HIV epidemic there and in sub-Saharan Africa more generally, showing how men and women navigate economic, social, and moral constraints and priorities, among which the perceived risk of HIV infection is just one factor. The reasons why married men are likely to engage in extramarital sex and married women frequently tolerate it are elaborated, and the degree to which the enduring importance of marriage and family are socially central to the context of extramarital sexual behavior is illustrated and explained.

Chapter 4, set in Vietnam and focusing particularly on the role of the State in mediating emerging economies of desire, analyzes extramarital sex in relation to the intersection of local and global consumer economies in a rapidly changing urban environment. Attentive to the political economy of sexuality, the chapter elucidates the way in which Doi Moi policies such as the "Happy Family" campaign have reconfigured the nature of sexual risk and facilitated and structured both men's possibilities for extramarital sex and women's acquiescence to their husbands' infidelities. Chapter 5 analyzes Huli people's ambivalence about companionate marriage—an ambivalence exacerbated by severe economic decline and the impossibility of achieving the middle-class lifestyle that Huli people associate with companionate marriage. This chapter also suggests that the history of Huli labor migration is simultaneously a history in which men's extramarital sexuality has increasingly become the norm. It concludes with a discussion of why Huli women do not keep "the secret" of male infidelity, but instead engage in public and often violent confrontations with their wayward husbands. Chapter 6, the final ethnographic chapter, focuses on Uganda, a country celebrated for its dramatic decline in HIV prevalence rates, in which risk for married women has nonetheless been shown to be persistent and is in fact increasing (Ministry of Health and ORC Macro 2006). This chapter links transformations of men's extramarital relationships to broader historical changes, including colonial marriage and adultery laws, missionary moral teachings, and shifts to a cash economy, which have gradually transformed the institution of multiple co-wives into a newer configuration of concurrent "informal wives." This study of Uganda, similar to the chapter on Nigeria, also demonstrates the iatrogenic consequences of HIV prevention programs, showing how public health messages about monogamy interact with the rise of modern marital ideas to drive men's infidelity underground. The chapter shows how these HIV messages provide women in Uganda with a moral discourse and platform to publicly air grievances about their husbands' extramarital sexuality. For wives who decide to "go public" with their husbands' infidelities, however, confronting the other women rather than their own husbands is pragmatically safer, partly because lingering gender inequalities mean that a woman still faces economic and social risks in challenging her husband's actions and reputation. Finally, the Conclusion builds on the framing we have provided here, articulating more broadly the importance of our work on extramarital opportunity structures, sexuality, and comparative ethnography. We also share some final thoughts on our work's policy implications and present a few possibilities for structural-level interventions that could help prevent marital transmission.

The locations where we worked were all physically distant and culturally distinct from the major twenty-first-century urban concentrations of wealth and power, so that our readers in those settings might be tempted to consider this only a story about a radically distinct "other." As we note in the Conclusion, however, the notions of extramarital opportunity structures, sexual geographies, and social risk ought to be every bit as applicable to analyses of sexual practices closer to home. They lend themselves to framing a deeper understanding of both our scandals du jour and the physical organization of the cities in which we live (such as how Atlanta's "lingerie modeling" businesses are clustered just north of the hotels where conventioneers so frequently stay, and New York City's slightly more upscale Hustler Club is positioned conveniently next to the entrance of the West Side Highway). More profoundly, we hope that the pages that follow will lead our readers to reflect on the nature of intimacy in their own societies and communities—on what is spoken and what is silenced, on whose pleasures are facilitated and whose forbidden, and on how the negotiations of love, emotion, sex, and trust provide windows into even broader questions about the lives we lead and those we might build.

1

From "Cultural Traits" to Global Processes

Methods for a Critical Comparative Ethnography

In stark contrast to anthropology's lone-wolf model of research and publication, we conducted the fieldwork for this project as a collaborative effort, sharing jointly developed research guides.[1] We hoped that the comparative ethnographic research design would enable us (1) to distinguish between the features of each field site that had wider theoretical and public health significance and those that were particular to each setting, and (2) to theorize about how complex processes—social, economic, and discursive—operate across different social levels and in different cultural arenas. For example, as marriages around the world move toward a more companionate ideal and structure, and as urbanization and integration with national or global economies (e.g., through wage labor) increasingly characterize many settings in developing countries, much can be learned from comparing how these processes are unfolding across diverse cultural contexts. In particular, the multisited structure of the project has allowed us to generate understandings about companionate marriage, labor migration, men's peer groups, and the social organization of infidelity that transcend the particularities of each case.

At the same time, we had been trained to be wary—and even highly dubious—about the very possibility of carrying out comparative research. Whether our reservations had been informed by postmodernism's influence on anthropology, by critiques of the culture concept, or by concerns about unwittingly falling into a neoevolutionary mode of thought in which each of "our" field sites would be mapped onto some teleological scheme, each of us entered the project with both enthusiasm at the prospect of becoming immersed in the others' data and skepticism about whether what we were embarking on was even possible. Anthropologists who read this text may be familiar with some of the debates surrounding the project of comparison, but the notion that comparison either as a method or an intellectual goal is problematic may be surprising to readers from public health or other disciplinary backgrounds where comparative projects are the norm and even encouraged as a way of creating generalizable conclusions and theories. Thus, in this chapter, we review the intellectual history of anthropological comparison and locate our approach to comparative ethnography in relation to the discipline's long conversation about the goals, methods, values, and flaws of comparative research.

We then discuss the methods used to carry out what we have come to think of as "critical comparative ethnography." In doing so, we demonstrate that comparative, team-based research can be particularly productive as a strategy for studying the intertwining of intimate subjectivity and global processes of inequality.

Historicizing Comparison within Anthropology

As students of sociocultural anthropology know, the discipline was founded with comparison as its raison d'être. Victor de Munck notes that for Sir Edward Tylor, one of social anthropology's nineteenth-century forebears, "anthropology had two complementary missions: ethnography and ethnology" (de Munck 2000: 279; see also Holy 1987b)—that is, the systematic description of individual societies, paired with comparison of societies. It was ethnology that was seen as giving anthropology its wider significance; ethnography was not an end in itself but rather the means to generate the cross-cultural comparisons that would reveal the nature and evolution of human society. As Ladislav Holy says, the comparative method "was seen as the means of formulating and testing hypotheses or generalizations valid not only for one specific society or culture but cross-culturally. . . . [It] marked the distinction between anthropology as a generalizing science and ethnography as mere description of one particular society or culture" (1987b: 2). Comparison was envisioned as the method for a science of human society akin to the intellectual project of natural history, and was thus sociocultural anthropology's "crucial justification" (Kuper 2002: 143). Much early anthropology therefore consisted of comparing societies according to particular "traits" such as type of marriage, level of technology, and political system, and categorizing them into "ethnologic stages" along a unilineal and progressive path toward greater complexity. J. D. Y. Peel describes the underlying logic: "The presents of backward societies were the equivalent of the pasts of advanced societies" (1987: 90).

From the very outset, however, the project of comparison was considered problematic. For example, in response to Tylor's presentation of results based on his (at that time) groundbreaking method of cross-cultural comparison, the statistician Francis Galton pointed out that seemingly distinct societies may have had a common origin and thus could be "duplicate copies of the same original" (de Munck 2000: 279). In other words, since Tylor was treating "cultural traits" as if they were independent variables that could be subjected to statistical hypothesis testing, he needed to be able to demonstrate that the variables were in fact independent. "Tylor had no way of controlling for the historical relationships between the cases in his sample" (de Munck 2002: 146), so his conclusions could not be considered statistically valid—a difficulty that has been referred to since as "Galton's problem." More significant, as students of anthropology learn early in their training, was

Franz Boas's assertion that the Victorian practitioners of the comparative method wrongly assumed that "the occurrence of similar traits in different cultures implies participation in a universal, orthogenic, evolutionary process" (Gregor and Tuzin 2001: 3; see also Silverman 2005). In other words, a singular, teleological evolutionary framework had been assumed a priori, and societies consequently evaluated according to this framework, with inadequate attention to the historical particulars of any individual society or to its cultural interactions with its neighbors. According to Boas, the "vain endeavor" (1940 [1896]: 280) of grand and fallacious theorizing had to be set aside while the "solid work" of thorough ethnographic and historical description took place.

The social evolutionists' conceptualization of societies as packages of stable cultural traits or variables has long been rejected by most sociocultural anthropologists, a theoretical shift we will discuss in greater detail. Nevertheless, the conviction that sociocultural anthropology only has value if it can make scientific generalizations beyond a single society—and the consequent urge to generate testable hypotheses based on comparison—remained robust in some strands of North American anthropological thought (despite the considerable influence of Boas and his students), and persists even today. During the mid-twentieth century, George Murdock created the Human Relations Area Files (HRAF) and the Ethnographic Atlas, both of which are data sets consisting of condensed and coded versions of a great number of ethnographic descriptions, to be analyzed by looking for correlations between the presence or absence of particular characteristics across societies. Drawing on these resources, or on other data sets produced through individual or team efforts, many North American anthropologists have attempted to establish cross-cultural causal explanations about the workings of human society. Perhaps most well known are the analyses stemming from or inspired by Beatrice and John Whiting's *Six Culture Studies*, which used observational data from a range of societies to generate theories about the relationships between household structure, childrearing patterns, and personality (Whiting and Whiting 1975; Ember and Ember 2001; Levine 2001; Munroe 2001). Despite persistent criticisms of this research genre, some anthropologists continue to assert that "cross-cultural researchers . . . can never reject the core axioms of a scientific paradigm: that cultures exist, that they consist of elements, and that these elements can be qualitatively as well as quantitatively compared across cultures" (de Munck 2002: 16).

In the British academic context, the project of comparison initiated by Tylor had proceeded quite differently and was more modest in its ambitions and scope. Focusing on sociological explanations (as opposed to psychological or environmental, for example) for the behavioral patterns observed, it eschewed universalist claims and typically restricted the comparative endeavor to a small number of well-researched and often related societies within one region (Holy 1987b; Peel 1987; Barth 2005). As Peel describes it, "This mode of comparative method did not just make use of ethnographies but . . . really arose out of ethnography and remained close to it" (Holy 1987b: 95). In other words, the British tradition rejected the statistical manipulation of cultural traits extracted from very different social, environmental, and historical contexts, and instead tried to theorize differences between societies that shared material environments and were often quite similar in terms of social organization, history, and belief system. An example often described as paradigmatic of this method is S. F. Nadel's research on witchcraft, which uses detailed ethnographic data from two pairs of societies. In his 1952 article, Nadel first establishes that the Nupe and the Gwari, neighboring groups from northern Nigeria, are very similar in that they live in identical environments, speak closely related languages, have an identical kinship system and political organization, and express very similar beliefs about witchcraft. However, Nupe witches are always women and their victims are most often male, while "witches and their victims are indiscriminately male and female" among the Gwari. The only other significant difference between the two societies is the fact that "marriage is relatively tension-free in Gwari, but full of stress and mutual hostility in Nupe" (20). Nadel thus concludes that witchcraft beliefs "are related to specific anxieties and stresses arising in social life" (28). This kind of regional "controlled comparison" (Eggan 1954) focusing on specific social institutions was carried out in a number of world areas, providing illuminating information, for example, about the organization of power and authority in Melanesia (Godelier and Strathern 1991) and about historical changes in the social structure of Plains and Pueblo Indian groups (Eggan 1950, 1966).

Critiques of Cross-Cultural Comparison

Both the American and British traditions of comparison were arguably aiming for a kind of scientific validity, but they proceeded based on very different epistemologies about what constituted scientific validity, as well as distinct ontologies about the nature of society, with the American tradition presuming that cultural traits from vastly different societies could be treated as independent variables, while the British tradition tried to control for confounding variables by choosing geographically proximate and culturally similar cases. The attempt to achieve scientific validity—however it was conducted—did not protect the project of comparison from being roundly criticized. These diverse critiques reflect larger theoretical shifts within the discipline of sociocultural anthropology; here, we briefly explicate the problems of place, analytical categories, culture, and globalization, all of which we particularly tried to bear in mind as we conceptualized our own comparative research.

The Problem of Place

Even for the regionally specific comparisons in the British anthropological tradition, the question of how to demarcate comparable sociogeographical units quickly became problematic. As Adam Kuper asks:

> How are boundaries to be drawn? Are the South African Bushmen one ethnographic case or several? . . . In what sense are the units that are constructed strictly comparable? Can the Bushmen reasonably be treated as a "case" alongside "the Bedouin," let alone Ming China? . . . Common ancestry was traditionally the usual basis for identifying an ethnographic unit. Evans-Pritchard's Nuer were defined as a single people because they claimed common descent. . . . [Many anthropologists have] ended up with units that have their own particular taken-for-granted quality. This is because they all correspond to political units established by colonial rule and legitimized by modern nationalist movements. . . . The boundaries of the nation or empire prescribe the framework for regional comparison. (2002: 145–47)

In other words, at best, the designation of sociogeographic units came to seem somewhat arbitrary—were boundaries to be decided on the basis of environment, on claims of descent and autochthony, or on linguistic criteria?—and not easily considered commensurate. At worst, the selection of particular units reinforced boundaries imposed through coercion and based on the negotiations between, and expediencies of, colonial powers. This issue was raised very early on in British anthropology. As Andre Gingrich and Richard G. Fox note, Max Gluckman "was among the first to challenge dominant assumptions about discrete, self-evident empirical units as starting points for comparative analyses. Through his own analysis of 'Zululand' as a product of colonial and capitalist expansion, Gluckman demonstrated that these units of comparison emerge, within fuzzy and volatile boundaries, at the intersection of wider and more encompassing processes" (Gluckman 1958; Fox and Gingrich 2002).

Further, not only do colonial and postcolonial projects construct and naturalize sociogeographical units, scholars themselves do so as well through their discursive accumulations about particular places and peoples. As Andrew Strathern and Michael Lambek point out, "The very constitution of 'region' comes into question. The region emerges not only from geographic proximity . . . but from the act of studying it" (1998: 22). As Richard Fardon puts it, "Each ethnographer enters 'a field' imaginatively charted by others" (1990: 24–25). Arjun Appadurai, discussing the intellectual history of the concept of caste hierarchy in India, similarly argues that an important reason why anthropologists have been able to sustain the fiction that sociogeographical places are units with self-evident boundaries is that "places have been married to ideas . . . whereby some feature of a group is seen as quintessential to the group and as especially true of that group in contrast with other groups" (1988: 39–40). Finally, again questioning the usefulness of conceptualizing peoples or places as bounded, comparable units, Fredrik Barth has repeatedly pointed out that (1) important sociocultural processes often take place at or across boundaries, and thus that treating places as autonomous units—whether they are regional neighbors or oceans apart—may blind a researcher to the most important dynamics taking place; and (2) contrary to Nadel's assumption that a society's own institutions (the nature of its marital relations, for example) are the most important sources of its cultural variation, it is entirely possible that "the most important mechanisms generating variation may operate across societal boundaries, and thus are not definitive of specific cultures or societies" (Bowen and Petersen 1999: 13; Barth 1987, 1999).

The Problem of Analytical Categories

Analogous to the problem of how to demarcate place—and whether it is an intellectually valid or productive undertaking—is the concern that the analytical terms used to describe aspects of society are not necessarily valid as overarching categories or independent variables for making cross-cultural comparisons. This problem is most relevant for the kinds of studies that are based on the Ethnographic Atlas or similarly derived data sets. For example, anthropologists may describe two societies as polygynous—and thus they may be coded as such in the Ethnographic Atlas—but that does not necessarily mean that polygyny looks the same in these two societies. In one society, wives may live together, and in the other, wives may have separate houses. In one society, the husband may be having sexual relations with his wives concurrently, while in the other, a man may cease having sex with his first wife upon marrying his second wife. In one society, the co-wives may have roughly equivalent social status, while in the other, they have quite hierarchical relationships. Polygyny is not polygyny is not polygyny. Depending on the questions asked in a comparative study, these differences will be profoundly significant, so that using "polygamous societies" as an independent variable and comparing it with "monogamous societies" will lead to spurious conclusions. "Polygynous" and other such broadly descriptive terms often operate (1) to mark difference in the "other"—in other words, all polygynous societies are "the same" only in the sense that they are assumed to differ from Western monogamous society, and (2) as a shorthand for signaling the kinds of questions that might be at issue in a polygynous society (e.g., how does a man allocate resources? do co-wives cooperate or compete?).

The Problem of Culture

This skepticism about whether a cultural trait in one society is in fact similar (or similar enough for any meaningful comparison) to "the same" cultural trait in another society is due not only to empirical facts, such as polygyny being variable from one place to another; these doubts also stem from profound shifts in the way that sociocultural anthropologists conceptualize culture. Beginning perhaps with Ruth Benedict, and then solidified by Clifford Geertz and what is sometimes called "the interpretive turn," culture came to be seen as dense, redolent with meaning, and highly integrated, so that one could not truly comprehend any particular dimension of a society (such as its religious rituals or its marriage system) without also understanding the larger context in which it was embedded. In one society, a particular ritual might be complexly tied to its economic system, whereas another society's social organization might only make sense in light of its religious ideology about purity and impurity. Thus, context was everything, and to decontextualize and isolate one particular cultural trait for the purposes of comparison with another society was potentially to strip it of its true meaning—that is, the meaning that it had for the members of that society and that it had in relation to other dimensions of that society. Thus, although ethnography has always referred to the description of a society, the very notion of description took on new meanings. The task of sociocultural anthropology became "thick description" (Geertz 1973), which included not only a detailed account of a specific practice of a society (for example, how people married in a particular society), but also a rich and rigorous interpretation of the meanings of those practices.[2] No longer merely the collection of data about preconceived categories, fieldwork for many anthropologists meant trying to immerse oneself in "culturally specific processes of meaning construction" (Holy 1987b: 8). Cultures came to be seen as integrated wholes that could not be dismantled into isolable elements. Perhaps comparison was possible, but only "on the order of comparing art styles or, common wisdom notwithstanding, apples and oranges" (Strathern and Lambek 1998: 21).

The idea that broader context is the key to understanding any particular dimension of society remains a—perhaps *the*—cornerstone of the discipline, and is the principal reason why anthropologists do long-term fieldwork and express skepticism about the validity of short-term survey research. However, the idea that culture is a highly integrated whole collapsed as the discipline yet again retheorized what culture means (see Smith's chapter in this volume). Particularly relevant to the project of comparison were the two related critiques about the holistic conceptualization of culture: that it overemphasized social consensus, and that it was ahistorical. Regarding the former, many scholars noted that "the interpretive turn" privileged the shared nature of meaning systems, thus obfuscating the fact that culture is often an object of struggle, that members of a society are differently positioned and experience their culture quite differently, and that social actors strategically resist, selectively practice, creatively reimagine, and otherwise negotiate the hegemonic social values and meanings of culture (Abu-Lughod 1991). At the very least, then, comparison *between* societies also requires the comparison of differently positioned groups *within* societies.

Regarding the second critique about the ahistorical assumptions of the comparative project, Peel points out that anthropology was initially conceptualized as "a natural science of society, in opposition to history as the study of unique sequences of events. So it has employed quite general sociological categories . . . and ethnographic descriptions of little temporal specificity" (1987: 88). In other words, written into the terminology and analytical repertoire of anthropology are inherently ahistorical concepts that reinforce the erroneous idea that cultures are unchanging except when altered by external forces such as colonization. Examining the intellectual history of sociocultural anthropology, Peel identifies five kinds of comparative analysis based on "the ways they handle history" (90). These range from the "single, universal, ideal" history of the social evolutionists to the kind of comparison conducted using the Ethnographic Atlas "where history is denied or ignored, as comparison is used to derive sociological universals or general laws," to the final (and, to his mind, best) mode of comparison in which "it is histories, or 'societies-in-change' rather than just 'societies,' which are compared" (109). Peel argues that differences between societies can only be understood "by means of a properly historical comparison . . . that is by relating the twentieth-century differences not only to other twentieth-century features but to their overall trajectories of change over several centuries" (88; see also Fox 2002).[3] Along the same lines, Appadurai notes that the failure to do this kind of historical comparison has led to spurious representations of many societies: "It is now increasingly clear that in many instances where anthropologists believed they were observing and analyzing pristine or historically deep systems, they were in fact viewing products of recent trans-regional interactions" (1988: 38–39). In sum, by noting the problem of culture, we call attention both to the critical importance of situating the objects of comparison within broader holistic analyses of the societies in question and to the profound shifts in how culture is theorized, which suggest that the historically embedded and internally contested nature of culture complicates the project of comparison.

The Problem of Globalization

The final issue that has problematized comparison—or at least forced scholars to rethink the goals, methods, and ontological assumptions of comparison—is globalization. In a sense, "Galton's problem"—that sociogeographic units held up for comparison are potentially historically connected in some way and thus not independent variables—has become the way of the world, so that the movement of people and ideas has made the project of comparison seem like the wrong methodology for the wrong questions. As noted above, particularly by Appadurai, many scholars would say that this is actually not a new problem, and that societies the world over have long been connected in ways that earlier anthropologists simply chose not to see. However, the intensification of these processes and their highly visible global reach has raised questions about what topics anthropologists should choose to study and how they should go about researching them. As James Peacock says:

[Globalization's] profound effect is the interconnecting and merging of cultures. In this regard, globalization poses a challenge for the comparative method, in so far as that method . . . emphasizes a certain integrity and distinctiveness of each [cultural] unit. . . . [Anthropologists have traditionally argued that] an aspect of a group or a culture can be understood only in its localized context . . . hence comparison is suspect . . . because it abstracts aspect A from context A in order to compare it with aspect B from context B. Globalism [poses an even greater challenge to comparison] . . . by denying the boundary between context A and context B; both A and B are part of a world system. Accordingly, A can only be understood as interacting with that world system. . . . How does one do globalistic fieldwork, tracing movement around the world, while retaining in-depth immersion in a localized culture? (2002: 45–47)

Arguably, as the paradigms and central questions of sociocultural anthropology have changed, so have its methods, from cross-cultural comparative methods (whether universalist or regional controlled comparison), to the exegesis of cultures-as-texts, to mobile and multisited research that traces the processes of globalization through "follow-the-thing," "follow-the-person," and even "follow-the-policy" methodologies (Marcus 1995). Each of these problems of comparison informed—and created some anxieties as we proceeded with—our discussions and plans for carrying out a comparative ethnographic study.

Some Important—and Not Always Acknowledged—Values of Cross-Cultural Comparison

Given the above history and critiques, it might seem that anthropology's founding impetus and "crucial justification" for the comparative project was a road that would have been better not traveled. However, before moving on to the ways in which the comparative project is being reimagined and reinvigorated—by us, we hope, but also by many other researchers—we want to discuss three domains in which we believe that the comparative project has both remained vital and been invaluable.

Feminist Anthropology

First, feminist anthropology, upon which our work draws, has benefited immensely from comparative ethnographic research. The early anthropologists of gender did not always stop to interrogate the epistemological assumptions underlying the comparisons they made. Nonetheless, the intensive research on women's lives that began to be developed in the 1970s provided a wealth of information about women's access to economic, discursive, and political resources; the cultural constructions of their reproductive roles; gendered myths about the origins of society; the gendered nature of public and domestic realms; and the relationships between kinship systems, systems of production, and gender inequalities (Reiter 1975a; Lamphere and Rosaldo1974; Sanday and Goodenough 1990). This ethnographic work helped to push forward important theoretical questions about the universality of male dominance—how to define it, whether it holds true ethnographically and historically, and why or why not—that continue to engage and preoccupy us today, despite the rapidly changing nature of the world and of men's and women's lives in it (Sanday 2002; Du 2002). Even though all the various theories for male dominance and female subordination have been critiqued (often through the use of comparative data showing that a theory was not in fact generalizable), those critiques themselves were—and continue to be—productive in pushing scholars to think about gendered agency and the structures of gender inequality. We tried to keep this mutually beneficial relationship between comparative research and feminist anthropology in mind as we conceptualized our own project's focus on gendered inequality and HIV risk.

Historical Materialist Anthropology

Second, sociocultural anthropology has never been a theoretically unified field. While one prominent intellectual branch of the discipline turned decisively away from the comparative project (because of the problems discussed earlier), another branch—informed by Marxist theory, and focused on structures of power and inequality—embraced it. This branch—typically associated with Eric Wolf, Sidney Mintz, and other students of cultural ecologist Julian Steward—advocated the historical comparison of economic processes (e.g., the development of plantation economies in the Caribbean, the growth of mining economies in Africa) rather than cultural traits. These scholars often demonstrated that seemingly timeless and defining cultural characteristics (e.g., the conservative values of peasant societies) actually emerged in response to the uncertainties and risks generated by encompassing economic changes. Wolf in particular is notable for maintaining a comparative perspective throughout his career from the 1950s to the late 1990s. He compared peasant societies within Latin America and between Latin America and Java; he compared the different patterns of family organization and inheritance between two geographically proximate Alpine villages, one Italian-speaking and one German-speaking (Cole and Wolf 1974); he identified similar processes of ethnic identity-making in groups as seemingly dissimilar as the Crow Indians and Rhodesian mine workers (Wolf 2001); and he compared the workings of ideology in societies again as seemingly unlike as pre-contact Aztec and Nazi Germany (1999).

What made these kinds of comparisons tenable within Wolf's analytical framework was his foregrounding, inspired by Marx's concept of "relations of production," of what he called the "mobilization of social labor" (2001: 61)—that is, how a people's capacity to work is organized, structured, and often coerced within different economic formations. In particular, he was interested in developing "theoretical constructs that would allow us to grasp the significant elements organizing populations not governed by capitalist relationships but contacted, engulfed, or reorganized by advancing capitalism" (337). Thus, for example, despite the myriad religious and other differences between peasant communities in Latin America and Java, Wolf was able to identify important similarities in both their structural status as labor reserves for urban industries and landholding elites, and in their strategies for survival (such as the emergence of community credit associations). Where some anthropologists saw unique, highly integrated, incommensurable systems of meaning, Wolf and his followers saw eminently comparable forms of labor exploitation and wealth accumulation. Indeed, in some ways, Wolf agreed with the early anthropologists about comparison giving sociocultural anthropology its raison d'être: only through comparison can anthropologists come to see how economic structures of power operate in analogous ways with similar consequences in vastly different areas of the world.

While our primary concerns in this book differ from Wolf's, the kinds of comparisons we undertake are informed to some extent by this branch of anthropology, which is commonly called "political economy." First, the way in which labor is organized—that is, how an encompassing economy shapes people's access to resources (e.g., land, jobs, money)—plays a part in the construction of cultural identity (Wolf 2001: 368). For our purposes, we focus particularly on how gender and class identities shape men's and women's marital and extramarital practices, but we try to emphasize that these identifications are often very much a response to encompassing and often rapidly changing economic formations. Furthermore, the organization of "social labor" also plays a part in producing what we call sexual geographies (see the Introduction), which again influence marital and extramarital practices.

Cross-Regional Ethnographic Comparisons and Conversations

Third, although much of the *statistical* research comparing cultural traits in vastly different societies has been problematic, there is a long history of richly *ethnographic* conversation and comparison between regions, such as Melanesia and Africa or Melanesia and Amazonia. These more ethnographic comparisons have sometimes taken the form of arguments and sometimes outright poaching of supposedly culturally or regionally specific paradigms, but in many ways these comparative conversations across culture-area boundaries have been tremendously productive. For example, early work on the kinship and social organization of groups in Papua New Guinea drew on notions of lineage and descent derived from research in Africa, but ultimately rejected these for approaches that instead emphasized the importance of reciprocity and exchange in producing kin relations (Strathern and Lambek 1998). These new understandings of kinship as something that was achieved and could change, rather than as a biological fact, subsequently reverberated back into the Africanist ethnographic literature, generating new questions and helping anthropologists notice phenomena that they might not have seen had they still been locked into regionally derived paradigms of how kin ties are constituted. Similarly, Thomas Gregor and Donald Tuzin (2001) explore the uncanny resemblances between societies in Melanesia and Amazonia: egalitarian social organization; societies organized around men's houses; men's secret rituals of initiation and procreation; and similar myths about the origins of men's cults and the cosmological importance of gender separation.

Just how to theorize such uncanny resemblances—socioenvironmental determinism? a Freudian-informed model of the male psyche? Lévi-Straussian transformations of underlying structure? anthropological fictions?—has been the cause of many scholarly arguments. Rather than trying to resolve these arguments, Strathern and Lambek suggest that it is the ongoing conversation itself that is valuable:

> We suggest that the fundamental goal of comparison is ongoing exchange, rather than the creation of distinct intellectual lineages. . . . There is no neutral universal framework, no objectivist language into which alternative theories, paradigms, or cultures could be set side by side, point by point. However, incommensurability does not imply incomparability. . . . To return to our Melanesianist model, what we exchange in the absence of common coin is not commodities but gifts. (1998: 21)

In other words, the ultimate goal of comparative ethnography is not to end this longstanding relationship via some final intellectual transaction, but rather to keep it going so that the exchanges, thefts, and cross-fertilizations will be of intellectual benefit to all. Appadurai acknowledges another potential benefit of comparative approaches: although he critiques the way in which "places have been married to ideas" (1988: 39)—such as caste hierarchies in India or exchange relationships in Melanesia—so that "ideas become metonymic prisons for particular places" (40), he also notes that being more consciously aware of the intertextuality between culture-areas might enable anthropologists to "develop an approach to theory in which places could be compared polythetically. . . . In such an approach, there would be an assumption of family resemblances between places. . . . This assumption would not require places to be encapsulated by single diacritics (or essences) in order for them to be compared with other places, but would permit several configurations of resemblance and contrast" (46).

It has been clear to us from the beginning of our collaboration that each of the contexts in which we worked was profoundly distinct from the others. No "single diacritic" could be used to make overarching comparisons. Therefore, we never sought to compare them in a way that would obscure those profoundly important particularities. With both the perils and values of comparison in mind, we ventured to develop a comparative ethnographic project that would serve our research goals and perhaps provide a model for other studies.

Critical Comparative Ethnography

We have taken great pleasure participating in the kind of conversation that Strathern and Lambek and Appadurai advocate—for example, in reading beyond the area literature to which we individually might have confined ourselves if we hadn't been working together on a comparative project. However, we are actually aiming for something more. Fox and Gingrich make the provocative point that "anthropology has a public responsibility to be comparative" (2002: 9)—that is, an obligation to examine how global processes generate similar inequalities, hazards, and violence, as well as responsive social movements, in and across different contexts (see also Peacock 2002; Levinson 2005). Although we hardly wish to dictate what anthropologists *should* be doing, we strongly agree that one way for anthropology to have a stronger public voice on world problems is through what we have come to think of as "critical comparative ethnography."

Much of what we are proposing is not new, and many anthropologists have used comparison to show that people everywhere are (unequally) affected by a shared set of global processes, as well as to illuminate significant similarities and differences in how this occurs and how people respond. For example, a recent special issue of the journal *American Anthropologist* examines indigenous rights movements in Africa and the Americas. Taken together, the articles "offer a critical, comparative perspective on . . . the complicated alliances, articulations, and tensions that have produced and transformed the transnational indigenous rights movement" (Hodgson 2002). Sally Engle Merry, taking a different tack, uses a multisited, comparative approach to examine how policies articulating violence against women as a human rights violation are produced in global conferences and then variably interpreted, implemented, and resisted in a wide range of places around the world (2006). Because comparative research necessitates engagement with a level of abstraction that will facilitate the identification of underlying regularities in social processes, some anthropologists use this approach to explore how power works at the state level. Jane and Peter Schneider, for example, compare the political structures of the Sicilian Mafia and al Qaeda (2002), while Rebecca Bryant conducted research with both Turkish and Greek Cypriot communities in order to explore the relationship between notions of kinship and the logics of nationalism (2002). More recently, Richard G. Parker, Rosalind Petchesky, and Robert Sember led a team of colleagues who conducted a comparative study of the politics of sexuality in eight countries and two multilateral organizations (the United Nations and the World Bank) (Parker, Petchesky, and Sember 2007), and Anita Hardon and colleagues used a multisited and comparative methodology to illuminate the challenges of using antiretroviral therapy in Africa (Hardon et al. 2007).

In short, the anthropological project of comparison is alive and well. Here we outline what we think is distinctive about our approach to anthropological research, as well as the ways that our study differs from the examples noted thus far. As we conceptualize it, critical comparative ethnography

- focuses on processes (not cultural traits), particularly the global processes that generate inequality (in our project, inequalities related to HIV risk). A focus on "traits" implies a local, bounded, and static understanding of culture, while a focus on processes implies attention to history, global-local connections, and the agency of local actors.

- subscribes to the idea that the best and most valid comparisons are based not on attempts to find statistical correlations between variables in society, but rather on rich, experience-near ethnography that is attentive to the relationship between large-scale social forces and individual experience, such as the connections between inequality and intimate human relationships (Nader 1994). Here we agree with Bradley Levinson (2005), who argues that if anthropologists are interested in broader processes such as nationalisms or labor migration, they must not cede the comparative field to survey research—precisely because anthropology is unique in its attention to context and its ability to analyze processes of meaning construction.

- is conducted with the intent to generate mid-range explanatory concepts or to refine the explanatory power of existing concepts. As Fox and Gingrich say, "Such medium range concepts . . . [have the] potential to identify and explain other dimensions of specific local-global processes and to situate local-global processes in wider contexts more effectively than 'thick' or 'finely-textured' descriptions and analyses alone were able to carry out" (2002: 244–45). Conversely, critical comparative ethnography can also be used productively to destabilize and undermine existing mid-level concepts: a central finding of our project was the variable meanings of fidelity and the instability of infidelity as a cross-cultural category. Thus, although "thick," reflexive, experience-near ethnography that Geertz proposed is desired, critical comparative ethnography does require a willingness to sacrifice some ethnographic detail.[4] Another way to think about this is that the turn toward political economy and structures of inequality (and the inherent shift away from entirely cultural explanations) has made global comparisons more possible.

- is attuned to the fact that culture is not unproblematically shared, that people are differently positioned (by gender, class, age, etc.), and that their different positions make for different strategies (when they encounter ideologies of love, for example). However, one thing that makes our project innovative is that we deliberately incorporated attention to inequality into the comparative research design, in part through a specific sampling strategy (which we will discuss). Obtaining a sense of people's variable ideals and experiences across gender, class, and generation was an aim of all the researchers. (There are, of course, problems with this: one of the most difficult aspects of designing the project, for example, was trying to create a sampling grid on which "low income and assets" in Mexico would be somehow equivalent to "low income and assets" in Papua New Guinea.)

- is specifically designed so that the results are comparable—or at least more comparable than those of ethnographies based on individually conceptualized and conducted research. For example, anthropologists interested in love and marriage can learn a lot by reading Laura Ahearn's *Invitations to Love: Literacy, Love Letters and Social Change in Nepal* (2001) and Linda-Anne Rebhun's *The Heart Is Unknown Country: Love in the Changing Economy of Northeast Brazil* (1999) back to back. However, although these books cover many of the same issues, they are not systematically comparable, since each researcher had her own conceptual framework, developed her own research design, and asked her own interview questions. Since we think that a significant part of the theoretical and persuasive power of anthropology comes from comparison, we were aiming for ethnographically rich results that were more systematically comparable, and we therefore used the same methods and interview questions in each site, modifying them to reflect local meanings and capture site-specific conditions when necessary. Even when our interviews and our participant observation took us into the many improvised and unexpected directions that are a hallmark of sound ethnographic research, our shared conceptual framework and the baseline of questions we all asked assured comparability across the sites.

This is not, to be sure, a rigid "recipe" for critical comparative ethnography—or, if it is a recipe, it is more a sort of recipe for a savory dish, which lends itself to experimentation, rather than a recipe for a cake, which if not followed to the teaspoon will fall flat. Indeed, we hope it spurs others' interest in developing alternative critical comparative ethnographies. We simply highlight these five characteristics of our project as elements that helped us find a place to work at the juncture of theoretically engaged anthropology and policy-relevant public health research.

Methods for Critical Comparative Ethnography

In the rest of this chapter, we discuss the methods we used, as well as some of the difficulties of trying to carry out research that aimed to be ethnographically rich but also systematically comparative. We begin by talking about the case study and interview sample, and then describe the methods of marital case studies and participant observation. The methods will be familiar to many, but some readers may be less aware of how ethnographic research differs epistemologically (and thus methodologically) from other forms of qualitative research, and so we try to spell out some of these differences.

We collected the data through marital case studies, participant observation, key informant interviews, and analyses of popular culture and HIV- or AIDS-related communication materials. Each of these methods was intended to capture one or several elements of the intertwining of individual strategies and experiences, the nature of intimate relations, and social, cultural, and economic contexts. As illustrated in Appendix I, each specific ethnographic method was appropriate for learning about particular elements of the overall problem.

Each method was designed to address the three principal aims of the project. To move from the relatively abstract research aims to actual research tasks, we articulated a series of questions that reflected the specific information we would need in order to address each aim. The first aim was to compare companionate marriage (in terms of relative penetration and associated local iterations of ideas and practices) and the specific forms of marital and extramarital relationships. The questions generated by that aim were: (1a) What are the specific local forms of marital relationships, including the gendered meanings of sexual intimacy and fidelity, similarities and differences in emerging forms of marriage, and sexual and HIV risk practices? (1b) How do marital relationships reflect the global ideas and practices associated with companionate marriage? (1c) What are the primary forms of extramarital relationships and what are the social aspects and sexual and HIV risk practices of each type of relationship?

The second project aim was to understand the ways in which these ideas about practices of intimacy have been shaped and constrained by gender-unequal structures and ideologies, local forms of economic organization, and cultural change. The questions to address this aim were: (2a) What is the specific configuration of gender inequality, economic structures, and cultural change? (2b) In what ways do these local aspects of social organization shape and constrain practices of marital and extramarital intimacy? The third aim of the project was to evaluate the implications of these ideas and practices for HIV prevention within and outside of marriage. The questions to address this aim were: (3a) How does the local organization of marital and extramarital intimacy contribute to women's risk of marital HIV infection? (3b) Under what social and economic circumstances is the risk of marital HIV infection greater or less?

Systematic Ethnographic Sampling: Axes of Diversity

A particular innovation of the study design was our use of a systematic sampling strategy to select the participants in the marital case studies and to prioritize spaces for participant observation. Ethnographic research is necessarily carried out with relatively small samples. Particularly when the research concerns sensitive and complex topics such as sexual behavior, it is possible to carry out multiple, in-depth, semi-structured interviews only with a relatively small number of people. Furthermore, a small sample size is necessary due to the time required to develop a level of trust and confidence with each informant so that they are actually willing to talk about private and sensitive issues.[5] In many ethnographic studies, however, it is not always clear how the people selected for the small samples relate to the range of experiences and diversity in the society as a whole. Having a clearly conceptualized sampling strategy, therefore, can enormously enhance the explanatory power and generalizability of ethnographic research. This is accomplished by recruiting participants who vary across theoretically and empirically determined social axes that reflect key aspects of diversity. Indeed, if anthropology is to contribute effectively to positive social change by making its findings persuasive to the public and to policy makers, it is hard to overstate the importance of incorporating a more structured approach to sampling. By including individuals whose access to critical economic, social, and symbolic resources is varied, but who share common cultural frameworks, we are more likely to see the diverse ways in which differently situated people use and interpret these frameworks.

The method we used borrows the idea of stratification from survey sampling in order to deliberately incorporate diversity into the small samples typical of ethnographic research. However, ethnographic sampling is fundamentally different than survey sampling because ethnographic sampling is concerned with capturing the range of experiences, behaviors, beliefs, and social types that exist, and with learning how these might map onto structures of stratification, rather than with making statements about their frequency or distribution within a population. Another way in which systematic ethnographic sampling differs from the classic demographic variables (race, sex, class) along which surveys are frequently stratified is that ethnographic sampling includes locally relevant manifestations of social structure. For example, in an early project exploring reproductive health among Mexican migrant women in Atlanta, Georgia, Hirsch wanted to explore how women's independence, power, and autonomy shaped their reproductive health practices. However, it was only after working in the community for several months that she knew enough about the women to conclude that this variation would be best captured by including diversity in terms of women's legal status, possession of a driver's license, access to consanguineal (as opposed to affinal) kin, and ability to speak English (Hirsch and Nathanson 1998; Hirsch 2003).

Because our goal in the current study was to explore how sociocultural factors intertwine with inequality to shape HIV vulnerabilities, it was critical to ensure that the samples reflected the locally relevant forms of social stratification that produced such vulnerabilities. In many ways, agreeing on a sampling strategy was one of the most difficult aspects of designing the project. It was difficult to determine in advance the three *locally* relevant forms of social stratification that would be significant in terms of HIV vulnerability in all five field sites. Should we choose level of education? Having a salaried job or not? One axis we considered was, in fact, education. But the question arose as to how meaningful a comparison education would be between, for example, Tari in Papua New Guinea, where few individuals have a college degree, and Hanoi, where a huge number do. We also briefly considered deliberately seeking variation in marital happiness, to address the potential bias in learning about marriage only from those whose marriages met local criteria for success, but it quickly became evident that this would be highly problematic. First, we realized that the decision to use marital happiness as an axis might well be based on Western assumptions regarding a causal connection between marital unhappiness and infidelity. Second, it was not at all clear how we could compare happiness or even satisfaction cross-culturally. Third, even if we could address the problems with comparability, recruiting according to individuals' internal psychological states would do nothing to advance our overall intention with the systematic sampling, which was to incorporate varying positions with regard to social factors. Another axis we considered was religiosity, or the degree to which people considered themselves religious. But although this was arguably relevant in many of our sites, further conversation revealed this too was also problematic, since it is only recently that the Vietnamese government has allowed its citizens to practice Buddhism openly, and it is primarily women who do so. Also, we wondered whether it would be possible to measure a person's religious commitment and differentiate between, for example, Pentecostal religion in Nigeria and Uganda and Catholicism in Mexico.

Ultimately, the marital case study participants across all five sites were selected to incorporate variation in (1) labor-related migration and mobility; (2) socioeconomic status (SES); and (3) duration of marriage—specifically, whether couples were recently married, well established in their family-building projects, or already grandparents. Labor-related migration and mobility was chosen as an axis of diversity due to its association with HIV transmission in all five sites. SES reflected differences in access to resources and actual wealth, both of which we thought might influence a person's extrafamilial leisure activities and ultimately shape his or her opportunities for extramarital sex as well as the types of relations in which individuals would engage. Duration of marriage enabled comparison across generations (capturing wider social change and location relative to emerging ideologies of companionate marriage) and reflected different concerns, experiences, and responsibilities across an individual's life course and marital progression.

Despite the use of SES as an axis, we remained aware of the (in)commensurability of inequality itself, and worried about the potentially false equivalence among the systems of social and economic stratification in these five quite distinct settings. Consider, for example, the differences in standards of living between a jobless and uneducated but landowning farmer in rural Papua New Guinea and a jobless, uneducated worker from semi-urban Mexico; each might be equally low on his respective social and economic totem pole, but the Mexican lives in a town with running water and electricity, is required by law to send his children to school through sixth grade, and can apply (if he is poor enough) for his family to participate in a government subsidy program through which they would receive direct cash benefits for attending health education classes and staying up-to-date on vaccinations. The landowning farmer in Papua New Guinea, by contrast, has no access to such resources or government-prescribed safety nets. The relative deprivation of greatest relevance to our informants, of course, was not that of some individual halfway around the world, but rather that of their position in relation to their neighbors. So, in the end, we decided to break the category into "higher assets and resources" and "lower assets and resources," making our use of the category one that would measure variation in ways relevant to each site, but that would not attempt to capture some absolute economic position across all five sites.

Determining SES was not always straightforward, and it sometimes led to other fruitful findings. For instance, after much discussion and debate, Parikh's research team in Uganda determined that the two socioeconomic categories would not adequately reflect the large and emerging middle class in their field site, and so they added a third category that included professional people who had entry-level or low-paying positions (such as secretaries or teachers) and wage laborers who had a steady stream of income. This three-tiered distinction was also adopted in Nigeria. In Hanoi, it proved difficult to determine the level of an informant's SES if he or she was not interviewed at home and was only asked about his or her assets. In addition, due to the rapidly changing economy, social status and economic status were not necessarily commensurate with or reflective of one another. Therefore, the Vietnamese team decided it was more important to interview individuals of different professions in order to capture socioeconomic diversity.

We relied on a sampling matrix to keep track of the extent to which the couples we recruited reflected these three intersecting axes of diversity (see Appendix I). In some cases, it was difficult to recruit enough marital case study participants to fill one of the boxes in the matrix. For example, in the Papua New Guinea and Uganda sites, it was almost impossible to find participants who were "high SES" but had no migration experience. However, this "problem" in and of itself counted as data, as it underlined the ways in which mobility and migration experiences are linked to economic opportunities.

Marital Case Studies

For the marital case studies, each member of a married couple was interviewed separately by either the primary researcher or by his or her research assistant (this was done in order to follow social conventions, where relevant, about not speaking with a person of the opposite sex about intimate matters). This method helped us learn about gendered differences in marital and extramarital experiences and ideals through two narratives (the husband's and the wife's) about the same marriage. This book's opening vignette about Chigozie and Ihunanya's respective accounts of their "modern marriage" clearly shows how this technique elucidated gendered differences and similarities in marital experiences and ideals. For the interviews, which took place over the course of several meetings and were tape-recorded for later transcription, each of us used a locally adapted version of an ethnographic interview guide that we had developed as a team (see Appendix II for our initial ethnographic interview guide template). The guide provided a framework for encouraging participants to tell the stories of their marriage, including how they met, why and how they married, and how their marriage had changed over time, including conflicts, expectations and obligations, and disappointments and satisfactions. Together with the participant observation, it was through these marital case studies that we learned in great detail about the primary phenomena we were seeking to understand: marital and extramarital experiences, and sexual practices. With their detailed information on men's and women's relationships with each other and with their kin and social networks, and on the gendered organization of labor, these marital case studies shed light on the strategic value of these social behaviors—so that we could see not just what people were doing, but why it might make sense to them, given their range of other options, to do what they did.

Once in the field, each of us adapted the shared research design to the local context. For instance, in Vietnam the entire project of data collection was complicated by the research protocol for foreigners, which required Phinney to be accompanied by a Vietnamese researcher or a Women's Union cadre and to work through official channels (e.g., the district Women's Union or People's Committee) to identify research subjects. Concerned with issues of flexibility, representation, and privacy, Phinney hired Vietnamese researchers to conduct marital case studies so that they could interview individuals on their own without the restrictions Phinney faced.

When there was a tension between the plans we had made as a group and the feasibility or appropriateness of those plans in the specific local context, context always won out—and the modifications usually served, in and of themselves, to shed light on the questions we were asking. In Papua New Guinea, for example, the idea of eliciting data from married couples on intimacy turned out to be not just difficult but downright dangerous. Huli men wanted to be interviewed first. Once interviewed, they refused to allow their wives to be interviewed, and a few were so angered by the request that Wardlow's Huli field assistants eventually became afraid to ask. (It was not surprising that the field assistants became anxious about potential threats to their own safety: because of ethnic conflict, election-related violence, widespread crime, and an ineffective (and often absent) police force, tensions were high in the Tari area at that time, and responding to insults with physical force is acceptable and fairly common behavior among the Huli.) Ultimately, the research team primarily interviewed men and women who were married, but not to each other. Again, although this kind of eventuality was disappointing, it led us to a deeper understanding of marital sexuality and power among the Huli through an additional set of questions that asked why Huli male participants were reluctant to let their wives participate in the study. Men said that no self-respecting man would permit his wife to participate in a study that included questions about sex and marriage because talking about sex automatically aroused a woman's desire, which would consequently make a wife more likely to stray (in other words, by permitting his wife to participate in the study, a man was potentially causing his own cuckolding). Also, a husband's authority might be undermined, since wives were likely to use the interview setting as a venue for airing complaints and even deriding a husband. Their responses suggest that the idealized model of companionate marriage—with its presumption of mutual trust—does not have much emotional purchase with Huli men, and that male authority continues to be central to their models of marriage.

Adapting a protocol developed by the team to the exigencies of daily life in five very different field sites was a constant balancing act. Traditionally, one of the great advantages of ethnography is its flexibility, with the research questions shifting to reflect emerging lines of questioning. As Liisa Malkki notes, "The living social context of ethnographic research is *expected* to transform one's original framing or animating questions. To hold on to the questions posed in one's original grant proposal when the context is continually teaching one how to ask better questions makes little sense in ethnographic fieldwork" (Cerwonka and Malkki 2007: 79; emphasis in original). Doing ethnography, Malkki continues, is "not a matter of the gradual accumulation of 'data' into a stable structure, but of moments of puzzlement and sudden realization, of making and unmaking" (175). The challenge to us as a team, of course, was that such individual moments of making and unmaking—or, in other words, unilaterally following new lines of inquiry suggested by emerging data—could have easily led us so far away from our initial questions that our final findings would have had little in common. We addressed this challenge by working together with a clearly articulated shared conceptual framework, by using very detailed instruments to organize the data collection, and by communicating via e-mail during our time in the field to provide each other with moral support, discuss emerging findings, and address site-specific modifications to the research design.

In Uganda, for example, the idea of articulating one's emotional feelings about a spouse to a stranger was so culturally unfamiliar to some of the older informants that they frequently took the question "How do you feel about your spouse?" to be an inquiry about a spouse's health (that is, how the spouse was feeling) or an inquiry about their overall appreciation of their spouse. Thus, common responses were "She feels well today" or "I feel good about her/him." The interview protocol allowed the researcher to rephrase questions and to add culturally meaningful follow-up questions in order to elicit the intended information. Creating probes to reflect local practices of articulating emotions and sentiments, the Ugandan research team eventually decided to ask, "If you were to write a love letter to your spouse, what would you write?" This revised question often generated lengthy answers as well as the emotional response about spouses that the original version had sought; it also revealed interesting gender differences in the complexity of the relationship between emotions toward a spouse and extramarital sexuality or treatment of a spouse. For instance, a man who recited a long, emotion-filled love letter about his wife might simultaneously have beaten or economically neglected his wife, or acknowledged various extramarital affairs. Such responses highlighted the fact that extramarital liaisons and love are not mutually exclusive; in other words, a man's participation in extramarital sex does not necessarily reflect a lack of love for his wife, and in some cases, as frequently discussed by men, a wife's tolerance and "patience" might in fact bolster a husband's emotions toward her.

Participant observation in households in Nigeria and Papua New Guinea spurred the addition of a new question to the marital case study guide that focused on whether husbands and wives "seek permission," "inform," or say nothing at all to their spouses when they leave their households for some kind of errand or social activity. In these two research sites—and to a lesser extent in Uganda and Mexico—this question elicited lengthy and sometimes surprisingly impassioned answers from both men and women, resulting in nuanced data that illustrated the specific nature of gender inequality with regard to mobility. In addition to demonstrating men's relative power and agency in this domain—which contribute directly to opportunities for extramarital sex—details about the processes (and domestic contestation) by which male and female mobility were negotiated served both to contrast different marriages and to illustrate the fine-grained aspects of marital gender dynamics. This question, however, yielded little valuable data in Vietnam, where informal rules of etiquette dictate that individuals inform others of their comings and goings regardless of status.

Participant Observation

Participant observation, which implies a structured manner of interacting with and observing people as they go about the daily business of living, is the central method through which anthropologists learn about social context and how people operate within it. Participant observation is an important complement to narrative data for several reasons. First, people are not always the best informants on how social structure shapes the options available to them: they may not notice how their options are constrained by social organization, or they may not wish to discuss it. Second, participant observation can help us gain access to what people *actually do*, rather than just hearing from them *what they say that they do*. This can include noticing spouses' verbal and nonverbal interactions, who is served first and more at meals, who interrupts whom and who is more easily silenced, and what people find unexpectedly—and, for the novice anthropologist, usually inexplicably—funny (Goldstein 2003). Third, unscripted moments of social interaction can—and indeed should—play a vital role in shaping the direction of ethnographic research. Fourth, participant observation provides information about local values and prestige systems in a fashion that can facilitate critical insight into how people shape the portraits they draw for us of their communities and their lives. People exaggerate, distort, and even outright lie, but they do so in systematic ways that reflect their underlying beliefs, and so participant observation can provide clues on how to critically interpret the narratives collected through interviews and focus groups. In rural Mexico, for example, some men claimed that they would never beat their wives, while others insisted on the importance of a man's "right" to discipline his wife physically. It would have been naïve to take either sort of statement as a perfect representation of actual behavior, but after spending time with the men and their families and watching them interact, Hirsch learned to read these statements as claims to a certain style of masculinity.

Our participant observation was focused on three domains of social life: (1) marital relationships as enacted in the domestic and public spheres; (2) extramarital relations, particularly in terms of the spaces where socializing among men and between unmarried women and men takes place; and (3) gendered interactions and ways of being in community public spaces such as markets, schools, religious services, and health centers, as well as at celebrations such as weddings. By spending time with couples and families, we learned about marital verbal and nonverbal interaction; consumption practices; the structure of private and public spaces in houses; the nature of marital communication; patterns of eating and socializing; men's and women's income-generating activities and contributions to social reproduction; how decisions about resource allocation are made; and gender and life-course differences in physical autonomy. Moreover, participant observation with those couples with whom we had also conducted marital case studies provided additional perspective on the lives and relations they had described to us, allowing us to consider for ourselves which aspects of their lives they might have chosen to highlight or deemphasize in the quest to present themselves strategically in the most flattering light.

To learn about the social organization of extramarital relationships, we conducted targeted exploration of the places where men typically meet potential extramarital partners, such as bars, pool halls, rent-a-room hotels, discos, nightclubs, and concert venues, and where they talk about these relationships with male peers. (The "we," to be sure, included our male field assistants, since only Smith, as a man, was able to spend much time in these settings himself.) For instance, the Uganda research team spent several evenings following what some men referred to as the "drinking route," in which groups of male friends would go from one drinking place to another, eventually ending the evening in one of the late-night bars along Main Street. At the final stop, a man might meet a potential partner for that evening or exchange cell phone numbers for a future rendezvous. Tracing men's evening drinking culture allowed Parikh's team to map out Iganga's sexual geography and observe how men's behavior changed as they navigated through it. We endeavored to explore the full range of extramarital relations, organized in every site into culturally specific taxonomies that varied widely in terms of duration, material exchange, emotional intimacy, relative secrecy or integration into semipublic patterns of homosociality, and marital disruptiveness.

Participation in the communal social and economic life of each field site, the third element of our shared plan for participant observation, was the route to learning more about how structural and cultural factors shape intimate relations. Paying attention to how the people around us supported themselves provided a window into the relative impact and form of labor migration in each field site, gendered opportunity structures, and how local systems of economic organization affect daily life. The ways gender and sexuality are mapped onto social space was another critical interest, as we observed where men and women spend time together outside the home and how the organization of these spaces shapes heterosexual, homosexual, and homosocial relationships. (In the Vietnam and Mexico field sites, we also learned how powerful ideologies of heteronormativity coexist with significant—and not very hidden—populations of men participating in various forms of same-sex sexual activity). We also explored the influence of religious movements; how the availability and use of relatively new forms of material culture such as lingerie and videos shape ideas about gender, sexuality, and desire; how images of family, gender, and sexuality are presented in television, popular songs, and print media; and how people understand and use these images.

Participant observation often generates moments of clarity about social organization. In a revealing moment in Mexico, Hirsch snuck into a cantina one night and hid in the kitchen with the cantina owner's girlfriend; they happened to come in just as a group of men wearing mustaches and cowboy boots were chanting "*beso, beso*," daring two males in their crowd to kiss each other. Particularly when exploring sensitive topics such as the vein of simultaneous intense homoeroticism and deep homophobia that runs through Mexican popular culture, participant observation opens the door to learning about these "public secrets" (Taussig 1999: 50)—the things that everybody knows about but nobody talks about.

Participant observation also helped us assess the reliability of information gathered via different methods. For example, few of the male informants from the marital case studies in Hanoi admitted to visiting sex workers, but they had remarkably good information about the circumstances under which men are encouraged to do so and where one should go to find sex workers. Phinney confirmed these accounts by employing one of her key informants, a motorcycle taxi driver, to show her these locations. To demonstrate the ease with which a mobile man can hook up with a sex worker, the driver stopped and made his arrangements with a woman while Phinney was still perched on the back of his motorbike.

Research Assistants

As many of the above examples suggest, we were all highly dependent on our local research assistants, both for conducting interviews and for participant observation. As women, four of us often could not even enter the male spaces where participant observation most needed to be done—because entrance would not have been permitted, because all typical activity would have ceased and attention turned to us if we had entered, because entering might have irreparably damaged our local reputations (and thus our ability to work), or because it would have been dangerous even to try. In the chapters that follow, we each discuss the nature of our research teams; however, because our research assistants played such a crucial role in this project, we also briefly discuss their roles here.

Our teams varied in terms of the number of field assistants, and their educational levels and social science research experience. Wardlow's four male field assistants in Papua New Guinea were all middle-aged married men who had completed grade ten at most, and had never conducted interviews before. Most important in her selection of assistants was that they differed in character and reputation: one was devoutly Christian and active in promoting divine healing for HIV; one was easily able to recruit participants from the drinking and gambling crowd; one was known as a wise and trustworthy elder; and another was known to have an unusually companionate marriage. In contrast, Hirsch's male field assistant was a Mexican physician and medical anthropologist in his mid-twenties who at the time was completing a master's degree in social anthropology; she supplemented the skills he brought to the project by seeking help—particularly help identifying prospective marital case study informants—from an elite, companionately married man, and a working-class woman who was also her closest friend in the field.

In selecting her research assistants in Uganda, Parikh considered age and kinship/social networks. Her team consisted of five assistants (two female and three male). She began with a male and a female assistant—both young, unmarried adults—who had been most helpful in her previous work on sexuality in Iganga, and were thus familiar with ethnographic research and comfortable asking sensitive questions about intimacy. Parikh then added a lead assistant who had a master's degree, a married woman from another ethnic group trained as a social worker, and a young man with a university degree in economics who skillfully navigated through diverse social landscapes. Discussions among this diverse group of assistants led to often humorous but insightful debates about the contradictions between modern marriage and infidelity.

Smith's team in Nigeria included two married women in the semi-rural site and an unmarried man and a younger married woman in the urban site. The assistants in the urban site found it easier to elicit sensitive information from people they interviewed than did his assistants in the rural area. The relative anonymity of the city appeared to increase candor: married women in the rural area feared that the women who interviewed them (women who shared their social networks) could use their responses in gossip. Phinney's team in Vietnam consisted of highly trained social science researchers with extensive experience conducting survey research but little (if any) experience conducting participant observation. As a result, they were adept at eliciting information, but tended to ignore the affect and emotion generated by the interview questions. Nor did they provide more than an outline of the locations in which they spoke with informants.

Our different strategies for recruiting and working with field assistants reflected, to some extent, the widely (indeed, almost wildly) different levels of socioeconomic development in the field sites. For example, Wardlow had been warned that in the context of Tari's severe economic deterioration and social unrest, paying just one or two assistants a high wage would make her and them objects of jealousy and potential targets for theft; hiring four men from different clans at lower wages was the wiser strategy. In Vietnam, in contrast, Phinney faced pressures and constraints due to the State's often strict regulation of foreign researchers, particularly Americans. In Uganda, Parikh had to be mindful of socioeconomic differences between participants and research assistants. For example, a rural, poor young woman might not have felt comfortable being interviewed by an urban young woman whose economic status and urban residence had allowed her to remain unmarried without any serious social consequence. Even if (or perhaps because?) they were the same age, their very different social worlds would have made our set of interview questions seem judgmental and unnecessarily nosy.

Asking field assistants to engage in participant observation in spaces the female authors could not enter was far more of a hurdle. Although field assistants who are men earn entry to male spaces by their gender (assuming that they can also afford the actual entry fee, if there is one), this does not automatically mean that they want to, that they feel comfortable doing so, that it wouldn't hurt their reputations, or that we have the tools and skills to learn from participant observation that we did not conduct ourselves. For Sergio Meneses Navarro, Hirsch's field assistant, the opportunity to spend every night in a bar quickly wore thin. Hirsch had joked during the hiring process that what she was looking for was someone who "liked to drink, but not too much," but in practice Meneses found it as tiresome to spend time in those spaces of masculinity as Hirsch found it frustrating not to be able to. Similarly, two of Wardlow's four assistants refused to set foot in *dawe anda* (rural brothels) for fear of compromising their reputations, and one would only go on condition that he was allowed to proselytize (a kind of participant observation that Wardlow was pretty sure would not result in useful data). In contrast, Parikh's assistants felt comfortable venturing to various places and were less concerned about whether being seen in certain environments would ruin their reputations. In fact, her two female research assistants were *excited* to have the excuse of research to enter spaces typically not appropriate for "decent" young women. On another occasion, the research team (excluding Parikh, who was in the capital at the time) decided to visit the local version of a strip club to see what really went on there.

(It turned out to be just women in ultra-mini skirts dancing provocatively for the audience, which was mostly men.) While hiring men as field assistants was critical to our ability to conduct this research, their masculinity did not confer on them a blanket privilege to easily go everywhere. Class, community of origin, reputation, religiosity, age, and marital status all complicated our field assistants' abilities to do participant observation. For Smith, the issues were reversed; as suggested earlier, particularly in the rural site, married women seemed uncomfortable revealing too much to the local research assistants, who were seen as potentially threatening because they shared the same social networks.

Finally, we should mention a kind of collaboration that we did not anticipate during the initial design of the project, but that we would certainly try to build into the design of any future multisited, comparative work—that among the assistants across the field sites. Several months into the project, Parikh's assistants requested contact with the research assistants in the other four locations. The assistants in Uganda wanted to know if what they were finding about marriage, intimacy, and infidelity was similar across the sites. Also, at least two of the assistants who had previously worked with Parikh had seen her come and go from Uganda, and they too wanted the excitement of transnational experiences, even if limited to virtual pen pal correspondence. The assistants wanted to communicate directly with the others (unmediated by the American principal investigators) not only about the research findings, but also about the process of actually carrying out the research, comparing experiences such as asking the sensitive interview questions. That we did not anticipate their desire for direct communication reflects our own internalization of the arguably colonialist, hierarchical model of the traditional relationship between anthropologist and field assistant. As it happened, *Born in Africa*—a film about Philly Lutaya, the international pop star who had been the first prominent Ugandan to go public about his HIV-positive serostatus—was being used in Papua New Guinea for AIDS awareness and was very popular among Huli men. Thus, the Huli field assistants were especially enthusiastic about the opportunity to connect with the Ugandan field assistants. Although the actual interactions among our field assistants were ultimately constrained by language barriers, the lack of Internet cafés in Tari, and other obstacles, we were struck by how the possibility of communication could potentially lead to comparative questions generated not only by us but by our local collaborators.

Iterative Fieldwork and Data Analysis

It is axiomatic within ethnographic research that analysis is an iterative process, which means that the insights generated by the data collection process are constantly being integrated back into the ongoing research project and design. This happens in ways that can vary significantly in scale, from refining or adding questions that reflect locally relevant concerns to adding entirely new lines of inquiry and categories of informants. Working iteratively in a multisited, comparative ethnographic project, however, meant the convergence of two very different field-work conventions: (1) the individual freedom and flexibility of individual anthropological ethnographic research projects that allow for changes in the field guides, the content of the questions, and even the specific topic under study; and (2) the logistical constraints typical of international public health research in which the field team who conducts the research may not have designed the research questions, nor do its members have the power to dramatically alter questions or change research direction while in the field. The shared conceptual framework that we developed as a team helped maintain the balance between improvisation and comparability, as did our constant communication, which included frequent discussions of how specific situations dictated the need for individual researchers to diverge from and change specific lines of inquiry in order to capture local meanings.

The "virtual chat room" we had envisioned prior to going into the field proved to be an invaluable source of intellectual and moral support for us, as investigators working comparatively on sensitive topics under sometimes challenging circumstances. After considering some of the more sophisticated technological options available, our group chose to go with a simple "reply-all" e-mail format (rather than, for example, an electronic mailing list or a password-protected discussion board). The fact that we could be in touch with each other at all allowed us to share revised instruments to maintain comparability even as we adapted them to particular cultural settings. For example, it became evident through our e-mail exchanges that in the Mexican field site, the marital case study method was proving less than ideal for collecting data on infidelity, because the couples who were most likely to agree to discuss the details of their marriages with an outsider (even separately from one another—they were not interviewed together) were the couples who were least likely to have been confronted with infidelity. In Uganda, the only extramarital relationship men mentioned was often the one they were least embarrassed about or most proud of, or the one that was the least threatening to ideas of moral propriety. As a result, no man mentioned having an affair with a sex worker (though we did not ask specifically if they had ever paid for sex) and when asked to discuss their most recent extramarital liaison, men tended to mention women whom they portrayed as socially and physically attractive and who were genuinely interested in them. And, as discussed earlier, the marital case study method was almost impossible to implement in the Papua New Guinea field site.

To address these problems but still maintain the comparative emphasis on love and marriage, the investigators agreed to reduce the number of marital case studies in the sites where they had proved problematic (slightly in the Mexico field site, and considerably in the Papua New Guinea site) and to incorporate individuals (without interviewing their spouses) into our samples who could teach us more about local opportunity structures for extramarital relations. Thus, although the specific research method was changed, the fact that we had initially agreed on the goals that motivated each question—rather than simply committing to a shared set of instruments—meant that we could obtain similar and comparable information through other means without reducing the overall comparability of the findings. It is hard to overemphasize the importance of this shared set of research goals and theoretical framework to our ability to carry out theoretically grounded comparative ethnography; since we each had a sense of why we were trying to learn about specific areas of social life, we all felt that we had the freedom to improvise in critical moments without risking the loss of fidelity to the group's overall project.

Working iteratively—in which there is a dialogue between the emerging findings and the evolving research questions—is itself an inherently analytic process, as the researcher is constantly filtering information, deciding what to listen to, which lines of inquiry to pursue, what social opportunities to explore, and which relationships to invest time and effort in developing. The "analysis," as such, began long before the fieldwork itself, with the process of elaborating our shared conceptual framework, which would help us see what our "data" were once we were in the field. Through articulating concepts such as "extramarital opportunity structures," we clarified for ourselves that what we would look for would be the social elements that enable men to participate in extramarital relations. Without establishing that concept or something similar, we might not have made the jump to seeing quite so clearly how social organization makes extramarital sex the sort of default behavioral option in many situations, including long-term migration.

An example of an analytic moment occurred when Phinney observed that perhaps the question we ought to be exploring was not why men engaged in extramarital sex but—given how common it was—why any men did *not*. Our answers to this question, which really underlines our interest in the social organization of extramarital sex, emerged during our first project meeting after we all returned from the field. At this meeting, the presentations about our fieldwork experiences laid the groundwork for many subsequent conversations about homosociality, men's alcohol consumption, the role of religion, people's engagements with globalization and modernity, wives' reactions to husbands' infidelities, the organization of marriage, and the varied nature of extramarital liaisons. In the chapters that follow, we have worked to make the resonances of those conversations clear, and to demonstrate how they challenged our thinking and deepened our analysis.

Conclusion

In recent decades, the comparative method has been thoroughly critiqued in anthropology, and ethnographic fieldwork has largely been naturalized (discursively and institutionally) as an individualized undertaking. Nevertheless, anthropologists engage in comparison all the time. They illustrate theoretical concepts to their students by comparing and contrasting case studies. At conferences and over coffee, they regularly compare notes about social organization, systems of meaning, and political processes with colleagues who work in different areas of the world. And, as myriad scholars have observed, anthropology originated not only in a fascination with the "other," but also in a preoccupation with "ourselves" and a compulsive desire to parse over and over again the similarities and differences between "us" and "them."

As we learned in the process of writing this book, comparative work is making a strong comeback, although the new comparativists may not necessarily recognize themselves as part of a new intellectual movement in sociocultural anthropology. We think of our own methodology and of much other recent comparative work as "critical comparative ethnography" because it employs rich yet structured ethnography to illuminate processes that generate similar kinds of inequality and vulnerability in different world areas. We hope that by reviewing the troubled history of comparison in anthropology, and by explicating the methods we used to carry out a newly reinvented comparative project, this chapter will speak to a variety of audiences about the intellectual and practical challenges of doing a study like this. The chapters that follow will illustrate, we hope, its intellectual and practical benefits.

To explain ethnography as a research practice, Malkki invokes the metaphor of jazz, asserting that "it is not the case that [in anthropology] there is an old, stable tradition with a fixed battery of methods. . . . Rather, improvisation *is* the tradition" (Cerwonka and Malkki 2007: 180). By comparing ethnography to jazz improvisation, Malkki asserts not only that fieldwork requires methodological resourcefulness, creativity, and flexibility, but also that it would be a mistake to regard it as ad hoc, unstructured, or unplanned. "There is, in fact, a lifetime of preparation and knowledge behind every idea that an improviser performs," she notes, quoting Paul Berliner (182). This metaphor resonates strongly with our own experiences of the ethnographic fieldwork process. At the same time, our comparative endeavor makes it clear to us that there is something missing from Malkki's exegesis of this analogy: jazz performers most commonly play as part of a group rather than alone. All the members of the group improvise, but all also agree to work within the themes that are structuring their collaborative effort. This is how we see the work of comparative ethnography. It is true that some improvisation—that is, the pursuit of some emergent lines of inquiry—may have to be foreclosed or only cursorily examined because of a commitment to the shared conceptual themes or framework. Nevertheless, given a compelling research question and a painstakingly constructed conceptual framework, the improvisation that characterizes ethnographic fieldwork is possible and can generate insights or new themes for the group as a whole.

2

The Geography of Desire

Social Space, Sexual Projects, and the Organization

of Extramarital Sex in Rural Mexico

Jennifer S. Hirsch

The geography of desire in Degollado is sharply divided between public spaces for the performance of sexual respectability and a semi-private backstage for illicit relations.[1] The meaning of each is mutually constituted, so that one makes sense only in light of the other; extramarital sex represents here not the negation of marriage but its complement. In exploring spatial aspects of sexuality in rural Mexico, I emphasize the complementarity of elements frequently viewed in binary terms: heterosexuality and homosexuality, marital and extramarital relations, and spaces of respectability and those of desire. In illustrating how social spaces incite sexual behavior, I show not just that sexual practices vary across locations, but also that space is an essential element of the social organization of sexuality. By moving across the social landscape, and engaging in the practices of meaning-making that distinguish a physical place from a social space, people produce sexuality in a way that is inextricably intertwined with the very constitution of that landscape. The notion of sexual geography provides a useful tangible articulation of structural elements of sexuality: the sexual geography through which men and women (but most notably men) navigate in and around Degollado can be seen as the product of the intersection of normative concepts of ideal masculinity and femininity with the gendered organization of the labor market and the family.

Sexual reputations depend on the agility with which people negotiate through this sexual geography, and in Degollado it is those reputations, rather than object choice, that are the most critical axis of sexual identity. Anthropologists of sexuality have argued convincingly that sexual identities vary cross-culturally (Herdt 1981, 1984, 1987; Carrier 1985, 1989, 1994, 1995; Parker 1985, 1991; Parker and Caceres 1999), so that, for example, practices that might signal "gay" in one context can signal "powerful adult man" in another. Unquestioned through most of this literature, however, is the assumption that partner choice is the critical axis of sexual identity. At least in Degollado, descriptions of sexual behavior—and, by extension, characterizations of people as particular kinds of sexual beings— emphasize whether appearances are managed appropriately in relation to contextually variable expectations, rather than what people actually feel, do, or exchange behind closed doors. This focus on reputation-based sexual identities holds true regardless of whether the subject is an unmarried adolescent girl, a married man with a female partner, or two men who have sex with each other. Adolescent girls, for example, are only *fracasada* (publicly ruined) when they become pregnant outside of marriage and their suitor fails to respond by marrying them, rather than if they are thought to have had sex before marriage but it cannot be proven (Hirsch 2003). So too in Degollado do people emphasize the distinction between flagrant and appropriately managed infidelity: a man will not provoke criticism from his peers for a fling during a night of drinking with his buddies, but he will if he drives down the street in broad daylight accompanied by a woman other than his wife. Similarly, the most salient criterion of men's sexual identities is not whether they have sex in private with men or with women but rather what their public gendered self-presentation is—whether or not they act and dress like *hombres normales* (normal men) (Carrillo 2001; Kelly 2008).

The overwhelming salience of appearances in Mexico's moral economy of sexuality does not mean that there is no stigma attached to same-sex sexual desire or activity. To the contrary, sexual inequality is a fundamental element of the spatial organization of desire, so that the heteronormativity that reigns (at least during the day) in the town's central plaza contrasts with the somewhat less compulsory nature of heterosexuality in the spaces where men relax together—and perhaps even in the plaza itself, late at night, when the town's nice girls are safely behind locked doors. Ideal "public" sexuality is (or ought to be) heteronormative, monogamous, and reproductive, while the sexual relations that flourish in private include possibilities for multiple partnerships, suspension of the need to demonstrate respect, the use of sexual jokes that would be considered disrespectful if told publicly in mixed company (Hirsch 1990), and a much greater flexibility toward object choice. The division between the spaces in which people strive to perform socially sanctioned sexual ideals and those in which they can let themselves be led by desire and the quest for pleasure is symbolized by the upholding of heteronormativity in one context and the possibilities for its abandonment in another. This spatial organization of sexuality, however, does not mean that people "control" themselves sexually in public and go crazy in private; rather, the range of meanings and behaviors in each set of spaces draws meaning from those of the other— and, in each context, men and women use sexuality both to generate pleasure and to nurture specific kinds of social relations. Just as the category of heterosexuality only emerged and drew meaning from the abject other of homosexuality (Foucault 1985; Weeks 1989; D'Emilio 1997, 1998), so too are marital and extramarital relations and the spaces across which they are organized mutually constituted and inextricably intertwined.

"Sex work" ordinarily refers to the exchange of money for sex, but here I play with a distinct notion of sex work by framing sex as a sphere of agency—the focus of concentrated effort in order to achieve specific goals. With an eye to how men and women use sexuality to build social relations, I explore the notion of "sexual projects," tracing out the range of goals men in particular have sought to accomplish through engaging in extramarital relations. Throughout this volume, we emphasize the structural nature of men's extramarital sexual relations, depicting them as produced almost inexorably by the intersections of gendered patterns of mobility, economic organization, normative expectations of gender, and patterns of kinship. Although the specifics differ for women, which makes the occurrence of infidelity either somewhat rarer or much more carefully hidden, it is possible to see the outlines of social organization in the scant information about those relations as well. This emphasis on the *social* production of infidelity provides a useful corrective to biologically based explanations. It fails entirely, however, to help us understand what it is, exactly, that men and women seek in extramarital sex, and falls short with respect to framing these practices in relation to tensions between structure and agency. It also runs the risk of implying that individuals have no choice but to seek extramarital sex—and since there were men across all the field sites who deliberately avoided extramarital relations, questions of agency cannot be ignored. Exploring what people seek out of sex means seeing sex at least potentially as simultaneously both a strategy and a goal—that is, something for which people strive for the self-evident reason of pleasure, but also perhaps as a domain through which they may access other key resources. The notion of sexual projects frames sexuality as productive of relations, identities, and even elements of social stratification, in addition to individual pleasure.

Men's love for their wives does form part of the cultural context of marital HIV risk, but not in any simple way. When a man hesitated to pursue a sexual opportunity, it was as likely to be as much out of concern for his reputation as it was for fear of emotional offense to his wife. In Degollado, young men across social classes shared with their wives a marital ideal characterized by emotional intimacy, trust, and warmth, in comparison to the men of older generations, who focused more on respect and the fulfillment of gendered obligations. The feelings that men held for their wives, however, were not always the primary determinants of their extramarital sexual behavior. Among the marital case studies, there were some older couples in which the men neither shared much warmth and intimacy with their wives nor avidly sought out extramarital sex. For these men, refraining from extramarital sex was a function of their desire to demonstrate a certain kind of public respectability and restraint. Sergio and I also met younger men who loved their wives, who took pleasure in their company as well as their bodies, and who felt close to them—but who continued to have sex with other women. For some men, love means that they are faithful because otherwise they could not face their wives; for others, it merely means redoubled efforts to be discreet—to make sure that their extramarital activities do not infringe on the companionate intimacy they are building with their wives. Although sexual projects can overlap with the marital project, they can also be in tension—a tension that is managed, I argue in this chapter, through keeping "the secret."

Women play a role, too, in keeping "the secret," by failing to ask, or asking in such a way that the question about whether a man would ever be unfaithful becomes an opportunity for the man to perform the role of a good husband. The mutually constitutive nature of marital and extramarital relations, however, should not be understood as a perfectly balanced static system in which what people do and think automatically reproduces social structure. Sometimes the humiliation becomes too much to bear: Juana, one of the few women who told her own story of infidelity, recounted being accosted on the main street by her lover's wife, who yelled at her, "Ya que tu señor no te llena, búscate un burro" (since your husband does not satisfy you, go find a donkey). I am not trying to reproduce here the image of an *abnegada* (silently suffering) Mexican woman; my point is more that the work men and women do together to keep "the secret" reveals something fundamental about marriage, gender, and the organization of sexuality. And, of course, women have their own secrets to keep: the much greater reputational risk that they run if they engage in extramarital sex hardly means that they never do it; it just means they must be extremely careful when they do.[2]

A Bit of Background on Degollado

The town's population of approximately fifteen thousand ebbs and flows with the seasonal migration of workers between Mexico and the United States. Located in semi-rural western Mexico, Degollado lies at the intersection of the Los Altos de Jalisco region (known for its traditions of horsemanship, its tequila production, and its relatively fair-skinned population) and El Bajío, which was at the heart of Mexico's post-revolution religious war, La Cristiada, and is still characterized by a fervently conservative practice of Catholicism (Hirsch 2008). Historically, the main sources of income in the region have been agriculture (especially the production of pork for regional consumption) and migrant remittances (the town has a history of migration that dates back to the early twentieth century), but the way in which the balance has tipped decisively away from agriculture is indicated by results from the 2000 census, which recorded only 30 percent of the population reporting agriculture as their main source of support.[3] The area's distorted age structure reflects the institutionalization of labor migration: the census data showed that there were 702 men for every 1000 women in the twenty- to twenty-nine-year-old range—traditionally the peak age group for labor migration.[4]

As the county seat, Degollado also provides opportunities for the commercial and professional classes: the town has two banks, a number of schools, many small grocery stores, a central market, and two modern supermarkets, as well as a small private hospital, some Internet cafés, and a number of other local businesses. Attempts at local economic development have included a clothing factory that promised many more jobs than it has been able to offer, the planting of agave in response to worldwide increases in tequila consumption, and the development of a regional stone-carving industry.[5]

The town's main plaza is planted with carefully tended rosebushes, as well as trees whose foliage has been pruned into orderly squares, their trunks primly painted white. After Mass on Sunday evenings, the plaza provides a stage on which young women and men court under the watchful eyes of parents and acquaintances. Groups of young women promenade counterclockwise, their arms linked. They may pause to chat with friends or relatives seated on the benches that ring the plaza, but the main objects of their attention are the young men walking clockwise or scattered around the plaza's outer edge. Eye contact and the flirtatious exchange of greetings occasionally lead to a pairing up, and the couple will then circle around together, talking quietly as they perform Degollado's central ritual of public courtship. When the activity winds down in the plaza around 10 p.m., they may walk hand in hand back to the young woman's home, and stand chatting—or embracing in the shadows of the quiet street—outside the girl's family's door. Increasingly, the disco has remained packed on Sunday nights after 10 p.m. (Thompson 2005), so clearly not everyone observes this traditional curfew, but nevertheless, it is known that as the evening wears on, nice girls ought to be at home—even if this knowledge is only honored in the breach.

When my husband came to visit during my first stint of fieldwork in Degollado more than a decade ago, he asked where we could go to drink a beer together and watch the bustling street life. "Married women don't drink in public here," I explained to him. We sat and had our cold Negra Modelo at home, chatting awkwardly with Doña Evita (in whose house I stay when I am in Degollado), and then stepped out to circle the plaza so that I could show off to friends and acquaintances the fact that I did actually have a husband. Although the new *terrazas* (open-air cafés bordering the plaza) Sergio, Brenda, and I sometimes visited during this period of fieldwork in Degollado bear witness to the rapidity of social change and the commercialization of leisure time in Degollado, homosociality remains a fundamental principle of social life. There are many places that good married women just do not go.

During the mid-1990s, very few women in Degollado even knew how to drive, much less had access to cars, and one almost never saw an unmarried woman in

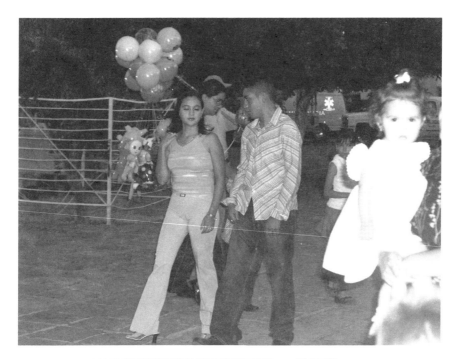

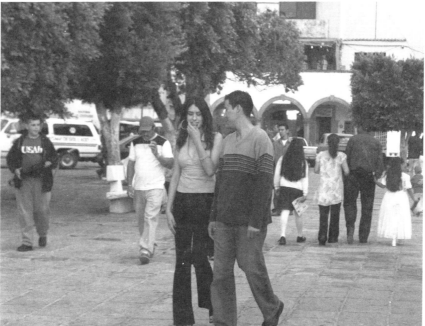

The plaza is the prototypical stage for the performance of respectable sexuality. Photographs by Jennifer S. Hirsch.

a car with a man to whom she was not closely related. The transgressiveness of a woman behind the wheel was underlined by the fact that one of the few other American women in town, a woman of Polish descent who had married a man from Degollado, was referred to as "la Jenny, la que maneja y fuma" (Jenny, who drives and smokes). Since then, some spaces that facilitate heterosociality have emerged, ranging from social institutions such as the disco and the indoor soccer leagues to the high school and professional workplaces where men and women study and work alongside each other. By 2004, the presence of young women in the streets had markedly increased: I saw them driving, being driven, and even zipping up and down the street astride ATVs, wearing revealing mini-blouses. Young women's access to cars reflects both their own incorporation into global patterns of labor migration (which provides some young women with the money to buy cars and excuses to learn how to drive) as well as the growing disposable income available to the town's wealthiest families.

Despite these changes, the patterns of social life in Degollado still reflect this division into spaces of sexual safety, such as the plaza and the home, and those of sexual disorder. The reputational risk a young woman runs by spending time alone with a man is reflected architecturally: all of the *terrazas* where younger couples sometimes meet are open to the elements, so that the public gaze can provide a brake on courting couples who might otherwise lose control.[6] This relationship between gendered prestige and mobility is mutually constitutive: men are more mobile than women because, reputationally, "El hombre no pierde nada, la mujer pierde todo" (men lose nothing, women lose everything), and that same mobility provides men with both the ability to earn money to spend on sex and the opportunities for relations that can be hidden enough to maintain the fiction of fidelity.

The Spatial Organization of Sexuality and Gendered Patterns of Mobility

Juan's journeys provide ample illustration of how men's lives are built around this gendered sexual geography. He learned early on about the special privileges of being a boy: as the oldest boy of a large set of first cousins, he was toted around by his older girl cousins as the "consentido" (the special little one), and as soon as he was old enough to do so on his own (age five or six, in his memory), he scampered about, herding his family's goats. Juan mastered the written word by reading the Bible and learned to add by working in his family's grocery. His time at what he calls "la escuela de la vida" (the school of life) served him well; he says he can still add faster in his head than most men can with calculators. He left home when he was barely eighteen. Arriving in Mexico City in the late 1960s, the pleasures of urban life quickly absorbed what little cash he had brought with him, but he was lucky enough to fall into a job as a construction worker on one of the major public works projects of that era, which led to the opportunity to work—and play—in towns and cities throughout the republic. After living in Mexico City, where he learned how to dance, Juan and his peers showed off their urban polish to girls in small towns across the country: "They all wanted to dance with us," he recalls, "because according to them, no one from the provinces knew how to dance, but the men coming from Mexico City knew all the latest steps." His agile footwork helped him realize his desire "to go around, to see things." He sees the story of his youth as one of mobility and exploration: the story opens with "Yo tuve mucho mundo" (literally, "I had a lot of world") and closes with "Ya me cansé de andar en el mundo" (I was tired of going all over the world). In contrast to today's men, who now seek soul mates, he sought a bride who was pretty, who came from a good family, and whose material expectations did not surpass what he thought he could provide; "Why," he notes, "would I look for anything more?" Indeed, his eventual wife seems almost incidental to the courtship, which had begun with his striking a bet with a friend that he could make the girl on the corner—whom they had both just noticed—agree to be his girlfriend.

Both before and after marrying, Juan worked as the manager of a local clothing factory outside of Degollado, a position that gave him constant access to young women who sought (at least as he tells it) his favors in return for jobs or promotions. After his marriage, one of his young girlfriends had said sadly that he could no longer "misbehave," but he told her, "Oh, can't I? Yes I can. Here, all our lives we continue." He was mostly careful to avoid liaisons with women who lived in Degollado, but he spoke of nights spent dancing in La Piedad and campfires on the banks of the Lerma River, falling asleep with a girlfriend to the strains of a guitar.

In contrast to the well-regulated sexual relationships on display in the plaza and on the stoops of young women's homes, less prestigious forms of sexual relations flourish in other spaces in town. In Juan's story, all of North America appears as the backdrop for his active sexual career—with the exception of his hometown, where he sought a wife and where he reports never having found (or even looked for) extramarital sex. This division of space into "licentious" and "respectable" characterizes daily life in Degollado. Men work hard to hide illicit sexual behavior in town, particularly when they are near the plaza; the farther men are from the plaza, the less careful they need to be.

From childhood on, boys can roam the streets in a way that their sisters cannot. As they grow up, young girls are taught to limit their interactions with men to whom they are not related lest they appear to be inviting a proposition. As a newcomer to the town, I was instructed not to speak to men on the street as part of the broader injunction not to engage in innocent behavior that could be sexually misconstrued. As is true in many other Latino and Mediterranean contexts (González 1974; Gutiérrez 1991; Rebhun 1999), home is the only space that is assumed to be free of sexual danger for women, and the farther that women go from home, the more sexual risks they are imagined to run—so that when a woman runs errands out of town, she frequently takes a child along as a sort of moral shield, to make it clear that she is not slipping away to meet a lover (Rouse 1991; Goldring 1996a, 1996b; Rebhun 1999; Hirsch 2003). These gendered notions of space and sexual risk constrain women's mobility. Post-secondary education only became a possibility for Degollado's wealthier girls when college-level courses became available in nearby La Piedad, from where they could return home daily before dark; the less-wealthy young women who flock north as labor migrants in increasing numbers (Cerrutti and Massey 2001) frequently safeguard the family honor by staying with older male relatives.[7]

Men's access to a homosociality well lubricated with alcohol is a fundamental component of Degollado's spatial organization of desire. Men socialize with their peers in a variety of spaces that their female relatives—wives, mothers, sisters—should not enter. Although not exclusively male spaces, they are known as places "donde las mujeres no entran" (where women don't go)—that is, where decent women do not go. These spaces offer varied pleasures with sexual partners of either sex, at a wide range of price points, as well as affective delights that may include both a woman's adoring and uncomplaining attention (for the price of a few beers) and the comfort of long hours of conversation and jokes with a beloved *compadre*.[8] The metal screen that stands just outside the entrance to each of the town's *billares* (pool halls) aptly captures the porous division between spaces of respectability and those of licentiousness: the screen demarcates the space while still allowing curious passersby to try to sneak a discreet glance inside. I had always been mystified by these screens, which so obviously (and, now I see, deliberately) fail to entirely separate the men playing pool and drinking beer inside from those outside. The billiard hall up the hill in Colonia San Gabriel was the regular haunt of one of Degollado's most sought-after young men, whom Sergio and I had first spotted talking animatedly to a group of older men in cowboy hats and boots during an evening street fair. With plucked eyebrows and a lithe grace, he was a fixture near that pool hall. The day I drove by to pick him up for an interview, he left behind a whole group of older men, clearly crestfallen at his departure. Rumor had it that on the other side of the screen, he did much more than talk with these men.

The billiard halls and cantinas, which serve beer and hard liquor to the accompaniment of a jukebox, are complemented by restaurants, discos, and *zonas de tolerancia* (red-light districts) in nearby towns and cities. A hallmark of many of these spaces is the same flexibility with regard to sexual object choice that Sergio and I noticed first outside the pool hall in San Gabriel: one restaurant in Degollado, for example, owned by a man widely known to have a long-term intimacy with a feminine-appearing man, has become a gathering place for other feminine-appearing men, some from the town itself and others from farther afield. On the road west of town, where several major cross-country highways meet, there are at least six "table-dance" venues where men can drink, watch women dance,

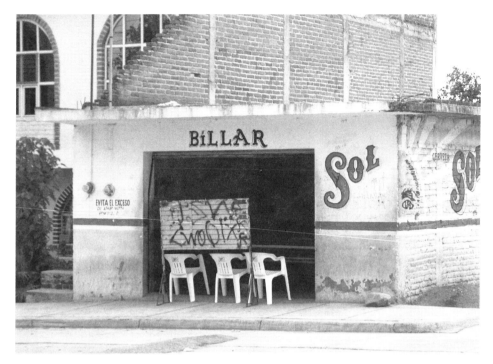

The entryways to billiard parlors and cantinas are always half-heartedly screened off from public view. The symbolic division between decent and sexualized space only serves to underline how they flow into one another. Photograph by Jennifer S. Hirsch.

and perhaps pay extra for a *sexy-privado*, which gives a man twenty minutes to spend in a small room alone with a girl of his choice. The man can pay a "penalty fee" to take her out of the bar for the rest of the night—or, if he prefers, he can cap off an evening of looking but not touching (or at least not touching for very long) by stopping by the all-night sandwich shop (with one of the few all-night liquor licenses in the city) that serves as a late-night gathering place for male prostitutes.[9] Nearby, one of the discos in La Piedad has reportedly begun hosting weekly *noches gay* (gay nights).[10] On Degollado's eastern side, forty minutes down the highway lies a red-light zone with perhaps twenty or so small brothels, including one known as the "bar Degollado"; as darkness falls, the street fills—particularly on paydays—with men whose worn clothes and calloused hands clearly mark them as manual laborers. They pay as little as one hundred pesos (about US$10 at the time) for sex with women. Ninety miles away in Guadalajara, a man can spend US$150 or US$200 on a massage and oral sex from the European beauty of his choice or wander through streets known for their selection of transvestite prostitutes. In all of these locales, men cover for each other: Leonardo, a successful business owner in his early thirties, failed to even notice the contradiction in his telling Sergio that when he and his girlfriend met regularly at a local cantina, "she would go there, and I would tell her to come meet me, but no one saw us—only the people in the cantina."

Degollado lacks the hourly motels that exist throughout Mexico as key spaces for hidden sex, but there are many in neighboring La Piedad. In a society in which men and women live at home until they marry, these motels provide opportunities for premarital sex, extramarital sex, and even marital sex. One man recalled how, as a bachelor, he and his friends would remind each other not to get Room #13 (where the toilet was broken) at the cut-rate motel they frequented with their girlfriends. They came to recognize the particular scent of the hotel's soap, so that they would tease each other, "Hueles a jabón chiquito" (you smell like those little soaps). One young married woman recounted how she and her husband visit the most expensive one once in a while to keep the spice in their relationship. Men bring their male lovers there as well: a young man in his twenties in La Piedad recalled to me how, before their stormy breakup, his lover (a senior official in the local police force) used to send a car and driver regularly to take him to that same luxurious motel.

Spaces outside of town are linked both in fact and in the social imaginary with sexual disorder and moral disarray. At a crowded rodeo about sixty kilometers from town in the spring of 2003, my good friend and research assistant Estela pointed out several married men dancing close in the main ring with young women in sexy Western wear who were definitely not their wives. Ever naïve, I was shocked to see these men cavorting in broad daylight, but the distance from town provided them with a cover that was apparently equivalent to nightfall, or to the screens in front of the billiard halls. The constellation of billboards along the highway outside Guadalajara underlined the way the ever-present possibility of betrayal looms over every family: at the rear is the ideal modern Mexican family, advertising some sort of processed food, and to the right, a bank calls out to those who triumphantly engage with the consumer economy, but in the center, overshadowing both, is a billboard for a private detective agency: "¿Sospecha usted algo?" (Do you suspect something?).

Men take advantage of their mobility to seek extramarital sex. Examples include "el cachimbero" (the truck-stop guy) who drove a delivery truck for his family's business but who reportedly knew every brothel along the way; an acquaintance of ours who came back frequently to Degollado to visit his aging parents, stopping in Puerto Vallarta for some socially risk-free sex before returning to the United States; the group of prominent businessmen from town who went together to Cuba on what was widely known to be a sex tour; and another acquaintance of ours, a restauranteur in the United States, who traveled frequently to Guadalajara to stock up on handicrafts and other items for his restaurants, using these work-related responsibilities as cover for trips to his favorite massage parlor in the city. At the farthest extreme, Mexican migrant men in Atlanta (interviewed

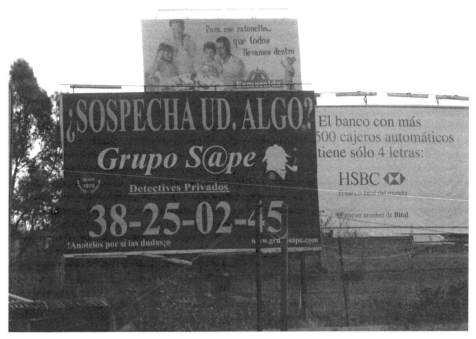

"Do you suspect something?" These billboards along the highway outside of Guadalajara in the spring of 2004 provided a striking juxtaposition of images. Below, a message advertising the services of a private detective agency. Above, a cheese advertisement presenting a well-dressed, fair-skinned, smiling nuclear family, with a caption that reads, "For that little mouse we all have inside." Little mouse, indeed. Photograph by Jennifer S. Hirsch.

as part of another research project) would sometimes jokingly respond to a question about their marital status by saying, "In Mexico, I'm married—but here I am single." Sexual geography is part of the national imaginary; one man in Atlanta, talking about the difficulties of remaining faithful to his wife back home, explained that the United States is, after all, "el país de los vicios" (the country of vices).

Gendered patterns of mobility are interwoven with and reflective of economic organization, which marks as masculine any sort of work that requires a significant amount of mobility. Because men bring home more money than women, they have more say in the disposition of resources, and therefore greater access to spending money for outside women. The gendered nature of the labor market comes into play in other ways in cases such as Juan's, as he sanguinely reports having taken advantage of the power he had over his young female employees to dole out work opportunities in exchange for sex. While some couples do manage to be faithful to each other over the course of long separations (one informant, giggling, recounted how a friend of hers had told her about having regular "phone sex" with her husband during their migration-related separations), the great distance from home lowers the reputational risks of infidelity. The alienation and loneliness of migrant life provide yet another motivation (Hirsch et al. 2009).

International labor migration also shapes the sexual landscape in Degollado. First, it distorts the population structure: imbalances in the sex ratios mean that young women see a reasonably high risk of, as they say, becoming one who "se le fue el barco" (missed the boat) and ending up as one of the town's many "quedadas" (leftover women). The acute sex ratio imbalance provides a backdrop against which to consider both the shifting norms about premarital sex and the ample commentary from married men about the surfeit of tempting young beauties. The increasing sexual visibility of available *muchachas* was evident in the marked sexual assertiveness of slogans on T-shirts in the town's Sunday market. The scarcity of young men can lead a young woman on the upper edge of marriageable age (anything older than her mid-twenties) to settle for a marriage with someone with whom she is not deeply in love, or else to elope with a man she barely knows; at the age of twenty-five, a potentially loveless marriage seems less terrifying than the life of a spinster.

Second, the perception of the United States as a land of sexual opportunity, common among young men, provides the consummate example of the spatial organization of sexuality.[11] Although men journey north for multiple reasons—among which economic reasons are usually primary—the temptation of easy sex with fair-skinned women figures prominently in tales of life on the other side of the border. Racialized notions of beauty are part of the erotics of migration; the persistent Mexican phenomenon of *malinchismo*—a devaluation of all things Mexican, accompanied by the simultaneous preference for the foreign, the northern, and the blonde—makes young men that much more eager to have sex with *las güeras* (the girls with light complexions) so much more available north of the border.

Men form several types of extramarital partnerships as they move across this cartography of desire and opportunity. Most common are brief paid encounters with women, usually in venues that sell alcohol. Married men sometimes develop long-term relationships with women they meet in this way, having children with them and providing the women with some of the economic, sexual, and affective benefits of marriage, although not the security and respect conferred by a publicly sanctified relationship. Occasionally there is talk of a married man or woman who forms a long-term sexual and affective relationship with another married person—there are, for example, endless jokes and the occasional bit of salacious gossip about an affair between a woman and her *compadre* or between a man and his *comadre*—but the risks of this sort of relationship are high and it is hard to know to what extent this exists other than in cautionary tales. (A *compadre* or *comadre*

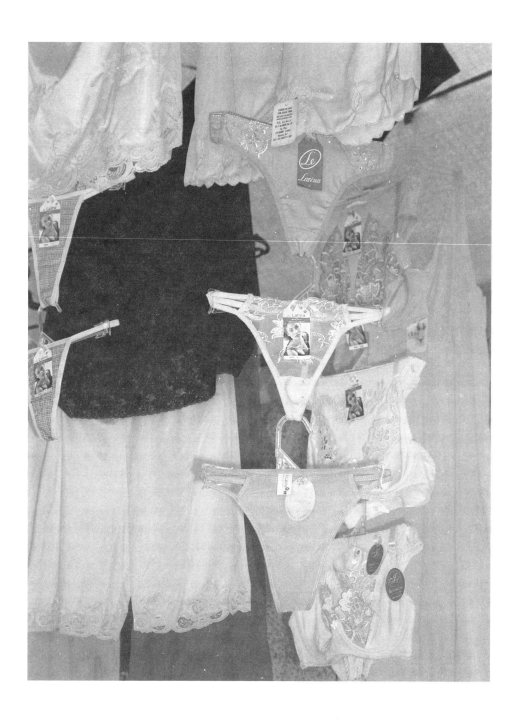

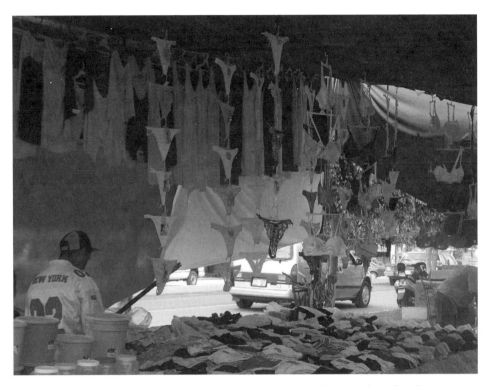

These items demonstrate a new assertiveness for women in the sexual marketplace. Other T-shirts (not shown) read, "My boyfriend is out of town"; "WANTED: Cute Boys for personal hands on services. Must be tall and good-looking. Respond only if you are hot!" and "So many boys, so little time." Photographs by Jennifer S. Hirsch.

is the godparent of one's child; *compadrazgo* presents one of the few social situations in which women and men who are not related by blood or marriage have opportunities to socialize frequently.) Men also engage in brief sexual relations with other men—sometimes paid, sometimes not—and occasionally these also develop into long-term affective relations. In Degollado, for example, there were at least two well-known homosexual couples of longstanding duration: one relationship consisted of a masculine-appearing married man and a very effeminate man, and the other affair was between two masculine-appearing men (mustaches, cowboy boots, and hats), both married. As the distance from Degollado grows larger, so too do the opportunities for sexual and social experimentation: men who spend time north of the border sometimes lead parallel but entirely compartmentalized lives, with families (or sexual identities) of which their kin at home know nothing (Carrillo 2004).

Geography, Social Risk and Sexual Identity

When asked to talk about their own or someone else's sexual behavior, both women and men classified their neighbors in reputational categories—but according to the visibility of their behavior, rather than for the behavior itself. Men, for example, would refer to themselves as "serio," "calmado," or similar adjectives, or else as "sinvergüenza" (lacking in shame). As with the sexual identities that divide men into "hombres normales" (normal men) and "jotos" (derogatory term for feminine-appearing men), these are based on appearances rather than actual behavior: a common response, when asked about infidelity, was to talk not about who does it and who does not, but rather about who is secretive and who is flagrant. As one man said, "Look, that it happens, well, it definitely happens. You hear, suddenly, about *fulanito* ["Joe Schmoes"]. . . . I'm sure it happens a lot. There are some who are clearly more discreet and they might do it, but you'll never know—no one knows—and there are others who are totally *descarados* [literally, "faceless"; shameless]: they go parading around town here with their girlfriends, without caring or having a bit of shame, and they are married men and all." To say that people distinguish between those whose behavior is visible and those whose is not, however, fails to quite capture the distinction that is being made—since, after all, the married men dancing in the middle of the rodeo ring with their girlfriends on that hot dusty afternoon were doing so in full sight of several hundred spectators. The distinction that matters is an individual's skill at containing practices that deviate from the ideal to spaces in which those practices will not count against him in the public calculus of sexual morality. For example, a migrant in his fifties lived principally in Chicago but traveled home to Degollado frequently to see to his local investments. When his wife recorded him and his secretary having sex in the marital bed in Chicago, and then parlayed this video into a handsome divorce settlement in a US family court, he became the laughingstock of Degollado. The mockery emphasized his inability to manage his affairs more appropriately. He should have known better than to bring his secretary into his home; as the saying goes, "Hay que saber dónde y con quién" (you have to know where and with whom). Many migrant men form long-term affective relationships with women while in the United States (similar in some ways to those described later in this book among the Nigerian men who migrate for work), but it is only when they bring these other women into spaces that form part of the transnational community (such as baptisms or weddings at which others from their hometowns are present) that they run the risk of rumors (or, even worse, video evidence) traveling home across the border.

People work to build or preserve their reputations: men who see themselves as "serious" or "calm" choose friends who will not undermine this public sexual identity. This can even mean finding others who will join them to go out for a couple of drinks and enjoy a "taco de ojo" (a tasty eyeful) at a strip club, but who will also want to be home in time to avoid causing undue suspicion, having walked a fine line between the creation of a private male sociality and their desire not to be "that kind of guy."[12] Reputation is also inherited, so that the reputational sins of the parents are visited upon their children. Parents worry when their daughters marry the sons of well-known adulterers, and a woman's own sexual misdeeds can poison her daughter's chances of making a good match.

A respectable sexual identity is a resource in which people invest and on which people draw in distinct and gendered ways. Men, for example, talked about resisting the temptations of extramarital sex out of a desire not to harm their local reputations. One man said that the reason he had never gone farther than flirting with the attractive young secretaries in his family business was "well, out of fear that someone would say, 'That damn flirt,' it would drag me into a damn problem, [so that someone might say,] 'Hey, your husband is coming on to me'—that is, more than anything, not to get a reputation. That is, I definitely notice other women, but *pueblo chico, chisme grande* [small towns have big gossip]."[13] This concern with reputation crosses class lines, and was expressed both by manual laborers and the business owners for whom they work. Through the construction of respectable sexual identities, men demonstrate their understanding of and appreciation for social hierarchy and their ability to control themselves. Although a man with a reputation for seeking liaisons with his secretaries might have a hard time hiring a girl from a good family to work in his business, some men who expressed this concern were far from being in a position to hire anyone, suggesting that they saw their own sexual identity as a sort of resource or capital that might serve them in other ways. For men, these sexual selves serve contradictory functions: they are a means through which men build relationships with other men, in part through demonstrating an assertive and sexually independent masculinity, but they are also a means through which men demonstrate their self-mastery, their social competence, and their respect (and sometimes their love) for their wives through carefully maintaining the appearance of fidelity.

For women, the lines are drawn between those who appear to conform to the expectation of one lifetime partner and those who do not. The absoluteness of this classification is indicated by the ease with which women can be reputationally dismissed by a pointed index finger, which is waved lightly in the air and accompanied by a raised eyebrow to indicate that a girl or woman whose reputation is under discussion fails the test. The implication is that even the slightest movement across the line can place someone in the category of sexually transgressive—as being "una de esas" (one of those girls). During courtship, young couples go through a ritual test of wills that involves the young man pressing for sexual intimacy—or perhaps even stealing a kiss—and the young woman heatedly responding that she is not that kind of girl. Sometimes couples even break up over these incidents, with a reconciliation predicated upon a formulaic apology from the suitor, where the crucial moment is his acknowledgment of her virtue. This will serve her later in the courtship—and potentially in the marriage—as a sort of moral ammunition.[14]

Women's reputations are so valuable that it felt dangerous even to talk about women who might have crossed the line: as we ran errands, visited friends, and attended social events, Estela and I developed a code through we could talk in front of her children about those women, both so that we could avoid impugning their reputations if we were wrong, and more generally so her children would not know we were talking about sex all the time. We called them "peluqueras" (haircutters), and we would joke about whose hair they would cut, how frequently they cut hair, and whether they provided haircuts only for friends or if they would also cut strangers' hair. We talked about men too, all the time, but it never seemed important to go to any particular trouble to keep the children from hearing those conversations. For a married woman, the maintenance of a publicly respectable sexual self is an ongoing demonstration of respect for her husband, as well as an investment in the marriageability of her children.

The classification of women into "good" and "bad" echoes throughout the organization of both marital and extramarital sex.[15] Men wryly comment that they seek women other than their wife because "para frijoles, hay en la casa"—that is, if they wanted to eat beans (i.e., something wholesome, basic, and not particularly spicy), they could do so at home, and that to really "coger rico" (for a really tasty fuck), there is nothing like a professional. Among older couples, men feared that to stray too far from the missionary position was to run the risk of insulting their wives, and women feared that showing a willingness to engage in more varied sexual play would move them in their husbands' eyes from being women of the *casa* to appearing to be women of the *calle* (street). Guadalupe's story, told through tears, underlines the reality of this risk: she did not bleed on her wedding night thirty years ago, and she ascribes all the suffering in her marriage—her husband's violence, his infidelity, and his emotional cruelty—to that moment, which they have never discussed since. The classification of women into *calle* and *casa* persists—although the definition of "good" woman has come to include the possibility of oral sex, thongs, push-up bras, and mutual consumption of pornography. As one of the young women I interviewed noted, "You have to be willing to be a little bit of a whore for your husband."[16]

Men's participation in extramarital sex in the context of homosociality also reflects this division of women into *calle* and *casa* based on their sexual reputations. In the past, men were free to enjoy the pleasures of the street and the night, and decent women were not, so that before marriage, it had been easier for a man to find sexual pleasure with a commercial sex worker, a buddy, or even a goat than it would have been for him to have sex with the woman he loved. These early experiences thus served as training in the separation of affect and pleasure—a way of learning to experience sex as something no more meaningful than a late-night plate of tacos on the way home from the disco.

The moral economy of sexuality leaves a woman who has erred with few options. Once a girl has ruined her reputation through a miscalculation, bad luck, or lack of access to male relatives powerful enough to force her boyfriend to *responder* (to own up to his responsibility), there is virtually no reputational salvation available to her and she is left with few social prospects. One young woman, for example, had a nickname that basically translated to "the horny one." Her story, as she told me, began when she fell in love with a man who had been a frequent visitor to the little store in which she worked. The small gifts and treats with which he romanced her soon turned her head; carried away, they began sneaking off to hotels together. She insisted that she had not known at the time that he was married, although in a small town this ignorance of a man's marital status would have been possible only if one had deliberately avoided inquiring. He left her after she became pregnant—and, in fact, she spoke admiringly of him for doing so, as she said that she never would have wanted him to leave his wife, to whom he had been married in the Church—and so, with a child to support and a reputation that closed off the low-skilled jobs that would otherwise have been open to her, she took the well-worn path of a fallen woman and began working in a cantina as a *fichera*, getting paid to keep men company and encourage them to buy beers for her and for themselves. Women's participation in commercial sex is often attributed to the plight of single mothers and women's limited options for supporting their children, but less frequently considered is how ideals of womanhood constrain women's options. A woman with a sullied reputation is virtually unemployable as a domestic servant—what woman would knowingly invite such a woman into her own home?—and is even problematic as a prospective employee in a small, family-owned business. Once a woman slips off the straight and narrow, she is virtually forced to specialize in being a bad woman. The virgin/whore dichotomy serves not just to scare women into preserving their sexual reputation but to ensure a steady stream of women with whom men can transgress.

The broad social consensus about the value of a respectable sexual self is indicated by the way even many of those who do engage in extramarital sex talk about being careful. Juan, for example, talked about how he has been "medio precavido" (somewhat cautious) in terms of never lasting more than a couple of months with a woman, to avoid developing the sort of affective entanglements that could come to haunt him. The most common strategy for preserving public face, however, is not to keep relationships short but rather to adhere to local conventions of sexual and moral geography; the way that physical mobility enables extramarital sex ultimately draws meaning from this shared distinction between spaces in which appearances must be respected and spaces that are beyond the reach of the wifely gaze.

The double standard is not just an ideological aspect of gender inequality; it is literally written into the streets and highways of Mexico. The idea of a double standard is frequently invoked as a kind of shorthand for cultural constructions of gender in which extramarital sex enhances a man's reputation but damages a woman's; this sort of explanation assumes the pre-eminence of ideology regulating sexual behavior. Conceptualizing the double standard, however, as something that merely permits men but not women to have extramarital sex implies a sort of hydraulic model of sexuality, in which desire bubbles up irrepressibly unless it is firmly socially tamped down, so that men engage in more (or more obvious forms of) extramarital sex because they face fewer penalties for doing so. This attention to cultural aspects of sexuality leaves a biological substrate of sexuality unquestioned and beyond the reach of critical analysis, overemphasizing the extent to which sexuality is a cultural (as opposed to social and economic) phenomenon. A spatial analysis takes us beyond this ideological approach by suggesting that normative ideals of masculinity and femininity and gendered labor markets intersect to create spaces that incite and facilitate extramarital sex for men, whereas no equivalent spaces exist for women.

The corollary of this reputation-based understanding of sexual identity is the realization that most rural Mexicans who engage in extramarital sex are fervently practicing "safe sex": for them, the most visible risk is a contaminated reputation rather than a viral infection. Seen from this perspective, a drunken quickie in a cantina bathroom with another guy is perhaps the ultimate in safe sex—condom or no condom—because the men would never tell their wives, there is no risk of pregnancy, and there is little acknowledged risk of falling in love. Compared to the dangers of a romance with a girl from one's own hometown, commercial sex is similarly perceived to be "low risk" as long as it is in a clean and sufficiently expensive venue. Commercial sex workers are perceived as women with nothing to lose; in spite of the fact that they are people's daughters, wives, and mothers, their reputations are already ruined and men can have sex with them without running the risk of incurring the moral debt produced by sex with a nice girl.

How "The House" Produces "The Street": The Intertwining of Marriage and Extramarital Relations

The best years of Santiago's marriage, he remembers, were early on, before the children came, when he and his wife were both living in Southern California; they would come home from work, shower and change, and then go out for dancing, for dinner, or to a party. He avidly studied pornography to make himself "más despierto" (more aware), wanting to school his wife in all the different ways of having sex—"dentro de lo que consideraba normal" (at least within the range of what is normal). They never planned to raise the children in the United States, so after their second child was born, Santiago's wife returned to Degollado to raise them there—which did not make him especially sad. He recounted how her attention turned more and more away from him and toward her maternal responsibilities.

Santiago migrated for years (first to Southern California, and later to Tennessee), returning to Degollado in the off-season to visit his wife and small children. Early in his sojourns north, he had been instructed by his peers in the fine points of men's behavior, including being given the advice that he should be careful about fathering a child because it could be, they warned, ten minutes of pleasure for which he would end up paying for the next eighteen years. Over the years, he developed a pattern of long-term relationships with women; he described his behavior as never being unfaithful—by which he meant he had never been unfaithful to his girlfriend of the moment by having casual sex! These women provided him not just with sex but with companionship during the cold winter months, as well as their domestic services—indeed, he highlighted the domestic nature of the relationships by comparing himself to a puppy, saying that all he wanted was to be treated nicely by someone. His calculated strategy of successive long-term liaisons included deliberately avoiding the use of each lover's name: "Nunca, nunca he utilizado nombres y así ya, mi mente esta acostumbrada a que va a decir nomás un cariño, un afecto pero no nombres, porque cuando menos acuerdes pues ya no te la acabas" (I never, never used names, so that my mind was used to only saying little pet names, sweet things, but not names, because when you least expect it, well, you've ended it [i.e., made the mistake of saying a lover's name to one's wife]). His routine of circular migration (and parallel monogamy) came to an end at last when he and his lover in Tennessee made the mistake of attending a wedding together; the neighbors from Degollado reported to his wife that they had seen him with a girlfriend, and she told him to come home or else she would divorce him and keep the house and their business. "Eso tiene que acabar, eso es normal" (It had to end, that's normal), he reflects, and now that he is back in town, "aquí no se puede, aquí no se puede, pa'mi no, o sea, lo que pasa es que eres conocido, y cualquier pinche movimientito, ¿sabes qué? si quieres vivir en paz, vive con tu familia nomás" (here you can't, not here, I don't think so—that is, if people know you, then any damn little intrigue . . . You know what? If you want to live in peace, then here you have to stay just with your family). He admits that he has had, however, several short flings, "una o dos esporádicas, así por buena suerte" (one or two, sporadically, just out of luck).

Extramarital relations and marriage are interrelated elements of social organization—but not in the purely affective sense, whereby an unhappy marriage results in infidelity. Rather, infidelity is an element of the gendered social organization whereby a man in Degollado can have a relationship with a woman organized around social reproduction along with another (or multiple others) to provide pleasure and diversion. Ironically, the very importance of marriage as an element of social organization is part of what makes extramarital sex so pervasive, so that infidelity can be considered the necessary corollary of relatively low (but rising) rates of marital dissolution.

Sayings such as "si no se lo dan en casa, se lo busca en la calle" (if he doesn't get it at home, he'll look for it in the street) suggest that a successful and well-functioning marriage should leave no room for extramarital sex, and the very nature of the opposition between the house and the street suggests that one is the total negation of the other. In actuality, however, the organization of marriage creates spaces and opportunities for men to develop extramarital sexual relations. In rural Mexico, marriage continues to be a vital form of domestic organization—it might not be too strong to label it a means for survival—in a way that it no longer is in the United States. Despite images and discourses that suggest that marriage exists as a structure for the realization of self and the satisfaction of the desire for intimacy, many people find their own marriages to be less than entirely satisfying emotionally.

There are, however, many reasons for men and women to remain together. A wife provides a man with a reliable source of domestic labor—not a trivial issue in a society in which wearing well-ironed clothes is a crucial marker of self-respect. The phrase men use to encapsulate the enduring commitment they feel to their wives in these cases is "Es la madre de mis hijos" (she is the mother of my children). Women stay with their husbands for the economic security, the respectability conferred by being under the moral protection of a man (even an immoral one), and because in spite of the emergence of the companionate ideal, most women still do not feel justified leaving a man just because of mutual incompatibility. Within these marriages of necessity, men have the option of finding pleasure and companionship with other women; married women can do so as well, but their more limited mobility and the constant burden of childcare make the logistics complicated and the risks higher. That marriage is the only route to leaving one's parental home—to becoming an adult—can force a man to marry a woman even if he prefers to have sex with men.

The importance of marriage as a system for social reproduction combines with intense heteronormativity to make it impossible for two adult men to live as a social and domestic couple. Residents of large urban centers such as Mexico City and Guadalajara can join growing communities of gay-identified men (and women), but these identities and communities barely exist at the local level.[17] The intersection of heteronormativity and a reputation-oriented system of sexual identity means that what matters socially is not whether men have sex with other men in private, but whether they dress and act in an appropriately masculine form in public. Both masculine- and feminine-appearing men who prefer to have sex with other men almost always marry women, both for cover and for convenience (otherwise, who would iron for them?). Sometimes they do so with the full knowledge of their brides. In one case, a man proposed to a young woman who was pregnant and had been abandoned, with the understanding that they would each provide cover for the other's socially unacceptable behavior. In other cases, these men's preference for men comes as a surprise to their wives, or is never openly acknowledged.

The extent to which couples fail to find a mutually agreeable frequency for intercourse—so that men look "in the street" for what they do not find at home—exists within a social world in which women face multiple demands in addition to the need to be their husbands' lovers: the gendered division of marital labor creates opportunities for men to form relations with other women regardless of how much they love their wives. Although women increasingly work for money even after they marry—most commonly in local commerce, as schoolteachers, and a few as accountants, lawyers, or doctors—parenting is still local women's real "career," in that it is the strategy through which they gain social advancement, public prestige, and secure family relationships. Changing ideas about fertility and the family (Hirsch 2003, 2004) have meant that couples have far fewer children than in the past, but lower fertility rates do not mean that women are spending less time parenting than their mothers did—in fact, if anything, the labor of parenting has intensified.

As I learned through having my own children with me in the field, women with young children invest vast quantities of time in feeding, bathing, dressing, and grooming them in order to keep up with the public demand for respectability—not to mention the overarching task of creating civilized people by teaching those children to kiss or shake hands to say hello and goodbye to adults, making sure they are trained to share any tasty tidbit of food (chips, ice cream, candy) with others in their presence without being asked, and ensuring that they know not to walk between two adults who are in the middle of a conversation. There is no formal day care available in the town. Even for those children who are in school, the school day (which begins at 8:30 a.m., unless it is raining very hard or the teacher is late) is interrupted by breakfast from 10:30 a.m. to 11:00 a.m., and ends at 2:00 p.m., by which time a woman must have the house cleaned, the laundry and ironing done, and lunch made. Only a slattern, furthermore, would give her children money to buy tacos at school for breakfast, or send the food with an older child or a maid; the time women spend together during the breakfast recess, leaning against the schoolyard fence, is crucial for both the interchange of gossip and the public performance of competent motherhood. I saw how schooling adds to maternal responsibilities in the volume of requests for presents for teachers, participation in school parties, costumes for pageants, and the like, over the course of even a single semester; in addition, the frequency with which school is abruptly canceled—for teacher trainings, bad weather, holidays, and even in one instance a teacher volleyball tournament—highlights the assumption of women's constant availability and supposed lack of any responsibilities that might supersede their maternal ones.

The all-consuming nature of motherhood—and the way in which it shifts women's focus from their husbands to their children—was exemplified for me during a Sunday lunch at the farm of a family with whom Sergio, Brenda, and I were acquainted. The elderly couple's daughters and daughters-in-law cooked, served, and cleaned up after lunch; in contrast, the adult sons, sons-in-law, and grandchildren spent the afternoon eating and then playing volleyball or swimming in the pool. In my fieldnotes after the picnic, I mulled over the possibility that once women marry, their fun is over.

Antonio, one of Degollado's leading entrepreneurs, expressed a certain wistfulness at his wife's complete absorption in the labor of parenting their three children. While praising his wife's commitment to them, he noted his own desire for the same "chiqueos" (babying) directed with such generosity toward the children. His frustration—which he expressed directly, as well as through struggling with the temptation of seeking some "chiqueos" from one of the town's lovely unmarried women—was shared by many men in our study: despite companionate discourses that emphasize marital affect and shared pleasure, the actual reward structure of everyday life turns women's attention to caring for the bodies of their children, not those of their husbands. Although the quality of the emotional and sexual intimacy between a married couple forms part of the panorama within which men seek extramarital sex, the extent to which couples are satisfied together is a product not just of affective factors but of broader social ones.

Material aspects of social class, of course, also shape men's extramarital sexual practices in critical ways, forming a key part of the terrain within which men negotiate or avoid extramarital sex. Middle- and upper-middle-class couples have access to patterns and spaces of heterosociality that provide alternatives to the infidelity-promoting homosociality of the cantinas and the billiard halls. They have larger houses and smaller families, so they are more able to host small gatherings of like-minded friends, as the town's young elite couples occasionally do. They also can afford to participate in couple- and family-type activities such as dining out on Sundays, trips to the movies, outings to local waterparks, visits to a zoo or a shopping center in one of the region's nearby cities, or even an annual vacation at the beach. Less wealthy families do on occasion travel to a beach (there are several annual bus trips from town, for example, that cater specifically to residents of the less wealthy *colonias*), but on those trips people sleep on the buses on the way there and back and while at the beach share hotel rooms with other families, so they hardly have the effect of promoting the exclusive togetherness of the nuclear family unit. Money gives men and women access to elite practices such as family travel, which enables heterosocial, family-oriented leisure time.

Structure, Agency, and Sexual Projects

The tone of Alejandro's marriage was quite different from Juan's. A construction worker in his early twenties, Alejandro and his vivacious wife Concepción were typical in some ways of what might be called a companionate marriage. Parents of a three-year-old and a set of young twins, they shared an easy joking relationship; one Sunday afternoon in my presence, for example, he cajoled her into helping him test out his brother's new shower, in which they had just finished laying new tiles. She blushed and swatted him when he said he needed her to soap up his back, but she joined him all the same. He spoke in the interview of sitting with his head on her lap to watch soap operas at night, and referred specifically to his love for her when explaining that since his wedding, he has not been unfaithful. What Alejandro meant by this, however, is that he has confined his extramarital sexual activity to professional sex workers in other towns, avoiding the risk of long-term relationships with women who could lay claim on his affective resources, and making sure that his liaisons take place outside Degollado, away from the social space he shares with his wife. His trips to these low-rent brothels outside town began during his early twenties; he told of being introduced to them by the men he worked with, in a sort of sexual apprenticeship reminiscent of his formal apprenticeship as a construction worker (and similar to the way migrant men in Papua New Guinea are tutored in these practices by those with more experience). He also indulged himself with local girls, but was careful to seek out those who had already been publicly sexually disgraced (who were, in the local parlance, *fracasadas*), so that he could not be forced to marry one in the event of a pregnancy. His appetite for one local red-light district grew to the extent that he sometimes took the bus there alone (men more commonly organize these field trips in groups), explaining that he had spent a great deal of time there right before his wedding:

> Pues cuando ya andaba con mi vieja, pues ya noviando en serio, ora si dije ya me voy a amarrar. Esos eran mis pensamientos. Yo 'orita quiero gozar para cuando me case me voy a calmar. . . . Si dije, ya por última vez voy a venir seguido. Yo cada, raro él . . . cada ocho días que no iba raro, pero sí cada quince días. Empezaba, yo, así iba solo a veces invitaba a alguien más. Veía una morrilla que me gustaba; "¿de a cómo es?" "no pues que de a tanto."

> (Well, when I had started going with the one I married, seriously courting, I said to myself, "Now I am really going to tie myself down." Those were my thoughts. "Now I want to enjoy myself, so that when I marry I will calm down." I said, "Now, for the last time, I am going to come here frequently." So every—it was rare—if I didn't go every week, at least every other week. I began, I, I'd go alone, sometimes I'd take someone else along. I'd see a girl whom I liked, and ask, "How much is she?" "Well, she's this much.")

This "calming down" meant confining the excursions to when his wife was menstruating or observing the customary forty days of postpartum abstinence. In a good week, Alejandro might earn two thousand pesos, and he recounted having spent nearly that sum in the red-light district while his wife was recovering from the birth of their first child, when money was quite scarce. Alejandro bitterly described the poverty he had faced as a child, wearing patched clothing donated by neighbors; thanks to Concepción's efforts, their children's wardrobes have not been quite so threadbare, but their money has never quite stretched enough to repair his truck (which has broken down repeatedly, occasionally stranding him in the red-light district and forcing all sorts of explanatory machinations to justify the resulting overnight absence), tile their own muddy bathroom floor, or buy much meat for his growing family. Alejandro, however, has to have sex every day—more on the days when he cannot find work and so is less tired out. Concepción manages on whatever he gives her, after taking out what he needs for cigarettes, beer, and his trips out of town.

Throughout the fieldwork, I found myself occasionally filled with rage upon hearing about yet another man who had gone on a bender, or one who had been very generous to his girlfriend—in both cases by using money that could have been spent on food or clothes or doctor's visits or schoolbooks for their children. Yet to see such men only as "wasting" this money is to fail to see that there is something about these practices that is so desperately important to these men that they pursue it despite the consequences—despite the fact that it means depriving the families they love of things they desperately need. Whether the man in question is a labor migrant who literally risked his life to work for ten hard months in the United States, or a brickmaker who sweated through a long, dusty Degollado summer as he formed blocks out of straw and horse shit, their money has cost these men dearly. That they spend it so freely on such brief moments of pleasure suggests that these men must be buying something precious.

A central point of this chapter has been to use the notion of sexual reputation to emphasize the interplay between structure and agency—that is, between the choices people make and the factors shaping those choices. Men and women deliberately work to craft particular sexual reputations as they move through the local landscape of sexual opportunity. Sexual reputation, however, captures imperfectly the agentive dimension of sexuality; although men and women manage their intimate lives with an eye to those reputations, building and maintaining a reputation as a sexually respectable person is hardly the only goal an individual can achieve through his or her sexuality. If nothing else, the ample cast of characters in town who depart significantly from reputational ideals suggests the importance of acknowledging a much broader range of sexual projects. In the final portion of this chapter, I trace how men use sexuality to define themselves as men, as middle-class, and as modern; to build relations with other men; and, at times, to protest the humiliations of poorly paid wage labor.

Identity building is a critical facet of men's extramarital sexual projects, in a way that stretches far beyond the question of respectability. Regardless of whether men assert that extramarital sex does or does not enhance their reputation, all the men interviewed saw it as a crucial arena through which they could assert what kind of men they are. The men who do not engage in extramarital sex made that choice deliberately, as a strategy through which they could demonstrate a modern masculinity. That these men and their friends were the primary audience for these performances (as has been demonstrated, a man could easily have extramarital sex without his wife finding out) underlines the importance of seeing masculinity as negotiated among men. Others have discussed how Mexican ideals of manhood are subject to dissension and internal critique (Gutmann 1996, 2003). These ideals are reflected in practice: men who are faithful articulate an encompassing vision of themselves as family men and the partners of their wives. This is an assertion not just of an affective and sexual companionship, but of a deep partnership based on fully knowing each other. That is, rather than focus on the presentation to their wives of a deftly packaged public sexual self for feminine consumption, such men insist on a seamlessness between their public and private lives that precludes the possibility of hidden sexual indiscretion.

A cursory reading of the media environment that people navigate suggests that men even in rural Mexico are surrounded by images of this alternative masculinity. For example, a portrait of a glowing father with his small child on the cover of *Padres* (Parenting) magazine emphasizes the intertwining of attentive fatherhood and success in consumer society, as does the extensive coverage of Father's Day in the regional paper. Luis, the son of a local artisan, was talented, hardworking, and bright enough to have secured a spot in one of the country's best residency programs in orthopedic surgery in a nearby city. As an up-and-coming young doctor who came home only twice a month, he had had ample opportunities to become involved with other women, both with other residents and with nurses, some of whom had quite openly propositioned him. He spoke disparagingly, however, about his colleagues who had engaged in this sort of behavior. His exhaustion served as a protective factor (he joked that instead of going out for drinks with his friends, he would have gladly paid them to let him stay home to sleep and study), but he also said that he could not live with himself if he had done something like that to his wife. Noteworthy is how he thinks of sexual intimacy with another woman as inherently injurious to his wife, whether or not she finds out about it.

Luis's masculinity ideals, self-confidence, and professional success—not to mention his long hours at work—may have made it easier for him to turn away from opportunities for extramarital sex. For other men, however, spending an evening at one of the local table-dance clubs provided an opportunity to demonstrate their independence to their friends, thereby protecting themselves from teasing accusations that "su mujer le mande" (your wife gives the orders). One evening, several young couples went out with Sergio and me for drinks at the relatively tony bar of a hotel in neighboring La Piedad. This was in and of itself an exceptional activity, as Degollado does not really have any social spaces of this ilk. While the other two women and I chatted about toilet training, costumes for an upcoming school pageant, and other scintillating issues, and tried to keep the children from breaking any truly irreplaceable *adornos* of the swanky décor, I found out later from Sergio that the men—under cover of the relatively loud music—had been making plans to go out another time to a striptease. The fact that they had used this ostensibly special moment of couple togetherness to plan an evening organized around the possibility of other women felt to me like a real kick in the ethnographic stomach—in spite of the fact that none of these men was even my husband! Part of the pleasure for them must have been the sneaking around—the simultaneous engagement with and rebellion against the structures of marital intimacy.

Men also use extramarital sex—and, in particular, commercial sex—to mark the intersection of masculinity and social class. Among the more working-class men interviewed, for example, a trip to the table-dance locale—where an evening can easily run into the hundreds of dollars—was a once-in-a-lifetime experience. It was most frequently a youthful rite of passage, but for wealthier men—and especially for returning labor migrants with dollars to burn (Hirsch and Meneses Navarro 2009)—more regular visits to the table-dance joints outside of La Piedad were a way to show off their more refined taste and greater disposable income. Some of those wealthier men contrasted the table dancers with the workers in the red-light district of Atotonilco, a nearby town, noting with disgust the corpulent figures of the latter.

Opportunities for commercial sex exist across a spectrum of age, beauty, ambience, and imagined practices of personal hygiene, so that when a man pays for sex, he receives not just sexual services but also a reflection of his position in the social world. Our acquaintances who waxed enthusiastic about being able to select from a parade of fair-skinned Eastern European beauties at the luxurious massage parlor in Guadalajara, for example, were simultaneously performing for us their worldliness, their *malinchismo*, their racism, and their access to disposable income. As with other forms of consumption, the goal is frequently not the possession of the item itself but rather what the ability to possess such items signals more broadly about the consumer. Men were sometimes ridiculed for seeking out sex with women who were not as attractive as their wives, with the gossips noting dismissively that these men "deja el maíz por los elotes" (leave the corn and take the cobs). The association between social class and categories of commercial sex was so strong that even Sergio had trouble managing to conceal the ways in which he found the women in Atotonilco not just unappealing but grotesque. Economic inequality shapes the context within which people navigate and negotiate their sexual selves, but the determination is not absolute. The fact that the only kind of transactional sex within a man's economic reach may be the degraded atmosphere of Atotonilco's Zona Rosa does not force him to seek it out. By turning up his nose at this emblem of local working-class masculinity, a man can show himself to be, at least in his own imagination, something other than the typical *albañil* (construction worker).

Men perform a modern cosmopolitan version of themselves by comparing notes on the sexual positions they have tried with women other than their wives. (That is why the porn they watch is foreign, not Mexican.) This suggests a way of jockeying for status among men that is based not on the exchange of women (Rubin 1975) but rather on their "consumption." Between a man and his wife, the discussion of sexual variety has a slightly different meaning, but likewise serves as a practice through which men can lay claim to modernity. That said, men do not talk among themselves about the explicit details of their marital sex life; they may joke about its frequency or even about a woman's enthusiasm (one man, for example, complained laughingly to Sergio about how tired he was because his wife would not let him sleep), but it would indicate a lack of respect for their wives were these men to go into more details.

Within a marriage, *una actitud abierta* (an open attitude) to the shared consumption of pornography symbolizes the trust and mutuality of a modern relationship, as opposed to the individual modern personhood indicated by a man's bragging about his commercial sexual exploits. Women's comments in interviews and everyday conversations with me suggest that anal sex and fellatio have figured prominently as the foci of marital negotiations about sexual variety. I heard much discussion of how men ask their wives for anal sex "a ver como se siente" (to see what it feels like). (Given how common sex between men appears to be, I suspect rather that they already know what it feels like, and that they like it.) One of the veiled threats behind this request—and the reason that Patricia told me that one has to be willing to be a little bit of a whore for one's husband—is that if the women did not allow them to have anal sex, they would look for it elsewhere. Oral sex seemed to have been more widely adopted into the sexual repertoires of younger couples—in the words of one wife, "Al cabo, bien bañadito, ¿qué tiene?" (after all, as long as they are well-bathed, what's wrong with it?).

Men use sexuality to form social relations as well as to create identities. Although the encounters between men and women sometimes lay the groundwork for affective relationships of some duration, a great deal of men's emotional focus is actually on their relationships with their male companions (Hirsch and Meneses Navarro 2009). These long boozy evenings can be about the pleasure of affect, of *cariño* (caring), of the touch of a true friend and the ear of someone who cares deeply—but (as in the Nigerian case, as Smith will discuss) this *cariño* is shared not between men and their hired girlfriends but among the men themselves. The sex is, in a way, incidental; the main project during these evenings is the construction and enjoyment of deep social and emotional bonds between the men, although the sex with women can help neutralize the almost sexual charge of the resulting intimacies, such as the way an arm around the shoulders can threaten (or promise) to turn into a deep and passionate kiss between two men with mustaches.[18] Organizing these outings around sex with women ironically keeps them safe from women, as the only women allowed into the charmed space are those whom the men can invite and dismiss at will—a much less complicated and intrusive presence than that of the women whose beds and tables they share during their daily lives. Similar to the Huli *dawe anda* described later in this book, these all-male spaces are hothouses for the propagation and nurturing of homosociality, and the homosocial relations that develop therein are critical channels through which resources are distributed and negotiated. Deals are made, bonds are forged or broken, *compadres* are chosen, and life goes on, one tequila at a time.

This is not to say, of course, that there is not an affective element to men's extramarital relations. In June 2004, for example, the atmosphere in the cantina on the western edge of town was funereal, with the jukebox playing song after song about heartbreak and betrayal. Pablo, the owner, stood mournfully behind the bar as the news circulated through town that his long-time lover, Rosa, was going to wed a widower who had returned to town over Christmastime looking for a wife. (Rosa explained to me that her responsibility to "buscar un porvenir" [find a future] for her children [one of whom had been fathered by Pablo] outweighed the depth of her love for Pablo.)

Sometimes, in fact, warmth and affection seemed to be all that men were seeking from these other women. For example, José, a young stone carver, shared a warm and sexually adventurous relationship with his young wife, yet spent a good deal of his free time (and money) with his friends at local bars, where *ficheras* joke and drink with them. *Ficheras* are paid by the owners for each beer a man buys while they talk, and so these women earn their living quite literally by providing men with the pleasure of their company. José spoke with wonder about spending time with these women—about the joys of flirting with them, and of speaking to them and touching them in ways he felt he could not with his wife.

Throughout this volume, the language of intention and motivation figures prominently. I end this chapter, however, with a final point that underlines the fact that sexuality is also a domain through which individuals embody longings that fit less readily into that sort of rationalist framework. Men frequently used food metaphors to talk about sex. In contrast to the oft-repeated "para frijoles, hay en la casa" (if you wanted beans, you could eat at home), which describes marital sex as something satisfying and necessary for survival, but also potentially monotonous, one man compared extramarital sex to candy several times. He spoke of "andar probando dulces de otra caja" (trying candies from another box), and explained the pursuit of extramarital sex in terms of both loneliness and curiosity, saying, "Nada más es como quien dice, para hacer un relleno [falta] un hueco. Por algo que les haga falta en un matrimonio, lo que buscan es desahogo, y a veces ya no solamente es desahogo, es un hábito de estar buscando siempre el dulce ajeno" (Sometimes it's, as they say, to fill a gap, because of something that's lacking in marriage, men look for relief, and sometimes not just for relief, it's the habit of going around always looking for another's candy). Seen this way, the pursuit and acquisition of sexual variety indicates that there is money to spend on discretionary pleasures, the refusal to be beaten down by poverty, and even a sort of resistance to the way structures of inequality threaten to confine people to their *canasta básica* (basic needs). The thrill in how men talk about this sex in Mexico is as much the thrill of running very quickly through vast sums of money as it is the sex that that money buys. "Me lo chingue" (I fucked it), men say with pride, using the word *chingar* to signal the transformation of hard-earned money into quickly consumed pleasure. I struggled not to see these expenditures as irrational—even cruel—because that same money could have bought a tank of fuel to cook with for a month, or shoes for their children, or a hearty meal of meat. Those who spend it, however, may be protesting that very rationality, asserting that they are worth more than the ten dollars per hour they are paid in Atlanta to work as undocumented construction workers or the five dollars per hour they are paid to pick berries, bent over all day under the Salinas Valley sun. What men are buying back, as the money runs through their hands like water, is their dignity—their claim to be more than laborers.

3

Gender Inequality, Infidelity, and the Social Risks of Modern Marriage in Nigeria

Daniel Jordan Smith

For quite some time, it has been common in anthropology to question the concept of culture. The discipline most responsible for popularizing culture as a lens for understanding human societies has grown increasingly anxious about its own foundations (Marcus and Fischer 1986; Clifford 1988; Abu-Lughod 1991). The reasons for anthropology's anxieties about the culture concept are manifold and include the degree to which a framework that privileges culture has contributed to a failure to examine adequately inequality and the political economies that gird it (Scheper-Hughes 1992; Farmer 1999); a relative myopia about history and the processes by which cultures are always changing (Comaroff and Comaroff 1992; Sahlins 1993; Donham 2001); and a growing recognition of the permeable and shifting boundaries of culture, accentuated by the current attention to globalization (Appadurai 1996; Hannerz 1996). The discomforts posed by these theoretical challenges to a static, bounded, and politically naïve concept of culture are exacerbated by the way that culture is frequently wielded in society as a form of explanation (and blame) that attributes to cultural practices outcomes that are better understood as the consequence of structural forces (Briggs 2003). This is evident with regard to the AIDS epidemic. Culture, particularly as it pertains to sexual practices that are dubbed as "traditional," is regularly invoked to understand and explain HIV risk and risky behavior. Nowhere is the concept of culture more commonly—and more perniciously—applied than in relation to HIV in sub-Saharan Africa (Caldwell, Caldwell, and Quiggin 1989).

The idea that traditional African cultural behaviors explain the continent's disproportionately large share of the global HIV epidemic is produced and circulated in media accounts, which document exotic beliefs and practices such as the notion that sex with a virgin can cure AIDS and the tradition that a widow must have sex with and perhaps marry a particular man in her husband's lineage.[1] These stories are presented as if they implicitly explain Africa's HIV problem. One need not dispute the existence of such beliefs and practices to point out that they are uncommon and that they serve to blame culture by suggesting that individuals with AIDS are themselves responsible for their suffering. Even if some traditional cultural practices do contribute to HIV transmission, their effects on the overall epidemiology of AIDS pale in comparison to issues of political and economic disparity, poverty, gender inequality, and what can only be described as normal sexual behavior. Unfortunately, these distorted representations sometimes find their way into social scientific accounts as well (Malungo 2001; Meel 2003; Schwandt et al. 2006). Even when researchers do not intend to depict these "traditional" practices as adequate explanations for the epidemic, the reproduction of these images has consequences. Global public health interventions designed to prevent HIV transmission frequently presume that inadequacies of knowledge and belief drive the epidemic.

In Nigeria, as in most of the world, the dominant public health strategy for preventing HIV infection focuses on educating people to reduce individual risk through behavior change, an approach that presumes that the locus of the problem lies in what people think and believe—i.e., in their culture and how it shapes what they do. This approach appears to have backfired, creating a situation where Nigerians—and arguably Africans in many societies—conceptualize HIV risk in relation to stigmatizing discourses from which they try to distance themselves. Partly as a result of local interpretations of globally circulating representations of risk and risk groups, ordinary Nigerians tend to connect HIV risk to social and sexual immorality, making it unlikely that individuals will conceive of their own behavior as risky (Smith 2003). As in many cultural contexts, the menace of HIV has become associated with a stigmatized "other" (Parker and Aggleton 2003). In these circumstances, it is not surprising that marriage is perceived as an environment of moral and sexual safety, making it particularly difficult for people to comprehend and accept—much less address directly—the fact that marriage is increasingly a primary pathway to infection. By targeting so-called risky or promiscuous cultural practices, public health programs make it virtually impossible for people who become infected with HIV through normative and "safe" sexual practices to acknowledge they have contracted the virus.

In Nigeria, as has been documented in other settings (Lurie et al. 2003), both married men and married women almost certainly infect each other with HIV. But women's risk of contracting HIV in marriage is driven by highly unequal gender expectations about marital fidelity, in which married men's—but not married women's—extramarital sex is relatively accepted, and in some situations even socially rewarded (Orubuloye et al. 1997; Cornwall 2002; Smith 2007, 2008). Indeed, as men and women navigate marital and extramarital relationships, anxieties about social expectations and reputation produce a locally dominant conceptualization of risk in which moral concerns about gender, family, religion, and social class trump conventional public health concepts of risk. Situating an analysis of risk and behavior in social terms rather than in epidemiological terms enables us

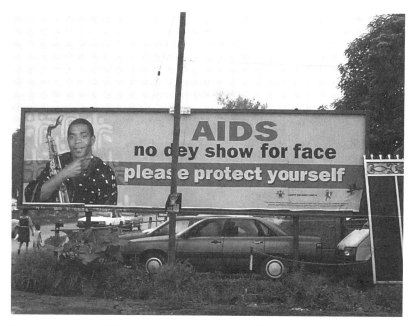

Warnings about AIDS are a common feature of the everyday landscape in Nigeria, but the effect of awareness on actual intimate behavior depends on much more than signboard messages. Photograph by Daniel Jordan Smith.

to make sense of actions that appear from a purely medical or public health point of view to be unwise, such as men cheating on their wives without using condoms, and women tolerating and having unprotected sex with husbands whom they know or suspect to be having extramarital affairs. In this chapter, I focus on the pragmatism with which ordinary married men and women in southeastern Nigeria interpret and negotiate social and moral risks in ways that can exacerbate the biological risk of HIV infection. In their actions, these men and women remind us that the social fields people navigate as they live in the era of AIDS involve priorities and challenges that can complicate and even outweigh more straightforward concerns about their health.

In particular, I examine men's extramarital sexual behavior and married women's responses to it in the context of a transformation of marriage. Characteristics of this particular transformation, which a growing volume of literature suggests is spreading worldwide (Collier 1997; Rebhun 1999; Ahearn 2001; Hirsch 2003a), and which the Introduction and other chapters in this volume explicate, include (1) a growing acceptance that a committed personal, emotional relationship between a man and a woman, crystallized in the idea of being "in love," is a suitable criterion for getting married; (2) the significance of spousal intimacy—communicative, emotional, and sexual—as a basis for the assessments of couples and other observers as to whether a marriage is good; and (3) the relative importance of the

conjugal relationship vis-à-vis other forms of social ties. The rise of what Nigerians call "modern marriage" would seem to suggest that extramarital sex should
become more problematic, as it appears to violate several key dimensions of an intimate and companionate conjugal bond. Yet, as in the other settings discussed in
this book, my research findings in Nigeria show that extramarital sex—especially
men's extramarital sex—is not only common but is in fact partly facilitated by the
nature and dynamics of modern marriage.

My argument is not that modern Nigerian marriage makes male infidelity
more likely—I don't think there are sufficiently reliable data for Nigeria (or elsewhere) regarding the incidence and prevalence of extramarital sex under different
marital regimes to draw any conclusions. Nor do I mean to suggest that by itself
modern marriage "causes" men's cheating. But I do argue that, similar to the cases
in Mexico, Papua New Guinea, Uganda, and Vietnam, men's extramarital sexual
behavior in Nigeria is shaped and perpetuated by a constellation of social forces
that enable, encourage, and even pressure men to engage in infidelity. I also argue
that the recent changes in marriage place men in specific positions vis-à-vis issues
of masculinity, kinship, generation, religion, and social class, so as to make their
extramarital sexual behavior both possible and likely (Hirsch et al. 2007; Parikh
2007; Wardlow 2007; Phinney 2008). Conversely, modern Nigerian marriage puts
Nigerian women in situations that make resistance to men's infidelity extremely
difficult.

To make matters more complicated, as men begin to participate in and accept
the changes in conjugal relationships characteristic of modern Nigerian marriage,
they face additional economic and moral pressures, symbolized respectively by
the burgeoning collective desire to participate in middle-class consumption (e.g.,
acquiring items such as cell phones, TVs, DVD players, and fashionable clothes)
and models of the family promoted by Christian churches (especially by the increasingly popular Pentecostal churches).[2] These growing pressures intensify the
burden of men's traditional role as family provider, even as economic realities
combine with cultural transformations to make men's positions more precarious.
The men I followed in southeastern Nigeria experienced tremendous ambivalence
about social change and its effects on their positions as husbands and fathers, and
this ambivalence shaped their marital and extramarital relationships, as well as
their navigation of both.

For women, even as modern Nigerian marriage promises conjugal bonds based
on greater intimacy and trust, potentially elevating the importance of the marital
relationship relative to other social ties, new challenges in navigating gender inequality and men's infidelity are posed. When husbands cheat in "love marriages,"
women find that the forms of leverage they can resort to are severely limited: the
possibility of appealing to kin and in-laws for help—a common strategy in more
traditional, arranged marriages—is less viable because it contradicts the dyadic
dynamic and intimacy-privileging image of a love marriage. Moreover, to confront

a man's extramarital violations in any public way not only signals to kin and community that the ostensible foundation of the marriage (love and trust) has been undermined, but it also weakens a woman's hand in negotiating with her husband using the terms on which the marriage was established.

The full precariousness of married women's positions can only be understood if one recognizes that the transformation of marriage in southeastern Nigeria is partial. While women are relatively free to choose whom they will marry, they are not nearly as free to divorce once they have married, especially if the marriage has produced children. The perpetuation of gender inequality makes opting out an unlikely option, as does the enormity of the social expectations and sanctions that enforce the paramount importance of parenthood and the permanence of marriage. As a result, many women with cheating husbands remain silent, at least in public, about their husbands' philandering. In so doing, they help cover for behavior that they find painful—but not nearly as devastating as it would be to reveal the violation to the world. As with men, although for quite different reasons, modern marriage is experienced ambivalently by Nigerian women, offering them new forms of intimacy and leverage with their husbands, even as these opportunities can become constraints in the context of men's infidelity.

After briefly discussing the opportunity structures and sexual geographies that enable and shape men's extramarital behavior, I aim to understand men's and women's ambivalence and the seemingly contradictory behaviors it produces. To make sense of these contradictions, I focus on the ways that men and women conceive of and respond to their perceptions of social risk in relation to marriage, infidelity, and HIV (Nichter 2002; Hirsch et al. 2007). This approach offers several important insights. First, it situates behavior in context, making sociological sense of people's practices rather than reducing them to some sort of primordial tradition or culture. Second, by allowing for ambivalence and contradiction, it depicts the subjects of our studies as living lives of the same degree of complexity that we intuitively recognize as integral to our own human experience. Finally, it recognizes the role of discourses about AIDS in contributing to the context of social risk, forcing those of us interested in responding to the epidemic to acknowledge our culpability in aggravating the arena of social risk by employing overly simplistic models of culture. In this way, anthropology's core concept of culture can be utilized in a form that engages human behavior in its sociological complexity—recognizing culture as a concept that requires explanation rather than serving as substitute for it.

Setting, Background, and Social Context

The settings where I conducted research on marriage and infidelity are in the midst of significant transformations that both frame and affect marriage and sexual behavior. One setting, Owerri, is a city of approximately 350,000 people and the capital of Imo State. Owerri has grown dramatically over the past decade through rural-urban migration, a trend that is broadly characteristic of Nigeria (and all of Africa, which is the continent with the fastest current rate of urbanization in the world [United Nations 2003]). In addition, the city has become something of a hub for higher education, with no less than five federal and state universities and well over 100,000 resident students. Owerri is a magnet for people seeking better opportunities. In local discourse, the town is also known as a bastion of extra-marital sex, symbolized by the scores of hotels that serve as rendezvous points for overnight trysts. The relative anonymity of city life protects both married men and their typically younger unmarried partners from attendant social risks—though as I will explain below, participation in extramarital sex can usefully be understood in relation to the social risks of *not* participating as well as in relation to the risks of doing it or getting caught.

The second setting of my research was Ubakala, a semi-rural community of eleven villages about five miles outside Umuahia, the capital of Abia State and an hour's drive from Owerri. Ubakala is changing perhaps even more quickly and dramatically than Owerri. Unsurprisingly, it mirrors Owerri in that it is a major source of rural-to-urban migration. If one includes migrants to other places who call Ubakala their real home, at least half of Ubakala's population lives outside the community at any given moment, most commonly in Nigeria's cities. Particularly striking is the large number of young people who have out-migrated. In addition, Ubakala has evolved from a primarily agricultural community into a peri-urban suburb of Umuahia. Just in the dozen years that I have conducted research in Ubakala, the commercial center of the community has grown from a sleepy out-post to a busy and vibrant center embedded in Umuahia's urban circuitry. Most households in Ubakala no longer rely mainly on agriculture; instead, they typically combine some balance of farming, wage labor, and small-scale commerce, not to mention dependence on remittances from migrant household members. Further, many married couples are separated geographically for extensive periods of time by economic strategies that require migration.

In both settings, I benefited from the help of four superb local research as-sistants: three women and one man. I relied on my female research assistants to conduct the interviews with married women, expecting that the women would be more likely to speak candidly about matters like sex, infidelity, and HIV with members of their own sex. By and large, this proved to be the case, although the married women's reticence about some topics, even with fellow women, proved instructive in its own right. I conducted most of the interviews with married men myself, but I also had my male research assistant conduct several interviews in Owerri, and he undertook participant observation in male-dominated social ven-ues there when I was working in Ubakala.

The populations of both Owerri and Ubakala are almost entirely Igbo, Nigeria's third-largest ethnic and linguistic group. In the scholarly literature and in popular lore in Nigeria, the Igbo are known for their entrepreneurial acumen, their receptivity to change, and their willingness to migrate and settle throughout the country in order to pursue their economic interests (Ottenberg 1959; Uchendu 1965; Chukwuezi 2001; Gugler 2002). As among other southern Nigerian ethnic and linguistic groups, formal education is highly valued, Christianity has become almost ubiquitous, and many aspects of what is too easily (and deceptively) called "Western culture" have been adopted, including capitalist-style consumption and globally influenced fashions, diet, music, and videos. As in much of the world, the average age at marriage in southeastern Nigeria has been rising, for both men and women. While the national averages are now above twenty years of age for women and twenty-five years of age for men, these figures are skewed by areas of the country that are much less developed than the Igbo-speaking southeast and still retain lower average ages at marriage. Among the population I was studying (albeit a population that was, even by Igbo standards, disproportionately affected by rural-urban migration, proximity to town, and city life), women tended to marry in their early to mid-twenties and men in their late twenties and early thirties. Perhaps the two most significant demographic facts for understanding the contemporary context of men's extramarital sex are (1) the relatively long period between the advent of a young woman's sexual maturity and her age at marriage (for most young women, this period covers at least five years, and frequently ten or more years), and (2) the high levels of mobility and migration, particularly to cities and towns, where young women are less subject to the regulation and surveillance of their families and communities, and where married men can engage in extramarital sexual relations in relative anonymity.

A final feature of Igbo society that helps contextualize the opportunity structures that influence infidelity is the predominance of sex-segregated social organization in much of everyday life. One must be careful not to exaggerate the degree to which men and women live in parallel social worlds—because, of course, they interact regularly in domestic and economic life, and contemporary trends such as increasing urbanization and coeducational schooling have eroded some boundaries of sex segregation. Nevertheless, it is striking how much of Nigerian everyday sociality unfolds in gender-segregated spheres.

The meetings of hometown associations, villages, and extended families are conducted with men and women sitting in separate sections. In many churches, men and women sit in same-sex pews, and church-related associations are organized as same-sex groups. At weddings and funerals—perhaps the two most important community and life-course rituals—men and women are generally spatially separated and interact mostly in same-sex tasks and activities. Even in southeastern Nigeria's busy and seemingly mixed-together markets, different commercial niches tend to be mainly male or female. Perhaps most important, the everyday contexts of sociality tend to be predominantly single-sex settings, at least relative to most Western or North American contexts. These include situations wherein people exchange gossip, cultivate patron-client ties, create and maintain friendships, and engage in the business of self-presentation through which reputations are made and status is asserted or exhibited.

Opportunity Structures for Men's Extramarital Sex

In previous work, I have described the main opportunity structures that motivate and enable men's extramarital sex in southeastern Nigeria (Smith 2007, 2008). Three sociological factors are particularly important for explaining the opportunity structures that facilitate men's participation in these relationships: work-related migration, the intertwining of masculinity and socioeconomic status, and the male peer groups that encourage and reward extramarital sexual relations.

Work-related migration features as a key factor in men's accounts of infidelity. Men whose work takes them away from their wives and families are more likely to have extramarital relationships, and they frequently attribute their behavior to the opportunities and hardships produced by these absences. Further, extramarital relationships in the context of work-related migration can be more easily hidden from wives, family, and neighbors. Every man I interviewed who admitted to having extramarital sex expressed the importance of keeping such relationships secret not only from his wife, but also from his extended family and his local community. Men are navigating multiple audiences and conflicting social risks when they engage in extramarital sex.

A second factor explaining men's infidelity is the intersection of masculinity and aspirations to display socioeconomic success. Men frequently view extramarital relationships as arenas for the expression of economic and masculine status as well as opportunities for sexual gratification. Indeed, it is necessary to understand the connections between masculinity and wealth (and gender and economics more generally) to make sense of the most common forms of extramarital sex in southeastern Nigeria. Men's desires to improve their class position and demonstrate their social status through consumption frequently intersect with the choices they make regarding extramarital relationships. Much of what goes on in the more public dimensions of men's extramarital sexual lives must be seen as a kind of social performance in which masculinity, sexuality, consumption, and social class are mutually implicated.

The prevalence and importance of all-male peer groups, a structural aspect of sex-segregated social organization, is a third key feature of the opportunity structures that motivate and facilitate men's infidelity. Male-dominated spaces for sociality—such as bars, pepper-soup joints, social clubs, sports clubs, and arguably even brothels—create or reinforce the male peer-group dynamics that reward men for what is perceived to be economic capability and masculine sexuality.[3]

Although men frequently bring their girlfriends to male-dominated venues, these settings remain sex-segregated in a fundamental sense. They offer men spaces to meet and entertain their extramarital partners out of the view of wives and other women, around whom they would be embarrassed to be seen with a girlfriend. Further, these social spaces are conversationally and behaviorally male. The talk is men's talk; the behavior is male behavior; the primary audience is other men.

Sexual Geographies and Gendered Social Space

It is obvious that extramarital sexual partners must meet, interact, and rendezvous somewhere; the fact that sexuality and sexual behavior are situated in social space offers another point of analytical leverage. As the previous passages about the significance of male peer groups suggest, social spaces have remarkably different valences and behavioral consequences. The same populations of people can, at least potentially, perceive and interact with each other completely differently depending upon the specific social space, with diametrically opposed meanings and consequences. The way the same men and women behave toward members of their own and the opposite sex are dramatically different in a nightclub and in a church, for example, with one venue privileging sexually explicit conversations and cues, and the other requiring a maximum of decorum. But many dimensions of sexual geography are less obvious, and noting them can add insight to explaining behaviors and their meanings.

The sex-segregated aspect of much Igbo sociality has been highlighted already, but based on my observations, it is hard to overstate the masculine quality of many of the social spaces that are conducive to men's extramarital sexual behavior. Men meet, entertain, and show off their girlfriends in places like bars, social clubs, and pepper-soup joints, where the younger unmarried women who tend to be the extramarital partners of married men are clearly supporting actors in a cast dominated by male-male dialogue and drama. In these environments, frequently lubricated by alcohol, the men's loud conversations feature discussions, debates, joke-telling, heated arguments, and other boisterous oratory. In contrast, the young unmarried women in these settings frequently sit quietly beside their animated male partners, sipping drinks and eating food—perhaps whispering occasionally to their men. If a woman is not partnered, she may talk quietly with other women or sit alone waiting for a man to invite her for a drink or a dance. Certainly not all extramarital relationships start in or involve these male-dominated social settings, but they are common, and they suggest the degree to which men are performing for other men when engaging in extramarital relationships.

If a key quality of southeastern Nigeria's extramarital sexual geography is the masculine tone of most public places where these sexual relationships are kindled, supported, and displayed, another significant feature of the socio-sexual landscape

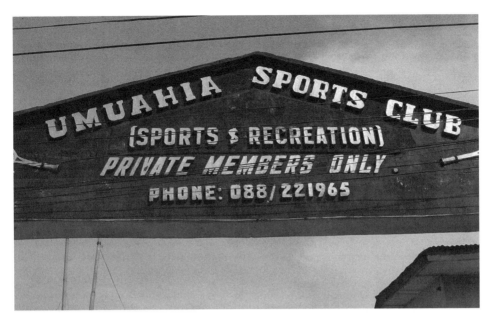

In southeastern Nigeria, venues like sports clubs are social spaces where married men entertain extramarital sexual partners and share their experiences with male peers. Photograph by Daniel Jordan Smith.

is the relatively strict separation of these places of infidelity from spaces associated with marriage, family, and community. When married men leave their homes to go to bars, eateries, or clubs, where they socialize with other men and possibly meet or meet up with girlfriends, they can reasonably expect that they will not encounter their wives (or any of their friends' or relatives' wives) at these places. The strength of this expectation is revealed in its violation: a tennis club in Umuahia where I am a member is one of these predominantly male spaces in which men frequently entertain their girlfriends. But it is also centrally located near the congested main market, and the wives of club members sometimes come to the club after shopping so that their husbands can drive them home. This is tolerated during daylight hours, but most men quickly shuttle their wives out of the club as soon as they arrive, and any man whose wife comes in the evening would hear about it from his peers. Her presence during those demarcated hours would violate the privacy of other men, not just that of her own husband.

Similarly, the younger unmarried women who tend to be men's extramarital sexual partners know that their claims on these men do not extend beyond the places where they meet. Young women know and follow these rules partly because they are economically dependent on the men, and partly because, as future wives to other men, they are invested in these same rules. Men do not have to fear that their lovers will show up at their houses, and certainly they would never take their girlfriends to church or to a meeting of age-mates in their village of origin. Young lovers who get pregnant almost always have abortions, even though abortions in Nigeria are illegal, clandestine, and dangerous. Men thoroughly separate these extramarital relationships from their marriages and families.[4] No man imagines divorcing his wife for a lover, or at least so it seems.

Indeed, if a man begins to allow the line between wife and lover to become too blurry, his male peers will strongly sanction him. In one case I remember well, an acquaintance was clearly falling in love with his girlfriend, to the point where he displayed public affection for her outside these masculine spaces, he spent multiple nights with her away from his family, and he apparently failed to provide expected economic support to his wife and children. All of these behaviors broke taboos that men enforce among themselves, and this fellow soon became the object of what one might call "an intervention" by his peers. They sat him down and made it plain that his behavior was unacceptable—primarily by threatening him with expulsion from the tennis club. The degree to which these gendered behavioral boundaries are socially recognized and enforced also contributes to the reasons why—and the ways in which—married women are often complicit in enabling men's extramarital sexual behavior. By observing these boundaries and tolerating their husbands' indiscretions so long as the men obey the rules, the women preserve the sanctity of their marriages—albeit a sanctity that does not dissuade male infidelity.

Finally, with regard to sexual geographies, it is important to acknowledge the fact that as an ethnographer, I do not have access to the most private aspects of extramarital sex. To the extent that I know anything about what Nigerians do behind closed doors and in bed, it is only based on what they say. Of course, many people choose not to share or not to share accurately this kind of information with others, much less with a prying anthropologist who wants to write about it. Even when people do talk about what happens in private, it reintroduces the notion of "a public," because these self-presentations are at least partly crafted with their reception in mind.

Nevertheless, based on many years of observations and conversations, I can report with some confidence that the private and intimate side of Igbo men's extramarital sexual behavior spans a wide spectrum of emotions, with some men developing or allowing themselves very little emotional intimacy with their extramarital sexual partners, and others finding significant emotional connection in these sexual relationships. Some extramarital relationships are brief and almost purely exchanges of economic support for sex, exemplified most starkly by liaisons with commercial sex workers. But many of these extramarital relationships are longer-term, involving greater intimacy and commitment. What is noteworthy, however, is how powerful the effect of public expectations is, both in encouraging men to believe that having extramarital sex is socially acceptable and in discouraging them from allowing these relationships to interfere with their social and economic obligations as husbands and fathers. Similarly, while it is hard to know how women who knew or suspected that their husbands were unfaithful reacted in private, the fact that the women we interviewed almost uniformly denied that their husbands were cheating speaks to the importance of a marriage's public face and the ways in which concerns with social reputation influence interpersonal dynamics, sometimes to the extent of putting women at risk for contracting HIV from their own spouses.

Social Risk: Making Sociological Sense of Extramarital Sex in Modern Nigerian Marriages

I use the concept of social risk, introduced at the beginning of this volume, to make sociological sense of behaviors that can otherwise be misunderstood as un-educated, irrational, or simply "cultural." While I am ambivalent about retaining the term "risk" in promoting a more sociological theoretical perspective, given that it suggests a particularly individualistic orientation to the world, I think that the costs of retaining the term are outweighed by the benefits of speaking to audiences that see public health in general and AIDS in particular through the lens of risk.

The concept of social risk enables an analysis that situates behavior within the complex contexts of economic opportunity and constraint, the shared (and sometimes contested) valuations of what merits social status, and the dynamic interactions between self-presentation and social reception through which reputations are forged and maintained vis-à-vis kin, community, peer groups, and other publics within which individuals' lives are enmeshed. I cannot, of course, account for every aspect of context that shapes behavior. I focus on key dimensions of contemporary social life in southeastern Nigeria that seem to be particularly salient at the intersection of modern Nigerian marriage, men's extramarital sex, and faithful married women's vulnerability to HIV infection.

In particular, I emphasize two features of contemporary Nigerian society that my research suggests are highly significant: (1) the interconnections among social class, gendered reputations, and identities, and (2) widespread ambivalence about extramarital sex in a context where the changing aspects of marriage figure centrally in transformations of and anxieties about family, kinship, and community. I conclude by examining the role of the AIDS epidemic and the interventions designed to combat it in inflecting moral discourses about sexual behavior. In people's real lives, these issues are not separate but deeply intertwined; however, for heuristic purposes, I discuss each issue individually, with the primary purpose of situating and understanding men's extramarital sexual behavior and women's responses to it.

Social Class, Gendered Reputations, and Infidelity

Put most simply, my argument about the connection between men's extramarital sexual behavior and economic inequality is that particular aspects of the performance of infidelity have become important markers of class position and masculinity for men in southeastern Nigeria. The ways in which men display their extramarital partners to other men and their ability to support and entertain their lovers can be usefully interpreted as forms of conspicuous consumption. I do not mean to suggest that all men's extramarital sex is motivated by this purpose or has this quality. Certainly many men keep their affairs completely secret, and some men who cannot afford to have extramarital relationships that serve as public economic performances still have extramarital sex. But the connection between infidelity and economic inequality is well recognized by Nigerians themselves (Smith 2001, 2002; Cornwall 2002). It suggests that there are important social benefits to men when they cheat on their wives. Conceived of through the lens of social risk, it means that in a context where people are increasingly anxious about and socially rewarded for proving their class position, the calculus for whether or not to have extramarital sex includes some degree of consideration, at least tacitly, of these factors.

In the sorts of venues where married men entertain their lovers and display them for their peers, it is not hard to see the connections between infidelity and the performance of economic status. In the popular bars and pepper-soup joints in Umuahia and Owerri where married men frequently socialized with their peers in the company of their girlfriends, these young ladies were lavishly supplied with food and drink. Men in the company of their girlfriends also seemed more likely to buy rounds of drinks for other men—a fact that a man's mates almost always managed to take advantage of, knowing that a fellow would be hard-pressed to forgo an opportunity to demonstrate generosity and financial buoyancy in front of his lover. No doubt men spent their money partly to impress their female partners, but they were also concerned with the impression they made on other men. Economic performance was rewarded by both fellow men and young women.

Over the past twenty years, I have had scores of conversations with the unmarried young women who accompany married men to bars, eateries, and social clubs. Indeed, it has been usually quite easy to do so, because in these male-dominated settings, the young women are mostly ignored conversationally (even though they are an obvious audience for the men's conspicuous spending). In addition, rather than being threatened by my talking to their girlfriends, many men (especially if they could count me as a friend or fellow club member) seemed to like it when I paid attention to their girlfriends. In a sense, I served as a further form of entertainment that these men could provide for their girlfriends, and with my expatriate/American identity, I offered yet another way in which men displayed their capital—in this case, their social capital, evidenced through their visible intimacy with a foreigner.

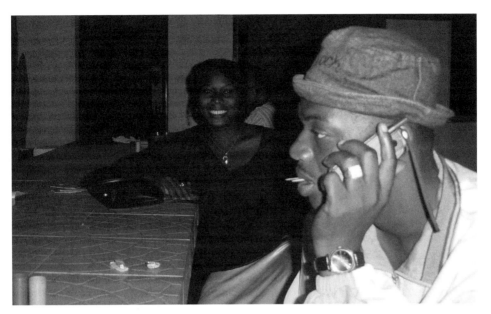

Cell phones have revolutionized extramarital sexual relations in Nigeria, providing a new means of communication and discretion, but they are also a new commodity that single women expect from their married male lovers. Photograph by Daniel Jordan Smith.

Young women have made it clear that economic support is a major reason why they seek the company of married men. Similar to what Hunter (2002, 2005) observed in South Africa, there are numerous idiomatic expressions in Nigeria that signal women's economic motivations. During the course of my research, I heard women describe their married boyfriends as "Commissioners for Transportation," a reference to the fact that married men frequently drove their girlfriends in their cars. Privately owned motor vehicles are a luxury of the relatively rich in Nigeria, and men are much more likely to own and drive cars than women are. I have never performed a systematic analysis, but it always seemed like the men with the most expensive cars had the prettiest girlfriends. Other allusions to boyfriends in terms of the political appointees who control Nigerian state government ministries included "Commissioner for Education" or "Commissioner for Housing," referring to the fact that many of the young women in these relationships expected and extracted money from their lovers for school or university fees and rent. Given the wide availability of cell phones in Nigeria after 2001, nearly every married man of means has been expected to become his lover's "Commissioner for Communication" by buying her a phone or providing her with calling credit; this now-standard demand has no doubt been augmented by the argument that cell phone communication can enable and enhance the relationships and help keep them secret from wives (Smith 2006).

The common expression among unmarried women in Nigeria (and, I gather, in much of sub-Saharan Africa) that there is "no romance without finance" signifies the economic foundations of what are widely glossed as "sugar daddy" relationships (Dinan 1983; Luke 2005), but the conventional focus too frequently draws attention only to the economic needs of the younger female partners. Less notice has been taken of the desire of the men to demonstrate economic capability as part of a larger masculine performance. The notion that these relationships can be reduced to men trading money for sex (with women wanting money and men wanting sex) misses much of their nuance and complexity. I can only focus here on the multidimensional character of married men's motives, but it is equally important to be aware of the complex and sometimes ambivalent intentions and desires of the women in these extramarital relationships (Guyer 1994; Smith 2002; Luke 2005; Pisani 2008).

Certainly married men recognize, both implicitly and explicitly, that part of what they are doing in their extramarital relationships is demonstrating economic prowess—to their lovers, themselves, and their fellow men. At the tennis clubs in Owerri and Umuahia, where I have been interacting with married men in male-dominated social spaces for two decades, men frequently give each other nicknames. These nicknames serve many purposes and draw on the Igbo convention of title-taking, wherein men are bestowed with honorary titles (and names) that signify social accomplishment and prestige (Uchendu 1965; Henderson 1972). Nicknames in the club are similarly honorific, but more playful and humorous. Often, they are directly related to aspects of masculinity such as economic achievement, political power, and sexual prowess. My favorite of these nicknames—because it signaled so obviously my clubmates' recognition of the performative nature of masculinity—was given to a man who was in his late thirties at the time. Married with three children, he was rich, good-looking, and very generous with his money: he was always buying food and drinks to go around, and contributed heavily every time the club tried to raise money for an event, an outing, or a building project. Not incidentally, he seemed to appear every week with a different (but always very beautiful) young woman. His nickname was "One Man Show."

The connections among economic means, extramarital sex, and the performance of masculinity were experienced not only by more privileged men with the capacity to attract and entertain relatively educated and fashionable young girlfriends, but also by poorer men who did not have such opportunities. The consequences of poverty and inequality were subjects of discontent for all sorts of reasons, and certainly poorer men's inability to attract extramarital sexual partners was only one among their many frustrations—though, among the younger unmarried men, the inability to afford to marry was perhaps their most aggrieved complaint of all. But even among poorer married men who either could not afford extramarital sex or who resorted to much cheaper partnerships (such as with prostitutes, or with less educated and less fashionable women who were less demand-ing but also less prestigious partners), the awareness of and desire for the sexual and masculine benefits that accrue to the wealthy were common.

I remember a poignant moment in an interview with an older man in Ubakala. At seventy-two years of age, he had been married for almost forty years. He had eight children, and he combined farming with a low-paying night watchman's job to eke out a living. When I asked whether he had ever cheated on his wife, he reported that he had not. Then, without any prompting from me, he added in Ni-gerian pidgin English, "E no be say I no want. Woman na money she want. You get for carry am go for restaurant, buy am food and drink, pay for hotel. Me na poor man. I no get money. If I been get money I been for want am" (It's not that I don't want it. But a woman wants money. You have to take her to a restaurant, buy her food and drink, and pay for a hotel. I am a poor man. I don't have money. If I had money, I would want it [extramarital sex]). Whether this man would have actually cheated on his wife had he been wealthier is impossible to say, but he clearly con-nected extramarital sex to economic capability.

For married women, too, men's infidelity involves issues of economics and gendered social reputation. From an economic point of view, married women's responses to men's extramarital sex typically must navigate two connected but competing realities. On the one hand, women are concerned that their husbands will shift economic resources toward their girlfriends. A woman who might ignore or tolerate her husband's suspected indiscretions is often more likely to confront him and even share her complaints with friends, family, and community members if she feels her husband is neglecting his spousal and parental economic obliga-tions in addition to cheating sexually. Indeed, a woman who seeks assistance in the face of a man's infidelity will find a much more sympathetic audience if she can show that her husband is failing to provide for his family than if she merely com-plains that he has failed in his promise of love and fidelity. As in the example of the intervention discussed earlier, even men who themselves cheat on their wives can be mobilized to scorn and sanction another man who allows his extramarital af-fairs to interfere with his economic obligations to his family. Similarly, a man who flaunts his infidelity too publicly—even if he has not failed his family economi-cally—can expect opprobrium rather than social reward among his male peers.

On the other hand, if women appear too strident in their confrontations with their husbands or in their complaints to kin and community, they may provoke spouses to withdraw support more openly—through divorce, by marrying a sec-ond wife, or simply by giving up any pretense of being a good husband, all highly undesirable results. Although divorce is relatively rare and polygyny is increasingly uncommon, the specter of each remains powerful in the patriarchal sex-gender system that dominates southeastern Nigeria, and they have certainly affected many women's calculations regarding potential conflagrations over infidelity. So too has the fact that some husbands brazenly flouted their economic obligations. In the communities I studied, such men were not well respected by anyone, but blame was sometimes allocated to the wives in stories that depicted the neglected woman as difficult, nagging, and impossible to manage. Conflicts over infidelity featured commonly in these accounts. For an Igbo woman, challenging a man's infidelity is a risky strategy.

Given these circumstances, one might presume (and I found some evidence to suggest) that women with their own economic means (mainly through running their own businesses, but also via formal employment) would be better able to prevent or minimize their husbands' extramarital sexual behavior. Certainly the few married men I interviewed whose wives had substantial (and occasionally even superior) economic resources appeared much more circumspect about their extramarital sex lives. But men who submitted too readily to wealthy wives were widely criticized in popular discourse. More common than a perceived association of women's wealth with male fidelity was the assumption that wealthy women were themselves more likely to cheat. Indeed, many stories about wealthy and powerful women suggest that they slept their way to wealth and power—a discourse that serves to reinforce male privilege and stigmatize female autonomy.

In addition to the ways that economic concerns and constraints shape married women's responses to men's infidelity, women's preoccupation with their own gendered reputations also figure heavily in their strategies and reactions. It is hard to overstate the importance of marriage and parenthood in the attainment of social status and full personhood in both Igbo-speaking southeastern Nigeria and West Africa in general (Fortes 1978; Smith 2001). To be unmarried or without children is to be socially immature or incomplete. For men, as demonstrated earlier in this chapter, social expectations about their roles as husbands and fathers establish strong boundaries with regard to acceptable extramarital sexual behavior.

For women, the social importance of wifehood and motherhood sharply circumscribes their options in the face of male infidelity. Few women seek divorce, even from egregiously bad husbands. The reasons are many, and they relate primarily to the social and reputational entailments of being a wife and a mother. In the Igbo patrilineal kinship system, children "belong" to the father and his lineage. A woman who divorces risks losing her primary parental role, including regular access to her children. In addition to concerns about ties to children, being married itself is a highly valued social position—one almost universally aspired to by women of all ages. Being an unmarried adult woman can be a stigmatizing and marginalizing experience, for widows and especially for the divorced or never-married. Even women of the highest status indicate the social importance of being married in the way they refer to themselves: female doctors, lawyers, and chiefs refer to themselves publicly and sign official documents as "Dr. (Mrs.) . . . ," "Barrister (Mrs.) . . . ," and "Chief (Mrs.) . . . " No matter their political, economic, and social achievements, women's status remains highly tied to marriage. In such a context, it is not hard to understand why women treat the problem of male infidelity carefully. In the language of social risk, wives often have more to lose by confronting their husbands' infidelities than by tolerating them.

Ambivalence, Anxiety, and the Contradictions of Modern Marriage

Much of the discussion thus far has portrayed men's extramarital sexual behavior and women's responses in instrumental terms: people making choices tied to their economic positions and gendered reputations. Analytically, there is much to be learned from this perspective. But for a more complete understanding of the social dynamics of infidelity, particularly as this relates to the institutional and intimate interpersonal aspects of modern Nigerian marriage, it is necessary to recognize that individual actors are often ambivalent about their situations and behavior. Further, these ambivalences relate to and are partly the result of anxieties about and contradictions inherent in social change, with the place of marriage and sexuality vis-à-vis the shifting dynamics of gender, kinship, religion, and social class

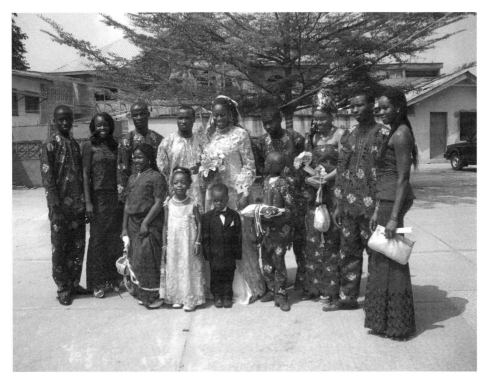

Weddings in southeastern Nigeria are events in which contemporary fashions and traditional ties to family are equally valued, symbolizing how "modern marriage" remains embedded in kinship and community. Photograph by Daniel Jordan Smith.

being central to this story. Much of what is hinted at here lies beyond the scope of this chapter, but I want to examine briefly how men's and women's understandings of and adjustments to contemporary marriage figure into the complexity of their feelings and behavior with regard to infidelity.

Most of the examples and discussion in the previous section would suggest that men who are unfaithful do not much believe in or willingly participate in the emotional and intimate interpersonal part of the project of modern marriage, symbolized most widely by the notion of being in love. This looks to be true if one considers things only from the point of view of men's relationships with their peer groups at places like bars and male-dominated social clubs, or simply by observing the prevalence of their extramarital partnerships. But I spent a lot of time interviewing individual men about their marriages and interacting with married people in their homes; in these settings, it was clear that men had multiple sides to them, and that they often felt real ambivalence about their extramarital sexual behavior. Assessing how much a man loves his wife is a nearly impossible task, even if one could somehow identify a culturally appropriate rubric. Further, the men I got to know in Ubakala and Owerri were unsurprisingly heterogeneous in both the style and degree to which they appeared to love their wives. But I can say without any doubt that many of the unfaithful men I got to know *did* love their wives. They overtly claimed to do so; further, many of the wives of cheating husbands said their husbands loved them, and both men and women provided countless examples of the loving things husbands did. I believed them. More important, I think they believed themselves.

To make sense of infidelity in southeastern Nigeria, it is necessary to move beyond the assumption that infidelity is incompatible with modern marriage (and hence love). Most of the men I interviewed identified their commitment to the welfare of their wives and children as the single most important expression of love. With this criterion paramount in their minds, very few men thought of their infidelity as categorically incompatible with loving their wives. It is worth reiterating that extramarital affairs rarely involved any intention to divorce and remarry. It would be a mistake to conclude that being a good husband—even from the perspective of the wife—maps isomorphically onto whether or not a man is sexually faithful.

In my interviews with the men, it was striking how frequently they talked about their wives and children in the same breath. Questions about their relationships with their wives drew from many men responses that talked about their wives *and* children. Despite changes in marital ideals, family structure, and residence patterns that increasingly privilege the conjugal bond relative to other kinship ties, marriage continues to be recognized by men as a means of social reproduction. For Igbo men (and for Igbo women), marriage remains in its essence a reproductive project.

That said, many of the men who married in the last ten to fifteen years spoke much more explicitly about emotionally intimate relationships with their wives than did men of older generations. I was struck by the descriptions men provided of helping their wives bathe, of talking with their wives about mutual sexual pleasure, and of finding times for intimate communication when kids were sleeping, chores were done, and kin were out of earshot. None of these things could have been predicted from listening to the men's talk about women and marriage among their male peers. Some men expressed an awareness of a certain degree of hypocrisy and a sense of guilt regarding their infidelities. Most commonly this ambivalence produced greater efforts to keep their extramarital sexual behavior secret in order to protect their wives and their marriages. It did not lead most men to be faithful. In these men's reckoning, their commitment to their marriages, if not their wives, was largely unaffected by infidelity.

Igbo women are at least tacitly aware of everything I have just described. They know that many men have extramarital sex; as I have already indicated, many women certainly know or suspect that their own husbands are unfaithful—and this was clear from our interviews with men, many of whom admitted that their wives knew of their extramarital relationships. Women are also well aware that male infidelity does not generally lead men to divorce their wives for their lovers. Nevertheless, we did not talk to a single married woman who approved of male infidelity. Women clearly viewed it as a violation and thought that husbands and wives should be faithful.[5] None of this seems surprising, but quite striking was the fact that it was nearly impossible to find any woman who would acknowledge openly that her own husband was unfaithful, even in the context of private interviews conducted by my female research assistants in which confidentiality and anonymity had been repeatedly assured. Nearly every woman concurred that male infidelity was rampant, but none would openly accuse her husband.

The women's unwillingness to discuss their husbands' extramarital sexual behavior during their interviews coincides with and must be understood in the same context as their reluctance to confront their husbands' unfaithfulness before kin and community. From our interviews with men, it was clear that women did sometimes confront their husbands in private about their suspicions or discoveries. They also sometimes shared their discontents with a close friend or relative. In contrast to Huli women in Papua New Guinea (see Wardlow, this volume), however, rarely did Igbo wives make a scene. Indeed, it was considered quite scandalous for a woman to publicly accuse her husband of infidelity. Women did of course sometimes resort to this, but it is instructive to realize that it was the woman who typically emerged from such actions with a more damaged reputation than her accused husband. The stain fell broadly on the marriage and family, so certainly men also wanted to avoid such scandals, but it was clearly the wife who suffered greater social stigma in the wake of a public accusation of her husband's infidelity.

Explaining why a woman is more shamed than her husband by a public airing of his infidelity requires connecting a number of factors. Above all, the situation is both a result and reinforcement of a patriarchal system of gender inequality. No matter how much one contextualizes it, there is no denying the fact that this circumstance is patently unfair to married women. In various ways, Igbo women lament male infidelity and recognize that its acceptability relative to female infidelity is a consequence of gender inequality. Yet, in subtle ways, women are complicit in the very dynamics that they also deplore.

Understanding how this particular aspect of gender inequality is maintained requires more information. As the discussion and examples provided earlier illustrate, women are highly invested in and accrue much of their status, satisfaction, and social reward from their roles as wives and mothers. It would be simplistic and inaccurate to dismiss women's desires for and participation in these arenas of femininity as imposed on them by men. Women genuinely value and are valued for their reproductive roles and will not easily give these up, which they risk doing should they confront a man's infidelity too boldly. Most Igbo women do not in fact think that male infidelity should result in divorce, and many tacitly agree that it is not worth a public fuss. They recognize that most men do not mean to threaten the permanence of marriage by having extramarital sex, and there is a certain amount of looking the other way if a man is discreet. Indeed, similar to what Parikh describes for Uganda later in this volume, most of the cases I observed of women who went public in one way or another (telling a pastor, informing her kin or in-laws, or simply yelling at her husband so that neighbors and passers-by could surely hear) involved circumstances where the woman felt the man had disgraced her by the blatancy of his behavior (often including the perceived neglect of his economic obligations as a husband and father).

All of this is complicated by the rise of the ideal of romantic love as a motivation to get married and as an element of marriage that is increasingly perceived to be important. If emotional, communicative, and sexual intimacies are a greater part of what men and women value in their conjugal relationships, it would seem that infidelity would be a more intolerable breach (for the Mexican parallel to this, see Hirsch et al. 2002). Indeed, the women we interviewed who were in self-described love marriages consistently and firmly expressed a view that infidelity was unacceptable. But these same women seemed the most resistant to acknowledging their husbands' infidelities and appeared to be as unlikely as other women to boldly confront an unfaithful man. This seeming irony, however, makes good sense. For women in love marriages, the public face of their relationships (and therefore their reputations as wives) depends even more on the perception of male fidelity than for women in marriages less committed to the romantic ideal. Further, in a gender-unequal context where divorce is not much of an option, a woman who openly challenges her husband's infidelity risks not only losing face, but she also faces the prospect of being blamed—the implication being that her love/sex/intimacy was not good enough to keep her man satisfied. Finally, in a love marriage, a woman who exposes and challenges her husband's cheating is saying that the supposed foundation of the marriage is broken, undermining the leverage she had based on the idiom of love. In these circumstances, it is not surprising that women are often silent about their husbands' extramarital sex, and even complicit in keeping it secret.

Conclusion: AIDS, Sexual Morality, and Social Risk

Using the concept of social risk as an organizing conceptual framework, the factors addressed in this chapter explain both the prevalence of men's infidelity in southeastern Nigeria and married women's relatively muted responses to it. Understanding the motivations and behaviors of both married men and married women is crucial to making sense of the epidemiological fact that for many married women, the greatest risk of contracting HIV is through having sex with their husbands. Perhaps the greatest irony and tragedy here is that modern marriage, with its promise of intimacy and the privileging of the conjugal bond relative to other social ties, does not seem to reduce the prevalence of men's infidelity. At best, it appears to require male discretion. At worst, it seems to make it even harder for married women to confront and curtail their husbands' behavior. Men's extramarital sex is a public secret. It is a secret that men are rewarded for sharing with their male peers as long as they do not disgrace their wives or neglect their families. It is a secret that women have been complicit in keeping hidden because their own roles and reputations depend so significantly on being married.

Part of what this research suggests is that people can be paradoxically aware of a problem in their society (or in their relationships) and able to talk about it in the abstract, but incapable of addressing it directly because of their personal stakes in the very circumstances that produce the problem. In southeastern Nigeria, people are well aware of HIV, its modes of transmission, and the practices that could reduce their risk. Yet as married men and women traverse Nigeria's contemporary sexual and social landscape, they must navigate a range of pragmatic goals and moral expectations related to marriage, family-making, and community reputation that frequently impinge on and sometimes completely overshadow a calculus for behavior that would privilege HIV prevention.

This analysis of the intersections among gender inequality, culture, infidelity, and the risk of HIV would not be complete without touching briefly on the ways in which medical and public health discourses about the epidemic have unintentionally contributed to people's failure to protect themselves. As I have written elsewhere (Smith 2003), AIDS is perceived in Nigeria as a problem of social morality. Partly as a backlash to the way in which globally circulated public health discourses about HIV implicitly or explicitly blame African culture for the continent's high prevalence of infections, Nigerians have constructed AIDS as something associated with the ills of too much Western culture (see Setel 1996 and 1999 for a similar argument about Tanzania). People's anxieties about underdevelopment, inequality, and unsettling social change are voiced through depictions of HIV risk as connected to immoral sexualities that then become the objects of stigma. In this context, few people want to imagine themselves as the kind of person (or as having the kind of sex) associated with HIV.

Perhaps the most tragic consequence of these anxieties is the widespread association of condoms with the spread of HIV, rather than with its prevention. Stories circulate of condoms infected with the virus, but even more commonly, people figure that those who suggest the use of condoms are signaling something about the morality of their own or their partners' sexual conduct. Condoms can be hard enough to introduce into any sexual relationship: evidence across the globe suggests that the more intimate a relationship, the less likely one is to use a condom (Preston-Whyte 1999; Kaler 2004). During my research, I found that married Igbo men cheating on their wives—men who did not want a pregnancy with their girlfriends and did not intend these relationships to be permanent—did not regularly and certainly did not always use condoms with their lovers. This seemed to be driven partly by a desire to separate symbolically their extramarital relationships from crude commercial sex; condoms were widely associated with—and widely used by—prostitutes. But public health discourses about the HIV epidemic itself seem to infect condoms with their own stigma: by not using condoms, men are symbolically asserting that their relationships are morally superior to promiscuous sex.

For a married woman, the notion of suggesting a condom for marital sex is almost unthinkable.[6] It violates the pro-natal mentality of Igbo society and contradicts notions of trust associated with marriage. It suggests a degree of female autonomy that would likely be extremely threatening to her husband. It implies that she feels sex with her husband is risky, casting aspersions on his sexual morality and insinuating that he has been unfaithful, which I have already shown is problematic. Worst of all, it could easily be twisted by a man to suggest that she herself is cheating. A woman suggesting to her husband that they use condoms, especially when the suspicion of his infidelity looms large, risks not only ridicule and anger but possibly even domestic violence. The specter of HIV only adds to the morally charged nature of these issues. For most women, the social risks of trying to protect their relationships with their husbands far outweigh the more distant prospect of HIV infection.

Examining married women's risk of HIV infection using the lens of social risk allows us to explain behavior in a manner that affords men and women agency and rationality while situating their actions in complex economic, social, and cultural contexts. It transcends a narrow conceptualization of risk that would discount reasonable explanations for why people do what they do. From the point of view of effectively combating the AIDS epidemic, in Nigeria and elsewhere, a focus on the sociological contexts and logics that shape behavior moves us away from a misguided conceptualization of culture as static, bounded, and apolitical, which is frequently deployed simply to cast blame. It privileges a concept of culture that recognizes the constraints people face *and* acknowledges their role in both navigating and reproducing their social worlds.

4

"Eaten One's Fill and All Stirred Up"

Doi Moi and the Reconfiguration of Masculine Sexual Risk and Men's Extramarital Sex in Vietnam

Harriet M. Phinney

As my family and I were being driven to Tay Phuong Pagoda, about fifty miles out-side Hanoi, I took the opportunity to question Anh Binh, our young male driver, about men's extramarital relations.[1] Although he spoke English, I conversed with him in Vietnamese so my children would not understand. Somewhat surprised by my question, he nonetheless proceeded to answer it. As part of his explanation, Anh Binh described how he and his male friends periodically drive to Hai Phong for the day to spend time with each other, eating and drinking in a restaurant in the company of young women. He said his wife does not know about these trips, and anyway, "It's not a problem."

"Are you and your friends worried that your wives will find out and be upset?" I asked.

Anh Binh answered, "No. . . . This kind of activity doesn't have much impact on your family. . . . Relationships men have with prostitutes are short and for fun only." He also indicated that his wife does not know when he goes to Hai Phong—just that he's away on those days.

On the way home from the pagoda, Anh Binh asked me if I knew what a *nha tam* was, because the section of the road we were on had a couple of them. I didn't. He pointed to a handpainted wooden sign with the words "Nha Tam" written on it. A *nha tam* (used interchangeably with *nghi tam*) is a "bath and rest-house": a room in or adjacent to a private house for drivers who need a bath and a rest. "Young women help them bathe," he added.

"Oh," I said, and asked if he would slow down so I could take a photograph.

"Do it quickly," he said. "The owner might see and get angry."

When I queried Anh Binh further on why men like to see sex workers, he said, "Vietnamese men, like all southeast Asian men, need and like to experience new and exotic things," and "men need more sex than women."

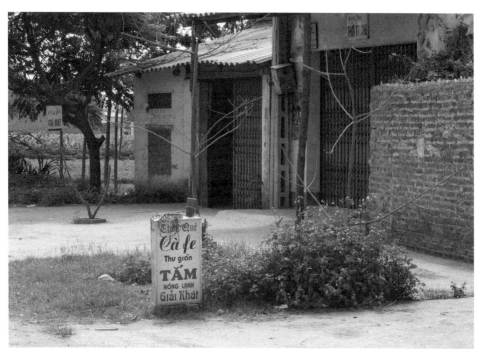

Nha tam (bath and rest-house) outside Hanoi. Photograph by Harriet M. Phinney.

Anh Binh and his friends were not alone in their desire to seek sexual relations outside marriage. His essentialist explanation for why Vietnamese men do
so was echoed by many other Hanoians I spoke to while researching marital HIV
risk in Hanoi in 2004—both men and women. Not everyone, however, held the
same opinion. Some dismissed such gendered and culturally essentialist notions
and instead retorted that the men having extramarital liaisons are newcomers to
Hanoi; they have money for the first time and don't know what else to do with it
so they spend it on sex workers. A well-known sociologist, focusing on the constructed nature of sexuality, thought that many Hanoians, women and men, were
experimenting with sex as a result of seeing new media images of romance and
sexuality from the United States.[2] The multiplicity of theories held by Hanoians
regarding the increase in men's extramarital sex and the fact that sex has become
a matter of public discourse and gossip in Hanoi reflect local concern about the
consequences of swift economic change, and in particular its relation to sexuality,
gender, and consumption. Indeed, Anh Binh's trips to Hai Phong and his beliefs
about masculinity, sexuality, and marriage point to a society undergoing rapid
changes in the way in which gender and other forms of social organization shape
masculine sexual risk, definitions of fidelity, and men's extramarital relationships
in and around Hanoi today.

Interested in the effects of globalization, and driven by concern with the emergence of HIV in Vietnam, social scientists have conducted significant research on the epidemiological, behavioral, and cultural attributes of sexual behavior in Vietnam.[3] Recent epidemiological reports indicate that the number of HIV infections due to sexual transmission is outpacing those caused by injecting drug use in Vietnam and is thought to be a key component in HIV's ongoing dissemination (VNMOH 2005). Many studies on HIV and on sexuality in general point to "Doi Moi" (Renovation), the policy the government began to promulgate in 1986 to transform the Vietnamese economy, as critical in shaping the HIV epidemic. The ethnographic research I conducted in 2004 found that although men and women had certainly engaged in extramarital sex prior to Doi Moi (Phinney 2003; see also Khuat Thu Hong 1998), Vietnam's government-led economic reforms mark a period in which men's opportunities to do so have multiplied quite strikingly.[4] Though the association between Doi Moi and sexuality is often articulated, there has been little explication of the processes through which Doi Moi's policies might structure men's access to extramarital sex.[5] What mechanisms are at work that would explain such an association? This chapter delineates the contemporary configuration of men's extramarital sexuality and seeks to demonstrate the way in which Doi Moi policies have had the unintentional consequence of facilitating opportunities for men's extramarital relations in Hanoi and women's acquiescence to their husbands' infidelity, and thus of contributing to marital HIV risk.

Rethinking Gender, Sex, Marriage, and Social Risk in the Vietnamese Context

The preceding chapter articulated the need to rethink notions of culture and risk in relation to HIV transmission and explicated the growing consensus among medical anthropologists about the need to take into account the social and economic factors that shape individual sexual behavior (Parker 2001; Parker and Gagnon 1995). Historical and anthropological research on Vietnamese families, reproduction, and sexuality, moreover, has demonstrated the extent to which people's intimate and private desires, sexual realities, and moralities reflect political and economic policies as well as cultural values at specific moments in time (Micollier 2004c; Phinney 2003, 2005; Rydstrom 2006; Nguyen-Vo Thu-Huong 2002; Pelzer 1993; Le Thi 1999; Werner 2002). This chapter builds on these insights by providing a particularly clear example of how political and economic change reshapes the terrain of sexual relations. This research also draws attention to the ways in which unequal gender relations are socially, economically, and politically organized. In order to understand how married women are at risk of contracting HIV from their husbands' extramarital liaisons, it is certainly necessary to focus on men's behavior, but it is critical to do so in a way that recognizes that men's extramarital relations are a gendered part of social organization and, in the case of

Vietnam, the unintended effect of state policies, rather than simply the product of individual decision-making or moral failings.

The decision to focus on men in this study is informed by two basic theoretical points. First, gender includes men (Connell 1995). Like many studies on gender around the world, studies conducted on gender in Vietnam have been considered synonymous with women's studies; the lack of academic articles and journals focusing on masculinity in Vietnam speaks for itself. Second, sexuality, like masculinity, is historically contingent; the manifestation of men's sexual desire is not solely rooted in their bodies. While contemporary anthropological theory regarding sexuality recognizes the importance of the social and economic forces and the inequalities that shape men's desires, consumption practices, identities, and sexual behavior (Parker and Easton 1998; Farmer 2001), such analyses are largely missing from sexuality studies on Vietnam. Instead, most studies on sexuality engage in tautological reasoning, attributing Vietnamese men's sexual drives to their Vietnamese culture or to southeast Asian tradition. Such analyses are problematic, given the extent to which consumer goods, technologies, and ideologies from the West and elsewhere have been circulating in Vietnam since it began to participate in the global economy. To date, few of the epidemiological, behavioral, and cultural analyses of men's sexual behavior in Vietnam have moved beyond such reasoning.

In these analyses, Doi Moi is conceptualized as a release valve on a pressure cooker of pent-up sexual desire. Sex is now everywhere. Although the analysis presented in this chapter also attributes the increased opportunities for men's extramarital sex to Doi Moi policies, masculinities and sexualities are not taken to be essential characteristics. Rather they are seen as products of changing social, economic, and political environments—an approach that enables us to look for factors in society that shape men's attitudes and behaviors rather than assuming that contemporary sexual desires and the associated activities have always existed. Thus, by focusing on the social organization of sexuality and its relationship to state policy, this chapter contributes to the small but growing number of studies on Vietnamese masculinities (Le Minh Giang 2007; Avieli 2007; Ngo Thi Ngan Binh 2007) that have been broadening understandings of male society and culture in Vietnam.

Informing these discussions of gender, sex, and marriage are shifting notions of what is considered appropriate or risky social behavior. Existing studies of risky sexual behavior tend to portray risk in individualistic terms. Yet, like sexuality and sexual behavior, risk is social and is shaped by larger social structures (Boholm 2003). How should we think about risky sexual behavior in the context of the contemporary HIV epidemic in Hanoi? Foucault's 1991 theory of governmentality is useful for thinking about the interactions between policy, social structures, and individual behavior as they pertain to men's sexuality in the Doi Moi era. Lemke's 2001 discussion provides an intriguing way of thinking about the ongoing process of Doi Moi and the Vietnamese State's logic of governmentality; based on Foucault's unpublished 1979 lectures on the genealogy of the modern state, Lemke writes about the manner in which neoliberal governments shift the responsibility for social risks to collectivities such as families and associations and ultimately to individuals (Phinney 2003). According to Lemke, the neoliberal government endeavors to achieve "congruence . . . between a responsible and moral individual and an economic-rational actor" (Lemke 2001: 201). It is not necessary to presuppose that the Vietnamese government is attempting to remake itself in a neoliberal mode in order to garner insights from this analysis. Instead of viewing Doi Moi policies in terms of the State's "withdrawal" from family life, we might view them instead as a "reorganization or restructuring of government techniques, shifting the regulatory competence of the state onto 'responsible' and 'rational' individuals" (202). By rendering economic the social domain, the Vietnamese State, like neoliberal governments, is able to "link a reduction in (welfare) state services and security systems to the increasing call for 'personal responsibility' and 'self-care'" (203), in the process shifting the locus of economic and social risk and the determinants of such risk for individual citizens.

Doi Moi was not simply a switch from a collective economy to market-based socialism. It was also a shift in governmentality—one that involved the reorganization and restructuring of government tactics. As I and others have argued (Phinney 2003; Werner 2002; McNally 2007), this has entailed a process whereby the State has shifted economic, social, and moral responsibility from itself to the family and to the individual. Prior to Doi Moi, risk involved eschewing Communist Party guidelines. Now, risk centers on one's engagement with the global market economy. It is within the framework of the market economy that the State, perhaps inadvertently, has restructured the risks of men's infidelity such that it now poses little social or political risk—only familial and economic ones.

Finally, what prompts wives to remain with husbands who are having extramarital sex, and what role does the larger society play in their apparent "willingness" to do so? Thus far, scholars concerned with marital transmission of HIV have said little about the factors that structure women's responses to their husband's infidelity. Contemporary qualitative research conducted on women, infidelity, and gender violence in Vietnam reveals the ways in which government officials such as judges and Women's Union officials appeal to gendered kinship ideologies, in particular women's obligations to their children and to the extended family, to encourage wives to remain married (Kwiatkowski 2008; Rydstrom 2006). In this chapter, I draw on this existing research as well as on my 2004 ethnographic research to elucidate the ways in which structural factors also shape women's acquiescence to their husbands' marital infidelity.

Focusing on the structural aspects of sexual behavior and risk has led me to argue that the contemporary nature of men's extramarital liaisons and their wives' response to it are shaped by three interrelated policies implemented by the Vietnamese government as part of Doi Moi: (1) the decision to shift from a socialist economy to a market-oriented economy, (2) the "Happy Family" campaign, and (3) the deregulation of public and private life. The focus of this chapter is not on the policies per se, but on the ways in which they shape men's opportunities for sex in Hanoi and inform men's efforts to be modern.

Doi Moi's Gendered Market Economy: Sex in the City

Doi Moi has instigated an iterative process within a global market economy that produces men's desire for extramarital liaisons (and supplies women for them), facilitates a notion of masculinity tied to commercialized and sexualized leisure (ensuring the demand for sex workers), and generates the means for men to engage in these activities. This process began in 1986 when the Vietnamese government initiated the process of moving from a centrally planned economy to a market economy with a socialist direction, with the larger aim of competing in global markets. In addition to dismantling agricultural-based cooperatives in favor of household production, the State removed most welfare subsidies, eradicating social safety nets such as health care, child care, care for the infirm, and educational support (Craig 2002). The State also began to downsize and close its factories, promoted private enterprise, and enabled the expansion of import and export markets.

The State's decision to integrate with the global market economy has led to a widening of employment opportunities, a profusion of household-based business ventures, and a multitude of private leisure establishments now accessible to Hanoi residents, whose standard of living has doubled since 1986. Integration has brought an abundance of consumer items such as DVD players, motorized vehicles, and cell phones, as well as access to the Internet and foreign films, literature, and news—items not widely available a decade ago (Marr 2003). Media from around the world, particularly the West, have provided new images of marriage, love, romance, sexual intimacy, and sexual relations.

Rapid economic and social transformation has had unintended consequences. Hanoi is becoming increasingly socially stratified, with the emergence of a highly visible moneyed class (Earl 2003; Drummond 2000), and now features a burgeoning sex industry through which, according to our research, many men move as enthusiastic consumers. We saw three ways in which the market economy shaped men's extramarital opportunities for, access to, and personal motivations for extramarital liaisons. First, the global market economy has led to the commercialization and sexualization (providing sex workers or other women as part of a customer's consumer options) of men's leisure in Hanoi. Compared to past generations, men today are more likely to spend their leisure time and disposable income at establishments that provide women as a way to attract customers.[6] Second, the market

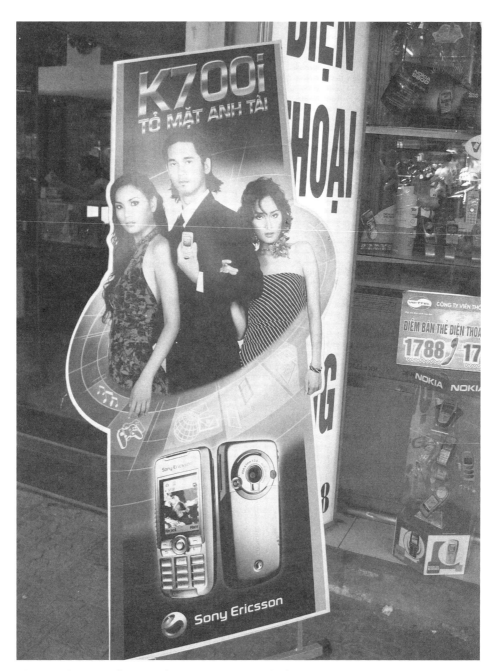

The sexualization of commodities is evident in cell phone advertisements. In addition to portraying a modern masculine identity in which men are surrounded by more than one woman, the advertisement serves as an example of how the State has turned a blind eye to what during the early and mid-1990s it would have labeled a "social evil"; it would have forced the proprietor to remove the sign. Photograph by Harriet M. Phinney.

economy has produced a new masculine identity that links consumption to sex. Third, Hanoians have more leisure time and money than they did before Doi Moi, providing them with new opportunities to consume the goods and services marketed to them.

Doi Moi has transformed Hanoi from a quiet city with little commercial activity to a city bursting with commodities. In the Hanoi of the early Doi Moi era, there were relatively few leisure establishments in which one was required to spend money, other than the circus, the zoo, amusement park rides, tea stalls, *bia hoi* (fresh beer) joints, and an occasional trip to a temple or tourist site. Beginning in the mid-1990s, a plethora of restaurants, karaoke bars, and cafés sprang up, enticing men to come spend their leisure time and money. As Lisa Drummond (2000: 9) points out, Doi Moi has "made possible and encouraged the commercialization of leisure space and the commodification of leisure itself. Leisure is now consumption, direct or indirect, where previously conspicuous or even moderate consumption of leisure was frowned upon and discouraged." The new leisure establishments provide private spaces for couples to meet, in contrast to the pre–Doi Moi era when the only places to go in Hanoi were people's homes, the park, or sidewalk stalls run by residents who more than likely knew one's identity.

With the aid of the emerging business sector, the sexualization of commercial leisure spaces in Hanoi that first developed in the late 1990s resulted in a radically altered sexual geography. Early in Doi Moi, male entrepreneurs from state organizations and privately owned businesses treated clients to food, drink, and the services of sex workers for the purpose of establishing personal ties that would facilitate economic transactions (Nguyen-Vo Thu-Huong 2002). Today, such practices have become obligatory in many industries, spawning a new set of enterprises geared to sexual services for men; the services range from hugging, kissing, performing stripteases, and fondling to sexual intercourse (Micollier 2004a, 2004c). These businesses offer men opportunities to engage in extramarital relations suited to their particular needs, incomes, work schedules, and marital situations. For example, while middle-aged businessmen with position and finances may have the connections, means, and mobility to dine with other businessmen for work purposes in fancy restaurants, low-level army cadres with limited incomes may choose to go to modest establishments to drink and enjoy the company of male friends and the caresses of sexy waitresses. An elderly man with little income and no motorbike or cell phone may tell his wife he is going out for a stroll to get some fresh air—and then head for certain streets with the aim of finding a low-cost sex worker with whom he can spend an hour in an inexpensive *nha nghi* (rest house). Married men who desire the intimate company of other men can now attend certain nightclubs where it is safe for gay men to gather.

Remarkable numbers of people, from families to small business owners, have sought to benefit economically from other people's desires by turning their homes or buildings into places that provide spaces for sexual intimacy. As a former

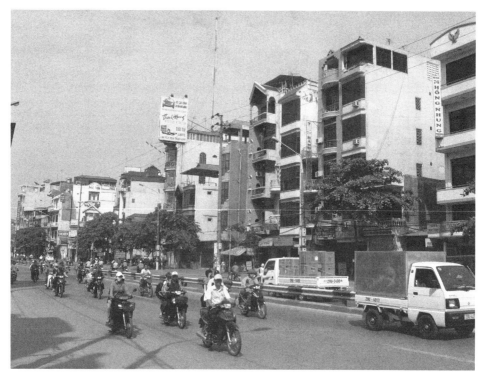

Nguyen Van Cu Street and the road perpendicular to it (running along the Red River) are lined with newly built "skinnies," most of which are *nha nghi*. Nguyen Van Cu Street is so infamous that men tease each other with the joke, "Have you been to see Ong Cu (Mr. Cu) yet?" Photograph by Harriet M. Phinney.

middle-aged manager of a mini-hotel told me, "We provided male guests the service of finding pretty girls so the men would not be lonely while they were away from their families. A lot of mini-hotels were built in the mid to late 1990s. Providing women enabled us to remain economically competitive."[7] The changing Hanoi landscape now includes a dizzying array of spaces where men can go to purchase sex, to seek privacy with a lover, or just to spend time with pretty women, including *nha nghi*, karaoke bars, *nghi tam*, hair salons, barbershops, nightclubs, *cafés om* (hugging cafés), fishing huts, bus stations, dancehalls, train stations, and the streets.

The most ubiquitous establishments are *nha nghi*. Easily identifiable by their neon signs, *nha nghi* provide rooms to rent by the hour or night, and some offer their clientele the company of a woman or man. Because *nha nghi* do not require personal identification cards, unlike Hanoi hotels, they provide a space for secrecy and anonymity. Karaoke has been popular in Hanoi at least since the early 1990s, but it was only really during the mid to late 1990s that reports began to circulate of

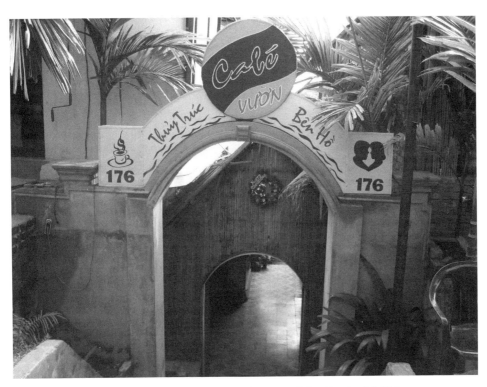

A hugging café where couples enjoy privacy. Photograph by Harriet M. Phinney.

sexual services also being provided.[8] *Nghi tam* located along the main thorough-
fares outside of Hanoi offer male travelers the chance to bathe with young women.
Flimsy fishing huts made out of thatch, wood, and bamboo perched on the edge
of ponds along the old road to the airport provide a pretext for engaging in other
kinds of activities. Nightclubs offer a range of sexualized leisure services that may
or may not include the opportunity to look up at women who are dancing and
gyrating on elevated platforms; private karaoke rooms for men to spend time as
they wish; the chance to critique the latest clothing fashions being displayed by
women and men parading up and down "runways"; sexy waitresses who will flirt,
touch, and sit in the laps of men in order to get them to purchase more drinks and
snacks; and the chance to meet waitresses interested in earning cash after hours.[9]

While most sexualized leisure services are oriented around heterosexual men
socializing with men, some businesses target other customers. For instance, *cafés
vuon* (garden cafés) cater to couples—particularly young unmarried couples—who
want a private place to hug, kiss, and pet one another while discreetly hidden behind tall palm fronds. Indoor cafés that appear only to serve coffee may also provide spaces for couples to be alone in the back. At one point during my research,
rumors floated around Hanoi about it being fashionable for young white-collar

workers to enjoy a little intimacy after eating lunch. Curious about these rumors, a male colleague and I went to a café known for providing private rooms for such purposes. We witnessed the start of two trysts that day: two separate couples arrived at the café, but instead of drinking coffee in the front room with the rest of the customers, they were furtively escorted by the proprietor past a doorway hidden by strings of wooden beads to private rooms in the back. As soon as the patrons were out of sight, the proprietor went outside to turn their motorcycles around so that the license plates did not face the street—a precaution against suspicious spouses or other lovers.

The forms of sexualized leisure offered by commercial establishments in Hanoi do not always involve sexual intercourse, but opportunities for arranging or engaging in sexual intercourse present themselves in these spaces. All of these establishments provide anonymous spaces for people to be alone—spaces that were neither visible nor available to the same degree prior to Doi Moi. The existence of commercial places to be intimate with someone is remarkable when contrasted to the late 1990s and even more pointedly to the 1960s and 1970s. One older male informant recounted how during the "American War," it had been difficult to kiss and hug one's girlfriend because there had been no place to go to do it; the Youth Union had patrolled the streets, keeping a lookout for transgressive behavior. He recounted having been told to go home by a Youth Union cadre while sitting on a public bench with his arm around his girlfriend. During the early 1990s, when I lived in Hanoi, I was told that one strategy for getting time alone with a lover was to arrange to meet at a friend's house and have the friend sit outside to make sure no one would come in. Now commercialized spaces abound.

As men's leisure options become increasingly commoditized, consumption has become a means for men to demonstrate their social mobility and class identity. For example, it is possible to buy an excellent cup of coffee for relatively little at a famous old café on Le Van Huu Street. However, young urban middle-class men sporting "polite clothing" (white-collar business attire) choose instead to buy coffee for themselves and their fashionably dressed girlfriends for three times the price at a fancy modern café not too far away on Ly Thoung Kiet Street. Whereas motoring about on a Honda Dream II gained one status during the 1990s, it was arriving on a Yamaha Mio or another motorbike manufactured outside of Vietnam (a Harley Davidson, for example) that demonstrated class and sophistication in 2004. As Truitt points out, "In Vietnam today, motorbikes . . . not only embody the freedom associated with the expanding marketplace and provide personal mobility, but they also signal a reordering of social stratification" (2008: 3). And, for those with real purchasing power, the ability to own a private car—necessarily foreign-made—is a true marker of modernity.

During our research in 2004 and 2005, men's ability to pay for food, drink, and sex workers also enabled them to perform a masculinity that was neither socially condoned nor available to an earlier generation. During the Second Indochina

War, masculinity was defined not in terms of consumption (indeed, consumption had been looked down upon), but in relation to men's devotion to the war effort and to the nation. After the Second Indochina War, men in the north demonstrated their devotion to building the nation by participating in communal work projects such as the construction of parks and the creation of man-made lakes in Hanoi. This public sector route to a male status defined in relation to one's contribution to communal nation-building efforts no longer exists in the way it did prior to Doi Moi. Gaining male status has shifted to the private sector and to private social networks. In 2004, a modern masculinity could be achieved by a number of different routes, including becoming a successful businessman, through artistic endeavors (Avieli 2007), and through one's sexual encounters. For example, an informant who worked for a United Nations agency told me that his Vietnamese officemates frequently boasted about their weekend sexual exploits. Another male informant recounted his boss's pride in having an affair with an attractive young secretary: she accompanied him on business trips since his wife had to stay home with the children.

Many different kinds of men demonstrate their masculinity through homosocial practices that include sexualized forms of consumption. The most common situations involve groups of men socializing with one another, whether in the context of work or, as was the case for Anh Binh, to gather with old friends (Tran Duc Hoa et al. 2007). Spending time with other men is nothing new to Hanoians. The ubiquity of men drinking beer and eating snacks with other men after work in *bia hoi* establishments scattered about Hanoi, or hanging out with other men perched on plastic stools at sidewalk stalls, smoking cigarettes and sipping tea or coffee, underlines the much greater social prominence of homosociality in comparison to heterosociality.

Such socializing demonstrates the quotidian nature of masculine homosociality in Hanoi—the daily events that enable men to perform a masculinity associated with a world beyond the family. What is new, post–Doi Moi, is the sexualized nature of men's leisure, particularly in their drinking activities. Anh Tran's business trips with his male colleagues provide a perfect example. When they travel, Anh Tran's boss and co-workers typically rent a private room at a restaurant where they can dine in privacy, usually with the men with whom they have come to do business. The proprietor of the restaurant introduces the men to a number of pretty women—one for each man—and tells each man to choose a woman of his liking. After they have eaten and drunk their fill, most of the out-of-town guests bring "their" women back to their hotel rooms.

Our informants believe that the economic expansion under Doi Moi has created an environment in which people now have the time to think about sexuality and the money to pay for it. One woman explained to me, "People are not starving anymore like they were in the 1980s; they have money and time to spend on other things in life like food and sex." The Vietnamese aphorism ("eaten one's fill and all stirred up") sums up this comment nicely. A retired male sewing factory employee noted that until relatively recently, he and his friends had had neither money nor places to go to spend money on women. Nowadays, he has more time and he has money, so he and his colleagues do go to places with girls (and karaoke or massage), especially when they are away on business.

Not all men go out looking for sex; a number of our male informants spoke of finding themselves in situations in which they merely responded to other people's prompting, or of other men who had been lured into situations they had not intended to be in. Speaking about a friend, one man said, "Men are negatively influenced by society, so he got caught up in a situation and went too far." Another man who traveled away from home a month at a time to teach and lecture said, "When a young woman invites me for coffee and karaoke, things go from there. It starts out innocent enough." A *xe om* driver explained that "from time to time, my friends encourage me to go, to be joyful." A private driver stated, "If a pretty girl sits on my lap and I refuse her, she will ask me if I am crazy or if I lost my penis or whether it doesn't work anymore."

The ubiquity with which men are offered opportunities to spend time with other women was reflected by a social scientist who told me how he had been offered sexual favors when he went to get his hair cut, and also how, a few months earlier, after he had checked into a hotel down south, a young woman had knocked on his door and offered to keep him company. Because of the way businesses and homosocial relations among men are structured and male status is constructed, men are led to engage in extramarital sex even if they did not begin with that intent; the social risks of refusing may outweigh the epidemiological risks of participating. Anh Tran said that during the business trips described earlier, any man who turned down the woman offered to him or declined to take her back to his hotel room would have been chastised and teased by fellow workers.

Rejecting the chance to be with a pretty woman is not simply a rejection of the woman, it also a rejection of the values of the larger group, and it disrupts the camaraderie that one's business associates, boss, or friends have tried to establish. It sets a man apart—something many men may not want to risk (Allison 1994; Ngo Thi Ngan Binh 2007). In other words, men risk losing both the appearance of virility and the chance to develop camaraderie with other men should they insufficiently demonstrate their desire for other women. This is particularly evident in Anh Tran's strategy when he was pressured by his colleagues to spend time with a young woman. On one occasion, rather than face the criticisms of his boss and colleagues, Anh Tran did take a young woman back to his room, but instead of having sex, he spent the time talking to her to find out how she ended up working in such an establishment; he chafed at the idea of having sexual intercourse with a girl his daughter's age. Another man, a police officer, said he avoided such situations with his male friends by leaving karaoke bars if women approached him and before he drank too much.

Clearly, the consequences of sexual risk have changed. In the past, the Communist Party's discovery that one of its members had engaged in extramarital sex could have caused a low-ranking party member to lose his job and party membership. But since Doi Moi, changes in state policy as a result of economic liberalization have played a role in shifting the valence of men's extramarital sex from being disruptive and penalized to being strongly (albeit indirectly) encouraged and fundamentally constitutive of male economic and social relations. Engaging in sexual risk is individually and economically productive (Zaloom 2004) because it enables men to produce modern masculine selves that are a critical asset in the market economy. In many ways, this is similar to the Mexican and Nigerian cases discussed in this book: all three contexts provide examples of the way in which men's extramarital sexuality produces modern masculinities and new social relationships. What makes the Vietnamese case distinctive, however, is that the State's economic liberalization policy has instigated the transformation of the social risks of men's infidelity. What we see is the emergence of a new political economy of sexuality. Old avenues to gaining status—being a good party member, engaging in communal projects—have been all but displaced by a focus on succeeding economically and demonstrating one's prowess through the consumption of modern material goods and sexualized leisure.

Happy Families: Women's Acquiescence, Sacrifice, and Silence

Although bearing and raising children has always been key to a woman's familial and social status in Vietnam (Nguyen Huu Minh 1998; Marr 1981; Gammeltoft 1999)—a consequence of the patrilineal and patrilocal kinship system—women's reproductive role has become intensified under Doi Moi (Phinney 2003; Pashigian 2002). This is a result of the government establishing the household as the primary economic unit, making the family rather than the commune or nation the focus of state-building efforts. Two Doi Moi policies in particular have intensified Vietnamese women's focus on motherhood and family: (1) the 1986 Law on Marriage and the Family, which garnered public discussion and acknowledgment that a woman's identity is first and foremost grounded in being a mother; and (2) the "Happy Family" campaign, launched in the early 1990s as part of the population policy that sought to link the nation's efforts to modernize with couples' ability to create "happy, wealthy, harmonious, and stable families."[10]

Together, the two policies represent a significant shift from previous socialist periods. First, by promoting women's maternal identity at the expense of other possible subjectivities, the Doi Moi state has reinscribed the traditional gender roles and inequalities of pre-revolutionary Vietnam, which also viewed women's maternal and familial responsibilities as foremost. Second, women and men had previously been encouraged to devote their energies to the war effort (by delaying love, marriage, and childbearing) and later to building the nation (by focusing on the commune or workplace) (Phinney 2008). Now the success of the nation is tied to the ability of couples to create economically successful households without the benefit of state aid.

In contrast to trends around the world, where companionship has become a marital goal, and "individual fulfillment and satisfaction rather than (or in addition to) social reproduction" the focus of the marital project (Wardlow and Hirsch 2006), the underlying criteria for the Vietnamese government's "Happy Family" policy are determined by the success of the marital project itself, a project our informants defined in terms of social reproduction and economic stability, not individual or couple satisfaction.[11] The unintended irony of this marital project is that it structures men's opportunities for extramarital liaisons and their wives' acquiescence in order to maintain economic and social status. It does this by encouraging a gendered division of marital labor and by reinforcing homosociality-promoting patriarchal norms that in turn provide opportunities for and structure the type of relations men seek outside marriage. As such, the "Happy Family" and marital fidelity are ultimately defined not in terms of sexuality but in terms of a couple's ability to raise healthy, well-educated children, and to survive and prosper in the increasingly global market economy. These concerns are reflected in our informants' notions of the ideal spouse and spousal communication, their gendered patterns of marital labor and how they spend their leisure time, and their definitions of marital fidelity.

The Ideal Spouse

While the "Happy Family" marital project emphasizes nuclear families' responsibility for their own economic success, this does not mean that love is not an important factor in choosing a spouse. Since the promulgation of the 1959 Law on Marriage and the Family, with which the Vietnamese State outlawed arranged and forced marriages and made voluntary love a requirement for marriage, Vietnamese couples have married for love. Yet, when asked what characteristics make an ideal spouse, economic stability and good character were foremost on our informants' minds. All but our youngest respondents felt that if a man provides for his family, he is fulfilling his familial obligations; regardless of whether he is having extramarital sex, he is being faithful to his wife and family.

In some cases, tolerance for a man's extramarital relationships was a husband's clearly articulated expectation. For example, when the middle-aged manager of a massage parlor told his wife she had better get used to his spending time with other women because it was his profession, she put up with it for the benefit of her children and the marriage. She did what many women are reputed to do, swallowing her anger at the infidelity. Acquiescence is not new to Vietnamese women: the Vietnamese State and family have long asked and expected Vietnamese women to sacrifice their personal desires for familial or national concerns (Pettus 2003;

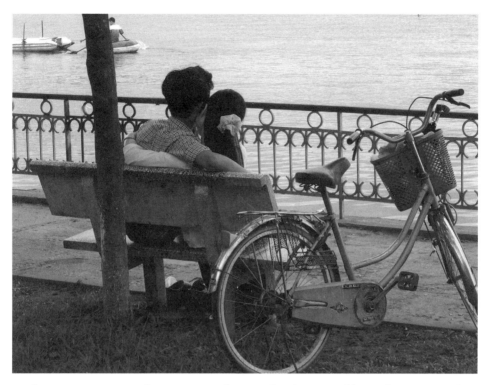

Looking out over West Lake in Hanoi: a chance to be alone in public. Today most couples use motorbikes to rendezvous. Photograph by Harriet M. Phinney.

Phinney 2003; Hue-Tam Ho Tai 1992; Marr 1981; Mai Thi Tu and Le Thi Nham Tuyet 1978). By remaining silent and continuing to take care of the children and the house, a woman fulfills her duties as a wife, a mother, and a citizen.

A wife's unwillingness or inability to discuss her husband's extramarital sexuality may be rooted in a number of factors in addition to preserving economic security and the marital project. First, because male sexual desire is typically characterized as a biological necessity, some wives and many men assert that men need to have sex outside of marriage if their wives are unwilling or unable to satisfy their sexual desires.[12] A male lawyer spoke of a postmenopausal woman who couldn't have sex anymore. According to the lawyer, "she secretly knows" that her husband has been going outside the home to satisfy his sexual urges, "but she does not say anything to her husband. This means that women are able to accept this matter, and moreover it has no impact on their marriage." In this case, not only did the wife recognize her husband's need, she decided to remain quiet about it for the benefit of her marriage. This was not the only case we learned about that featured an older woman who no longer wanted to have sexual intercourse and who consequently turned a blind eye to some of her husband's extramarital activities.[13] It is worth noting, however, that our informant (the lawyer) was clearly also expressing his own views on the matter, in his own way legitimizing the wife's silence.

For some couples, there appeared to be a distinct relationship between the husband's extramarital sex and reproduction. One newlywed husband did not see the point of having sex outside of marriage when he was trying to get his wife pregnant. His reason for not having extramarital relations was based on his reproductive desires. However, another newly married man got caught having an affair with a market vendor while his wife was pregnant with their child. When the young wife went to her father-in-law to complain, he dismissed her concerns and told her it was to be expected. This was not the only story I heard about a husband seeking sex outside marriage during his wife's pregnancy or the period of abstinence following birth, which can be for up to nine months.[14] The third case is that of couples who have completed raising their children. Many men and women spoke of cases where women who had borne all the children they wanted or who were postmenopausal no longer wanted to have sexual intercourse with their husbands. For these women, the primary purpose of sex had been to reproduce, and having done so, they no longer wanted sexual intercourse.[15]

That women and men would conceptualize marital sex principally in terms of reproduction is not surprising, given Vietnam's patrilineal and Confucian roots. With regard to Confucian ideology, Evelyne Micollier points out that "in the context of matrimonial exchange, sexuality and sexual life are reduced to reproductive behavior in order to obtain sons. This idea explicitly denies erotic desire" (2004c: 16). Yet, while a number of women we spoke with did seem to echo this belief, other women did not; they and their husbands considered sexual satisfaction to be a key to a good marriage. Nonetheless, that did not necessarily stop the husbands from seeking sex outside marriage.

The belief that Vietnamese men are capable of having sex with women without loving them has circulated in the media since at least the mid-1980s and was shared by many of our informants. It renders moot a wife's concern that her husband's sexual relations with sex workers will shatter their family happiness (should she find out about them). For example, during the late 1980s and throughout the 1990s, discussions took place on whether married men should help older single women (ones unable to marry) get pregnant so they could bear a child to take care of them when they aged. The Women's Union supported this stance and ran a series of articles to dispel concerns that men having sex with unmarried women would shatter family happiness (Phinney 2008). While there were many components to the Women's Union argument, a key element of it was based on the notion that since the men did not love the women and would not maintain relations with them, there was no danger. While younger married women are likely to take issue with this rendering of male sexuality, the Women's Union line of reasoning suggests that wives have nothing to worry about and hence nothing to discuss should their husbands visit sex workers.

Spousal Communication

In order to learn about spousal communication and its role in spousal sexual relationships, we asked couples to tell us what they talked to each other about. While some husbands talked to their wives about issues beyond the family such as their work, few discussed their social activities, the places they patronized, or their conversations with other men. A *xe om* driver who frequently went out with married male friends to drink and to find women explained, "It would not be appropriate." A private driver said it would "not be interesting." One young newlywed said she has no idea what her husband does at work or with his friends: she does not ask; she just has to trust him. When we inquired about shared topics of conversation, all our informants responded that they principally discuss family issues: household finances, upkeep of the house, children's education, and extended family members. Romance, sexuality, and their relationship are typically not discussed, although some did discuss the importance of *tinh cam* (sympathy and understanding) for one another. As Robin Sherrif (2000) has pointed out, silence is not necessarily an individual choice; it can be a "shared silence" that is socially organized, expected, and recognized. This shared silence enables the couple to maintain the semblance of a "Happy Family," upon which their economic and social status rests (Ha Vu 2002; Phan Thi Thu Hien n.d.).

Not all women remain silent. Divorce is on the increase, with domestic violence and allegations of infidelity and incompatibility the most commonly cited reasons. Yet, this increase needs to be placed in the larger sociohistorical context, recognizing that prior to Doi Moi, the state limited the number of divorces it granted each year. Probably the most important determinant of whether a woman will seek divorce is whether she is economically independent and socially secure; this tends to limit the option to middle- and upper-class women. Thus, women who may have argued and fought with their husbands about seeing sex workers or taking lovers may in the end decide to remain with their husbands for economic security. I was told the story of an "attractive" middle-aged woman—one whose children had grown and moved out of the house—whose husband had fallen in love with a younger woman. He asked his wife if she wanted a divorce. When she said no and the younger woman got pregnant, the man built a small house for the younger woman and her child in a prominent section of town. The man moved back and forth between the two houses. The neighbors who lived near the younger woman were apparently sympathetic to her situation and did not treat her with disrespect. The wife had not wanted to divorce her husband because it would have meant a significant loss in financial security, a nice place to live, and her social status as a married woman. According to the woman who told me the story, the wife had had no choice: "She would have had nothing, despite her stable salary, without her husband's income."

Gendered Patterns of Marital Labor

Gendered patterns of labor structure husbands' and wives' time differently, ultimately providing men the justification for spending time away from home in situations where they encounter opportunities to engage in extramarital liaisons. By tying women's identities and status to reproduction and the family, the 1986 Law and the "Happy Family" campaign have reinvigorated traditional patterns of household labor, making women more responsible for domestic work than men. This trend has been augmented by other economic policies that have caused women to be laid off from state-sector jobs more readily than men and have lead to an increase in women's household-sector employment, which in turn keeps women closer to home.[16] Married women with children do most of the domestic work, leaving them with far less leisure time than their husbands. When wives do have free time, they spend it with the family and with other women who have children near home.

A husband's role, on the other hand, as *tru cot* (pillar of the family) requires him to have a good understanding of society, and encourages and enables him to explore the urban environment and to socialize with male friends in new gendered social spaces. When I asked our informants how they spent their leisure time, men said they spent it at home or out with other men eating or drinking tea or beer. Countless times I have socialized with men whose wives could not join us because they were taking care of children. It is not surprising, then, that we rarely observed married women enjoying time together or older married couples spending time alone in commercial leisure spaces in Hanoi, aside from the lunchtime break.

As Ngo Thi Ngan Binh points out in her research on modern masculinity, contemporary male homosociality often derives from men's need to socialize with other men outside the home for business purposes. Drinking "is popularly used as an effective social route to upward mobility where business dealing is lubricated, social power is negotiated, potential connections are created and personal gains are exchanged" (Ngo Thi Ngan Binh 2007: 8). Indeed, some wives encourage their husbands to go out drinking with other male friends and acquaintances in order to make sure their children get into good schools (2007). A wife's lack of mobility and her husband's ability to be mobile enable him to engage in extramarital relations. Thus, whereas Doi Moi policies drive men into the commercial economy for status and leisure activities, they tend to reinforce women's domestic orientation, allowing men greater access to extramarital liaisons without the risk of being caught by their wives.

Definitions of Marital Fidelity

The emphasis Doi Moi policies place on economic fidelity structure the type of extramarital sex engaged in by married men. Eight of the nine men in our study who reported engaging in extramarital sex said they had had liaisons with sex workers.

They consider this type of liaison less risky than taking a lover because visiting a sex worker is "finite, temporary," and need not require a large commitment of time and money. Recall that this was Anh Binh's reason for why it was okay to visit sex workers. He also noted, as did many people when referring to men's extramarital sexual liaisons, that a husband's job is to provide economically for the family—to make sure his children are well brought up. According to these men, a sex worker poses no risk to family stability, in contrast to taking a lover, which risks draining a man's affective and financial resources should he become emotionally involved with her or get her pregnant. In this case, as was true for some of the men in Hirsch's and Smith's chapters, love and infidelity are not necessarily incompatible.

Because state-sector jobs are no longer as highly valued as they were prior to Doi Moi, engaging in extramarital sex has taken on a new meaning: rather than posing a risk to one's job, it poses a risk to the success of the family—at the same time as it can be a crucial strategy through which men seek that same economic success. Having set up the household as the primary economic unit, the State now relies on the economic success of its citizens and families to achieve its own success in the global market economy. The social risk of men's infidelity becomes acceptable as long as it does not threaten the economic stability of the family and, in turn, the success of the "Happy Family." Risk is redefined and recategorized: the redefinition and recategorization of risk benefits the State's projects even though it might produce some marital discord. The productivity of "Happy Families," now responsible for their own welfare, is necessary to the economic success of the country, and thus to the progress and prestige of the State.

More than a decade after the promulgation of the "Happy Family" campaign, the Women's Union has begun to recognize that the sex industry poses a danger to the "Happy Family" campaign and a risk of HIV infection. Particularly note-worthy about the State's initial response was its decision to place the responsibility for men's extramarital liaisons on their wives. When the Hanoi Women's Museum first opened in 1996, it offered women classes in cooking and cosmetics in order to teach them how to be attractive women, good cooks, and attentive wives. These values were instilled in one middle-aged wife who in 2004 said, "According to my thinking, it is a wife's lack of care for and attention paid to a husband that prompts men to go outside the house." In addition to her salaried work, Chi Nhung devoted her free time to her husband's needs: she always inquired when he came home whether he was tired and about his work "to show that I love him and value him." Her husband (with whom we spoke separately) agreed that if a wife got old and failed to take care of herself, her home, and her husband, then her husband would become bored with her. He also was adamant that all men, regardless of what they say, like "new and strange things." He asked, "Who wouldn't want to go out with some young woman?"

More recently, in order to counter the pull of the sex market, the Women's

Union has encouraged wives to remain sexually alluring to their spouses in order to keep them faithful.[17] One man echoed this message: "A woman should look very pretty so her husband will value her." This notion also is reflected in market developments: beauty parlors, beauty contests, aerobics classes, dancing and fitness clubs, and fancy clothing stores—including sexy lingerie shops—have sprung up throughout Hanoi to cater to women's new concerns about body image and to help them respond to their new government-mandated responsibility to keep their husbands faithful.[18] The burden placed on women to keep their husbands faithful is paradoxical, given the gendered sex roles among our informants: all our informants, female and male, stated that it was the husband's role to initiate sexual activity, not the wife's. One husband said it would be a turn-off if his wife initiated sex; he would lose interest. Thus, while wives are now held responsible for arousing their husbands' sexual desire (and maintaining it over the course of their marriages), it is not considered appropriate for wives to initiate sexual activity. Vietnam is not the only place where society places the blame for men's sexually errant behavior on a wife's failure to be erotically or emotionally satisfying; as the chapters on Nigeria and Uganda indicate, women there are also blamed for their husbands' infidelities. The Vietnamese case is distinctive, however, for institutionalizing and actively promulgating this discourse through a state agency.

This strategy, which places the responsibility on wives to remain sexually attractive, also makes wives more likely to acquiesce to their husbands' infidelities and provides implicit social tolerance of extramarital liaisons. A number of our male and female informants spoke of a husband's right to seek sex outside marriage if his wife could not satisfy him. A *xe om* driver joked that sometimes when he left the house, his wife would jokingly tell him, "Don't bring anything home." While all of the wives we interviewed were well aware of HIV and AIDS, to the extent they did discuss it with their husbands, such discussions were about HIV and AIDS in general, not about men's extramarital sex per se. The account of the driver's wife was one of the few instances we saw of a wife openly addressing with her husband the relationship between his extra-familiar leisure activities and the marital risks of HIV transmission. It is likely many wives do; their decisions not to publicly discuss or expose their husbands' transgressions should not necessarily be construed as indicating they do not privately question or seek to change their husbands' leisure activities. Indeed, it was only from our male informants that we learned that their wives might be aware that their husbands had engaged in extramarital activities. Publicly, women, more than men, tend to remain silent.

By failing to address men's responsibility for engaging in risky sex, the government and society uphold the continued conceptualization of marital fidelity in economic rather than sexual terms. The State's ability to relieve men of responsibility could well be informed by the types of essentialist assumptions regarding masculinity and male sexuality discussed earlier.

Deregulating Public and Private Life

"Rice is essential but tiresome; you should get some noodles." This joke implies that one's spouse is rice (*com*), which is bland and gets tiresome, so one should go out for some noodle soup (*pho*). *Pho* is sweet and delicious. Like men's opportunities for new kinds of sexual experiences, *pho* became more available outside the home during the mid-1990s, when this ditty began to circulate in Hanoi.[19] This joke foreshadowed the increasing economic freedom and modern masculinity that for some would become increasingly linked to the global economy, consumption, and sexuality. It also spoke to shifting marital ideals and a changing urban environment.

These social changes have been shaped by the State's decision to loosen its direct control over population movement, public and private spaces, and the kinds of activity that take place in Hanoi (Drummond 2000). In the process, and despite efforts to the contrary, the State is losing command over moral issues. These factors contribute to the ease with which married men seek sex outside marriage.

In contrast to the prior era, when migration was limited by the State, the opening of the economy has been accompanied by an increasingly mobile work force. White-collar Hanoi residents frequently travel to other parts of Vietnam or overseas for work or educational purposes, leaving their families behind for extended stays. Large numbers of migrants seeking economic opportunity have moved to the cities, dramatically changing the urban landscape and the social dynamics of city life.[20] Among these migrants are young women from rural areas who go to Hanoi to seek employment in the sex industry. The state's passive accommodation of this industry has led to a dramatic increase in the number of sex workers in Hanoi and men's corresponding opportunities for extramarital sex.[21]

In addition to permitting rural migrants to move to Hanoi to work and live, the Vietnamese government also lifted restrictions on foreign visitors and foreign residents. As a result, Hanoi has become a much more diversified and open society. Describing the change, one male Hanoi native said, "It used to be a small town; we knew everyone and everyone knew what we were doing. Now you don't even know the person living next to you; the social connections between people are looser. As a result, you can pretty much do anything you want and no one will know." This anonymity, coupled with the ability to furtively make arrangements by cell phone and get across town quickly via motorbike, has contributed to the ability of men and women to engage in affairs unbeknownst to their friends, neighbors, and spouses.[22]

For instance, my favorite *xe om* driver showed me how easy it is for a man with a motorbike to locate sex workers and contact them later by cell phone to determine what time to meet. One night, while I was on the back of his bike, he spoke with three different women on the street, negotiated a price with the third, and

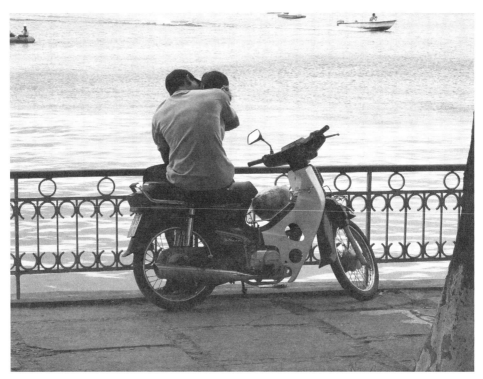

West Lake motorcycle romance on Thanh Nien Boulevard in 2004. During the 1960s and 1970s, such public displays of intimacy were frowned upon; couples spotted by the Youth Union would have been reprimanded and sent home. Photograph by Harriet M. Phinney.

logged her cell phone number into his, promising to call her after he dropped me off. He was not the only man out looking for women: we saw an older man who could not walk very well trying to wave down a sex worker on a motorbike; we watched a middle-aged man go up and down the same street, evidently trying to find a sex worker he knew; and we saw men hanging out on park benches negotiating with women. He also mentioned how, since becoming a *xe om* driver, a few "lonely women" whom he had given rides late at night had invited him into their homes to stay a while. Another driver recounted how having a motorcycle enabled him to maintain relations with an old lover who lived on the outskirts of Hanoi. His wife, on the other hand, did not leave home as frequently; she was occupied with the children and selling *pho* out of their house.

New forms of geographic mobility and labor migration provide men with frequent access to extramarital sex. According to our findings, professions that present men with the most opportunities for extramarital relations are white-collar jobs (state and private enterprises), and the entertainment, hotel, and transportation industries.[23] What the men in these industries have in common is mobility in a manner and to an extent that their wives do not share. Of the seven men in our marital case studies who had had extramarital relationships, four were in the transportation business. One informant who drove a passenger car for a private company described how his boss always provided food, drink, and women for his work associates when traveling out of town; the driver was included in these "business meetings" when he wished to be. Another informant, a truck driver who transported goods around the country, maintained a relationship with a woman en route down south to Ho Chi Minh City.

In addition to increased mobility, many of our informants attribute men's extramarital sex to the influence of foreign media that portray alternative ideas and images of sexuality, intimacy, and marital relations. When I asked him about the impact of these media, one male informant said, "They stimulate desire for so many things. Not everyone can gain access to material goods, but they can have access to sex because it does not cost a lot." Until the mid-1990s, most consumer goods were purchased in governmental department stores or brought in by relatives living overseas; this was due to the state's desire and ability to maintain strict control over imported commodities. Since then, however, the State has lost the level of control over imported commodities it once had.[24] As a result of seeing new ideas in the media, several of our informants have been experimenting within marriage with novel forms of sex, but far more men are choosing to experiment outside of marriage. Similar to Hirsch's research findings in Degollado, one recently married man said that he and his wife watch porn videos together and then try to imitate what they have seen on film. Other men, however, said they would not dare experiment with their wives because their wives would become suspicious, wondering where they had learned to do such things. This was one reason men said it was better to go outside marriage for something "new and strange."

The State no longer has direct control over the kinds of activities that take place in Hanoi. The tours of downtown Hanoi I took revealed to me the ubiquity and openness with which men of different ages and socioeconomic backgrounds look for sex workers in clubs, restaurants, on the street, and in neighborhood parks. Ironically, a well-known place to find prostitutes at night is across from the Hanoi Women's Union. Almost all of our older informants commented on the ease with which men are able to engage in extramarital relations with sex workers today. This is remarkable, given that prostitution remains illegal.

Prior to 1959, men went to Kham Thien Street (then known as a red-light district) in Hanoi's Old Quarter to find prostitutes. At that time, prostitution and polygamy were legal, but commercial sex work was principally confined to a single locality. In Hanoi today, men can find and are offered sex throughout the city as opposed to it being located on just one street. Yet, from its founding in 1954, the Democratic Republic of Vietnam has tried various methods to rein in extramarital sexuality. In 1959, the government revised the Law on Marriage and the Family to promote marriage based on free will, mutual respect, and love. Prostitution and polygamy already having been outlawed, monogamy was to become the locus for satisfying men's sexual and reproductive needs. During and after the Indochina wars, the Party enacted punitive measures for party members who transgressed socialist marital ideals. State employees who engaged in extramarital sex put themselves at risk socially, economically, and politically.

It was not too long after the reunification of the country and the failures of the socialist economic policies that the Vietnamese State realized it had lost its moral authority and command over the hearts of its Vietnamese citizens (Giebel 2001). Doi Moi and governing tactics such as the 1986 Law on Marriage and the Family as well as the "Happy Family" campaign were efforts to reassert its economic and moral authority (Phinney 2003, 2008a). Rather than directly intervening in the lives of its citizens or policing individual moral behavior as it did prior to Doi Moi, the Vietnamese government instead seeks to create responsible, moral economic actors; individuals are now entrusted with personal responsibility and self-care (Lemke 2001). Thus, more recently, the State has embarked on a "civilization" campaign to encourage people to become refined and cultured individuals in order build a civilized nation.[25] One aspect of this effort is to encourage marital fidelity. This plea for men to change their individual behavior fails to recognize the social nature of sexuality and sexual risk—the construction of which the State itself has inadvertently helped to create. As in Iganga (which Parikh will point out in her chapter), monogamy in Hanoi is promoted in a socioeconomic context that provides abundant opportunities and rewards for men who decide to engage in extramarital sex. It is worth noting that there are few opportunities for men to engage in alternative types of commercialized leisure—for instance, those that target and encourage heterosexual sociality (i.e., for married couples to spend time alone or with other couples).

Although it failed to see that its own policies contributed to the situation, the Communist Party did become concerned with what was happening to Vietnamese culture due to the increasingly rapid movement of people and foreign ideas, technology, media, and consumer goods throughout Vietnam, especially in the cities. In an effort to assert control over what it saw as "negative foreign influences," the government embarked on the "social evils" prevention campaign. Initially, the government tried to use it to restrict non-Vietnamese cultural images, the importation of Western media, and access to certain Internet sites. Though it is still trying to control Internet sites, it has largely abandoned the effort to control the importation of Western media and images. While not necessarily doomed by the effects of Doi Moi and globalization of the economy, the government's ability to control Vietnamese citizens' access to foreign cultural productions was certainly rendered more difficult by the nation's integration into global economic markets.

Now, having all but abandoned the effort to deny access to foreign images, the key focus of the campaign against "social evils" is geared toward eradicating deviant behaviors by condemning drug use, pornography, and prostitution. According

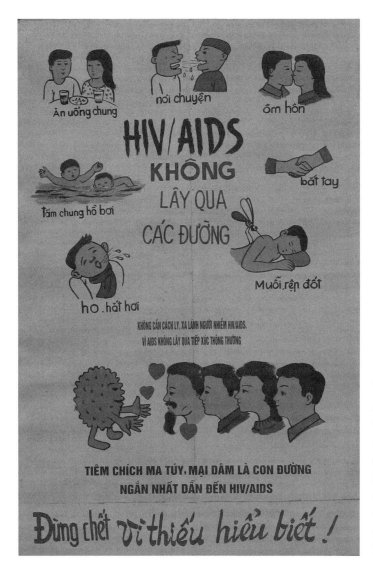

"How Not to Get HIV/ AIDS." Billboards scattered throughout the city and surrounding environs are geared to improving knowledge, reducing fears, and eradicating the stigma of people living with HIV or AIDS. Photograph by Harriet M. Phinney.

to McNally (2007), the HIV prevention campaign engages in two different methods of outreach. The first is moralistic and discriminatory: it targets individuals who are categorized as prostitutes or drug users, the two recognized risk groups. These individuals are dealt with in a negative fashion: they are given mandatory HIV tests and some are sent to reeducation camps. The second strategy is geared to those who do not identify as a risk group. They are targeted through an Information Education and Communication (IEC) campaign that encourages condom use by creating "caring and responsible" individuals. However, because most people perceive the epidemic to be located in risk groups (groups with which they do not identify), few people believe that their sexual practices and behaviors could put them at risk of contracting HIV. This individualized approach to IEC fails to address the gendered social organization of men's extramarital opportunities.

The ensuing criminalization of sex workers has resulted in government and social discourse portraying sex workers—not their clients—as the source of the problem. This has led the State to turn a blind eye to men's behavior (despite the occasional reprimand of an uncouth official) and society to accept it, enabling men to engage in extramarital sex with relative impunity from wives and society. Thus, while the government has made prostitution illegal, it has not addressed any of the underlying social and economic causes that led to the development of the sex industry and that are in fact the result of the State's own economic liberalization policies.

The State's loss of control over "immoral" behavior could equally be seen as a loosening of control; the State may simply not be as concerned with its citizens' sexual activities as it is their economic productivity. Either way, it is more useful to view it in terms of a restructuring of risk, where certain kinds of sexual activity are no longer seen as threats to the socialist agenda now that the family is embedded within the larger global economy. Risk has been reconfigured such that it is okay to have sex with a sex worker because it does not pose a serious threat to the productivity of the Happy Family.

Conclusion

Ethnographic and epidemiological research from around the world indicate that married women's greatest risks for contracting HIV are from having unprotected sexual intercourse with their unfaithful husbands and from the differential power relationships between husbands and wives (UNAIDS, UNFPA, and UNDP 2004; UNESCAP 2003; VNMOH 2005; Glynn et al. 2003 and 2001; O'Leary 2000; Mayer 2004). In Vietnam, married women are at risk of HIV infection because of their husbands' sexual infidelity and inconsistent condom use. Indeed, public health officials in Vietnam recognize married men to be a bridge between sex workers (one of the three populations in Vietnam with high HIV/AIDS prevalence) and their wives (Trung Nam Tran et al. 2004).

This chapter, in order to shed light on marital risk of HIV infection, has examined the political economy of sexuality in Hanoi and the way in which sexual behaviors are shaped by social processes. In Hanoi, the commercialization and sexualization of men's leisure and societal pressures to engage in a masculinity based on the demonstration of extramarital virility is placing men at risk of contracting HIV from sex workers and other young women positioned to attract men to commercial establishments, and thus at risk of transmitting HIV to their wives.[26] Not only do the unequally gendered consequences of Doi Moi policies provide opportunities for and structure the type of sexual relations men seek outside marriage, they also promote the idea that women are responsible for their husbands' extramarital transgressions. Men do not always use condoms, and so their trysts put them and their wives at risk of HIV infection.

The issue is exacerbated by the unequal power relations between men and women. The nature of spousal communication, centered as it is around domestic concerns and off-limits to discussions about a husband's leisure time, renders it difficult for a woman to ascertain if her husband might be putting them both at risk. The striking aspect of women's sacrifices and the silence surrounding men's extramarital sex is that both are expected and both are socially shared. Sexual infidelity becomes a secret to be maintained for the benefit of the couple, their marital project, and the success of the "Happy Family."

While the Vietnamese government has made serious and concerted efforts to combat the spread of HIV and AIDS in the general population, the State has undermined its own efforts with the Doi Moi policies discussed in this chapter—policies that structure and shape the contemporary nature of the household division of labor, that facilitate men's opportunities for extramarital sexual relations and women's acquiescence to it, and that redefine marital fidelity and the recategorization of the social nature of sexual risk since the socialist era. Without addressing both the contradictory processes that encourage men's opportunities for extramarital sexual relations and the cultural and essentialist reasoning associated with such behavior, it will be difficult for men, sex workers, and married women to change their sexual behavior and reduce their HIV risk.

5

"Whip Him in the Head with a Stick!"

Marriage, Male Infidelity, and Female Confrontation among the Huli

Holly Wardlow

Miriam only had a sixth-grade education, but she had become relatively well-off: her husband was a coffee buyer, purchasing green coffee beans from families in the Tari area and selling them to a roasting factory in a distant town. He had saved enough money for them to set up a small trade-store, selling the few goods that can be found in all such stores in Papua New Guinea: salt, cooking oil, soap, canned mackerel, and packages of instant noodles. Hers hadn't been an arranged marriage, but he hadn't been her first choice either. As she put it, "Before I got married, I had four boyfriends. I married the fourth one, but my true love was the very first one." (Her "true love" was a much older man, and when her parents found out about the relationship, they had sent her away to live with her mother's brother's family.)

Unlike her first boyfriend, who had surreptitiously given her money enclosed in love letters, her husband had gone about things the proper way: he had asked an older male relative to approach her parents and negotiate the amount of bride-wealth he would have to give; he had spoken to her in public, but only when his sisters were present; and he had agreed to pay a *manayi* (an older man who is an expert in traditional customs) to teach Miriam and himself about sex. Miriam described the ritualized sex education they had received: "It was just the three of us—me, my husband, and the *manayi*. We killed, cooked, and ate a pig together, and when we were done, the old man instructed us. He said, 'Our custom is for husband and wife to have sex like this. This is how you will get pregnant.' And then he explained what to do. [*Interviewer*: So he was very direct?] Oh yes, they are very candid and direct. He said, 'You, woman, you will lie on your back. And then your husband will put his penis in you and move it.' Very direct. We were so embarrassed listening to him. And we were embarrassed again the first time we had sex. But by the second or third time it was not so embarrassing. We had been taught the proper way, so there was no reason to be embarrassed."

In point of fact, her husband was actually quite a bit more knowledgeable about sex than he had let on. Buying and selling coffee kept him on the road much of the time and brought him to large towns, where he often went out drinking with other coffee buyers or treated his less well-off male *wantoks* (literally, "one talk"; people from the same ethnic group) to nights of carousing, including sex with women they met at bars. Most of the men in the Papua New Guinea sample typically asserted that they only did "traditional" sex with their wives but would try "style style sex" with other women (Wardlow 2008a); unlike them, however, Miriam's husband had chosen to share his sexual knowledge with her, initiating her into erotic language and practices that their *manayi* had not taught them. In answer to my question, "Can you tell me about a time when you were newly married and your husband did something that made you really happy?"—a question to which most women responded with stories about gifts or about a husband praising them in front of his family—she told me about the time he introduced her to mutual oral sex. As she described it, "He just about died—he expressed so much pleasure. And he said things to me like, 'Oh Miriam, my love, this is too much. I am dying.' And I felt the same way, and we both finished our worries [a Huli euphemism for orgasm]. We were really joined. And we did it a lot after that. Sometimes I would even say to him, 'Let's do that other sex and not the kind that makes babies.' . . . He is living in Port Moresby now, but I believe he still thinks about me and the sex we had together. It really joined us. What we did together was against Huli custom, and I don't think that other spouses do the things we did together. We were really joined. But then that second wife came along and did her magic and got me kicked out of our house."

Miriam had thought she had what anthropologists and historians of love and marriage sometimes refer to as "companionate marriage" (Hirsch and Wardlow 2006), and in many ways her marriage did correspond to the way this marital form has been described in the scholarly literature: she and her husband had chosen each other based on mutual attraction and affinity; they had established a new residence together; their relationship with each other had been more emotionally intimate than the relationships they had with other people; the quality and degree of their intimacy had been important criteria for assessing the success of the marriage (or, at least, this is how Miriam characterized her own feelings); and they had made decisions together in a relatively egalitarian way (e.g., it had been her idea to start the trade-store, and he had trusted her to run it when he was away). And, as Miriam described it, mutual sexual pleasure had been a kind of "emotional glue" (Hirsch 2003) that had joined them together—though it wasn't just the shared pleasure that had generated this intimacy. For Miriam, their intimacy had also been created through their transgressive decision to have sex in ways that fundamentally contravened Huli custom—a decision that people of their parents' generation and many in their own would have considered imprudent at best (Wardlow 2008a). She described it as their secret that they had kept from the world.

That he was having sex with other women—not only when he was away, but also when he was in Tari—and that he intended to use his coffee profits to take a second wife had come as a rude shock. And although their marriage (as Miriam described it in retrospect) was somewhat atypical for the sample, Miriam's response to her husband's sexual infidelities—violent confrontation—was not:

I was pregnant with my first child. It was the middle of the day, and my husband had bought coffee beans, put them in a storage building, and come home. He gave me twenty kina for dinner, and I bought two chickens, some greens, and plantains. While we were cooking, my husband said, "I'm going to go buy some betel nut and cigarettes." So I sat and waited for a while, but he was gone a long time, so I went out to the road. He wasn't at the nearest store, so I became very suspicious. I left everything and I followed him. . . . I got to a crossing in the road and saw his bicycle—he had hidden it behind some long grass. So I hid there and waited. . . . Then I saw him and this woman I'd seen flirting with him before. The two of them entered a long drainage ditch all overgrown with bush.[1] I was out of breath from running to catch up to him, so I didn't follow them immediately. I wanted to be able to sneak up on them, but I was breathing too heavily. So they went into this ditch, and then a minute or so later I followed them. I had a knife—not too long and not too short—and I had a stick in my other hand. And I crept up on them, and there they were—naked! They were busy kissing and touching each other, and I stabbed the woman in her side, pulled it out, and then jabbed her in her thigh. And before my husband could stand up, I whipped him in the head with the stick. He grabbed his trousers and tried to put them on, but I kept whipping him with the stick. He ran away and left the woman sitting there in the ditch. . . . The woman had to go to the hospital, and then her kin came to me and said, "Your husband is going to have to marry her. The two of you will have to give bridewealth for her." And I said, "Fuck—I'm not the man here. I didn't fuck her. He's the man—talk to him." But I didn't like her, and I didn't want her as a second wife, so I told them to take her back home. I said I'd rather pay compensation for her injuries because I didn't want my husband bringing that woman into my household. When I saw her again, I said, "Don't try to fuck my husband again. Watch out. If you do it again, I'll kill you." [*Interviewer*: Did your husband give compensation to her family for having sex with her?] Yes, and he also had to give compensation to me for stepping over me. ["Stepping over" a wife is a Huli idiom for adultery; it is meant to convey the disrespect and polluting consequences of illicit sexual behavior.] And I said to him, "We get along so well, and we were so in love, so how could you go and fuck another woman?" [*Interviewer*: And what did he say?] He said, "You are pregnant and we can't have sex. [Abstaining from sex during pregnancy is a custom almost all Huli women follow.] . . . What I was doing with her—it meant nothing. It was just because I felt the need for sex. Don't be angry. I'll give you K300 so you won't be angry with me anymore. You are pregnant and it's hard for me to go without sex for so long."

On that occasion, Miriam had accepted the money and the explanation. She managed to prevent the other woman from becoming her co-wife and went on to have three children with her husband. But like most Huli men who can afford to, her husband had eventually insisted on taking another wife—an emotional betrayal that had driven Miriam into having her own affair, which had then resulted in her husband divorcing her. As she described it,

> I was really angry with my husband, and so I went out and had sex with another man. . . . But my father found out and he hit me and broke my nose. He hit me, and then he informed my husband. And the two of them hauled me to the house of this other man. My husband wanted to fight with him, and so a lot of my husband's male kin came with us, carrying bows and arrows. They wanted to start a tribal fight, but this man gave my husband K1000 and nine pigs. . . . I didn't want to leave my husband, and I tried to explain that I did it because I was angry about him taking another wife. But he kicked me out and insisted that my family return his bridewealth. So I had to leave him.

Miriam's story encapsulates many of the issues that I discuss in this chapter: men's and women's often conflicting ideals and expectations of marriage; the continuing prestige for men of polygamy; the extramarital opportunity structures—such as men's work-related mobility—that make men's infidelity very likely; the gendered spaces and sexual geographies—such as bars—that enable and incite extramarital liaisons; and the way that the social risks of extramarital sex are constructed so that husbands face few penalties as long as their liaisons are with women who are perceived as "not belonging" to any particular man (e.g., sex workers), while wives often pay the heavy price of divorce or even death.

I end this chapter with a discussion of Huli women's typically public, confrontational, and often violent reactions to their husband's sexual itinerancies. Much like the Ugandan case in this book, this chapter asks, "What are the social risks and rewards associated with going public or remaining willfully ignorant of a husband's extramarital sexuality?" One of the ways in which the Huli sample most differed from the other four field sites in this project was the women's refusal to feign ignorance of or maintain silence about men's infidelities (see also Wardlow 2002b). This refusal, I argue, is in part due to the ambivalence that women feel about the companionate marriage ideal. Although women long for this ideal in many ways, there are aspects of companionate marriage in its Huli incarnation (specifically, a kind of bourgeois, Christian, patriarchal ethos about not "airing dirty laundry" and about preserving the appearance of family harmony and respectability) that Huli women resist. Confrontational reactions were especially common among women of low socioeconomic status whose husbands did not have salaried jobs. A couple of women married to civil servants—that is, men with relatively secure, middle-class salaries—responded differently. In other words, unless a woman has risen into the middle class and has much to lose in terms of social prestige and economic security (which was not the case for most of the women in this sample), violent confrontation is the best means she has of securing public support and salvaging her own dignity in the face of her husband's infidelity.

The Research Setting

The research for this chapter was conducted among the Huli in the town of Tari, Southern Highlands Province, Papua New Guinea.[2] Little wage or salaried labor is available in Tari itself; thus, in addition to growing staples like sweet potato, most people make money by growing coffee or selling produce to local teachers, health workers, and civil servants. Remittances from family members working outside of Tari are important, as is the Porgera Joint Venture (PJV) gold mine located in Enga Province, north of Tari. Many Huli make the two- to three-day hike to Porgera in order to look for work, visit family members who have some connection to the mine, dig through the mine's waste rock for unprocessed gold, or engage in illegal mining in PJV's open pit (Wardlow 2009; see also Jacka n.d. for harrowing descriptions of the latter two practices). Moreover, in a rather unusual arrangement, PJV is almost completely powered by a natural gas plant located to the south of Tari, and is thus dependent on the seventy-eight-kilometer-long electrical line that runs through Huli territory. Families who own the land on which the electrical pylons are built receive annual "occupation fees," and the communities that abut the pylons receive some services from PJV, such as road maintenance and school renovations (Lavu 2007).[3]

In the spring of 2004, the Tari area and much of Southern Highlands Province was at a dismal and sometimes violent low point. At the national level, the Papua New Guinea currency (the kina) had experienced a precipitous decline, falling from US$.85 in the mid-1990s to US$.30 in 2004. The costs of store-bought goods had risen accordingly, but wages and the prices that people could command for their agricultural products had not. The economic decline was a constant topic of conversation in Tari, with many people asserting that they could no longer pay their children's school fees and could now afford to buy only cooking oil and salt (the rice and canned mackerel that they had purchased in the past now financially out of reach). Not surprisingly, crime had increased: households each had to have at least one person home at all times in order to deter the theft of pigs, chickens, and even laundry hanging out to dry. The longstanding problem of armed hold-ups of public buses on the road between Tari and Mendi (the provincial capital) had worsened to the point that road travel was almost impossible. The one bank

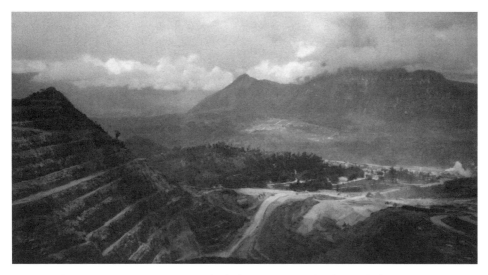

Many Huli men migrate to Porgera to look for work or to dig through the mine's waste rock for gold. Photograph by Holly Wardlow.

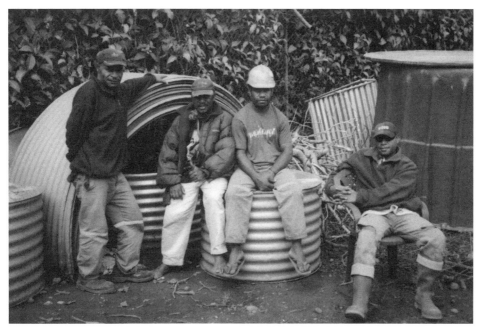

PJV hires some Huli men as security guards, community liaison staff, and laborers on community development projects. Photograph by Holly Wardlow.

and the one large store that had sold electronic goods, clothing, and groceries had been looted by armed gangs in 2002 and had subsequently closed. The increase in violent crime had prompted many salaried employees to flee the area, leading to the closure of primary schools, health centers, and the post office.[4] The phone lines were down and the hydroelectric project that powered Tari town was broken.

Attempts to remedy this chaotic situation had been stymied by the fact that the 2002 elections had been plagued by the intimidation of voters and the theft of ballot boxes, and thus had been declared a failure, which meant that the province had no government, an unprecedented situation not anticipated by the national constitution. Provincial government offices in Mendi had been looted and left empty. Finally, in a good example of community divestment being a vicious cycle that results in further divestment, many development organizations, including the National AIDS Council, had declared Tari a "no-go zone," asserting that it was too dangerous to send their employees there.[5]

Changing Ideals and Experiences of Marriage

Many Huli women aspire to what they sometimes call "the new kind of marriage" (hereafter referred to as "modern marriage"). Importantly, women almost always describe this new ideal in a totalizing way—that is, as a coherent and indivisible unity of emotional, economic, gendered, and religious characteristics and conduct. In other words, when women talk about modern marriage, they talk not only about marital intimacy, trust, laughter, and affection, but also about living in a *haus kapa* (literally, "a house with a copper roof," as opposed to a house made of locally grown materials); having a husband with a salaried job; attending church together; and spending one's days sweeping the house, planting decorative flowers, strategizing how best to budget money, and buying household goods and new clothing for children. Thus, for many women, modern marriage is as much about a move into the respectable Christian middle class as it is a sentimental act of love (Wardlow 2006a).

Moreover, because the ideal of modern marriage is associated with being a good Christian and with progress, many men recognize it as the marital form to which they should aspire, even as they tend to be more wary about it than women. Thus, even as they expressed doubts about this marital form, many men described themselves as working hard to achieve more companionate marriages than their own parents had had, and they spoke of this endeavor as evidence of their own moral enlightenment and orientation toward progress compared with pre-mission generations. For example, almost all of the participants' parents had lived in separate houses, but most of the male participants themselves had decided to share houses with their wives.[6] Even men who continued to live in their own houses declared that their marriages were more intimate than those of previous generations had been. As one middle-aged man said, "My mother's house was in one area, and my father's house was in a different area quite far away. They only came together to make children. They didn't sit down and talk. My wife and I also sleep in separate houses, but our houses are on the same area of land, and I come to see her every day, and we go to the market together, and we work in our fields together. We sit down and talk to each other every day."

One telling generational contrast emerged in answer to the interview question, "What do men need to do so that they will have good marriages?" This quote from a seventy-two-year-old man who had three concurrent wives at the time of the interview was typical of the older generation of men:

> Women expect that a man will have enough land to divide evenly amongst his wives, enough pigs so that they all have some to raise, and that he will provide protection for his wives and children. If a man does this equitably, his wives will think he is a good man.

In contrast, the quote below was characteristic of most men in the younger generation and some in the middle-aged generation:

> I think before I speak to her. I think about what I need to say to her that will make her happy, how I should express something in a way that she will understand and accept. . . . If I do this, then she will have empathy for me and I will have empathy for her. Even if I can't give her money or food, we will still get along if we are communicating well and if I speak kindly to her.

Men in the younger and middle-aged generations were also more likely than older men to say that if they learned a joke, some gossip, or some important news, that they would most want to share this with a wife rather than natal family members or male friends, another indication of the increased emotional centrality of the marital relationship.

However, "modern marriage" is a dramatic change from precolonial practice, and many people—male and female—expressed some skepticism about how communicative and emotional intimacy could possibly be the basis for a successful marriage. As one middle-aged woman said, in answer to the question of whether she thought love was important for a happy marriage:

> No, it's not important. You can have love, but what if you don't have food or money? My husband can eat the food I've grown in the fields or the pigs that I have raised. And when my family is in trouble, if he helps them, then I will really be happy with him. But just showing love, that's no good. I mean, expressing your feelings, or talking about your feelings together, or talking about desire— that kind of thing. That's not important.

A generation ago, Huli men and women lived quite separate lives (Goldman 1983; Frankel 1986; Allen 1995). Husbands and wives cooked, ate, and slept in different houses—ones that were sometimes quite distant from each other—and while women were and are highly valued for their agricultural and domestic labor, traditional discourses about women tend to be quite disparaging, describing them, for example, as "nogat mana" (without knowledge), a phrase that implies ignorance and lack of self-control. Even aphorisms that are not explicitly denigrating to women tend to support male dominance—asserting, for example, that women should be "fenced in by men" or "under the legs of men."

Men were and are taught to avoid too much contact with women, and in the past, the social organization of space facilitated this avoidance. Boys over the age of six lived with their fathers, and many young men joined "bachelor cults"—camps in isolated mountain areas where they were taught skills in hunting and battle, as well as rituals for enhancing their physical appearance and maintaining their vitality. Martha MacIntyre has described Papua New Guinean ideal male embodiment as "both beautiful and dangerous" (2008: 181), a phrase that corresponds well to Huli men's descriptions of themselves as fierce and alluring warriors. Importantly, a man's strength, charisma, and good fortune were thought to stem from his physical purity; thus, part of learning to be a man was learning protective practices for slowing the inevitable aging and deterioration said to be caused by excessive contact with women. Men were taught to cleanse and purify their bodies by drinking water from remote mountain springs, and they learned to stave off bodily decline by avoiding food prepared by women and by limiting marital sex to days eleven through fourteen of a wife's menstrual cycle (Wardlow 2008a; Glasse 1974; Frankel 1980). (Many men in our sample stated that they still try to follow the last practice, while also conceding that it is far more difficult now that husbands and wives live together in the same house.)

Because many of these customary practices are conceptualized as "health promoting" for men, it is perhaps not surprising that men express more reservations than women about renouncing them in favor of the modern marriage ideal. However, men's misgivings are motivated by more than fears about the dangers of female fluids and essences. First, many men share women's Christian, middle-class vision of modern marriage, and since most men will never be able to obtain a salaried job or to install a wife in a *haus kapa*, they are apprehensive and sometimes resentful about the way in which the man-as-cash-provider model of masculinity is becoming normative. Intersecting with this apprehension is the fear that modern marriage means abdicating male dominance and privilege (though, in fact, this had not occurred among the couples in the sample who had achieved a relatively middle-class lifestyle and appeared to have "modern marriages." A couple of women of high SES stated, for example, that they loved their husbands, but also that their husbands had burned their high school diplomas so that they would be unable to get jobs).

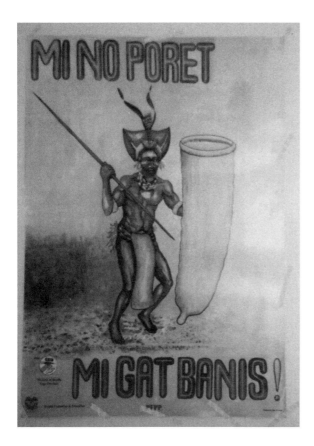

This poster attempts to use images of traditional masculinity—the brave tribal warrior protecting his family and clan—to encourage condom use. The caption says, "I'm not afraid; I have a shield!" In fact, many people told me they were embarrassed by this poster and even found it offensive, precisely because it mixes two symbolically opposed domains—warfare, which has noble associations, and sexuality, which is considered private and shameful. Photograph by Holly Wardlow.

Men's resentment about what they perceive as a loss of dominance is exacerbated by bridewealth inflation (from nine pigs in the 1960s to twenty-seven pigs in the 2000s) and the increased pressure to pay at least half of bridewealth in cash (rather than in pigs). Many younger and middle-aged men in the sample spoke heatedly of the hardships they had endured (digging illegally for gold at Porgera, for example, with the risk of being shot by security guards) and of the debts they had incurred while trying to accumulate enough cash to get married. In return, although they did not seek to be tyrannical in marriage, many felt that they were owed a wife's deference, hard work, and obedience. In a sense, men's fear and anger about disenfranchisement in the modern global economy is expressed as a sense of male entitlement within marriage, and arguably this is part of the reason why polygamy continues to be highly prestigious (at least among men). Thus, some men said that what they wanted more than anything else was renown and power in their local community, and the only foreseeable way to achieve this was to be "a man who has many pigs, many wives, and many children." A hard-working wife who was willing to sacrifice her own desires (for monogamous intimacy, for example) was essential for achieving this goal.

Finally, for some Huli men, decisions about whether to live in the same house, sleep in the same room, sit side by side, or have an egalitarian conversation with a wife are as much about an increasingly politicized ethnic identity as about desires for a particular kind of marriage. In an era when many Huli feel that their integrity as an ethnic group is being threatened (by the abysmal failure of government services and by a national media that often vilifies the Huli as particularly uncivilized and violent), some men assert a profound cynicism about practices such as marital monogamy and co-residence that are promoted by religious missions as the only moral way to live, or are represented as self-evidently normal in state discourse. It is significant that during the time of this research, many Huli were advocating strenuously for seceding from Southern Highlands Province and forming what was described as a cosmologically ordained new Hela Province, in which they would be the dominant ethnic group, Tari would be the provincial capital, and Huli cultural practices would be valorized and promulgated (Ballard 1994; Haley 2007). When specific family forms and affective practices (such as marital cohabitation and intimacy) are associated with an abortive modernity (that is, a sense that modern progress has failed to materialize and that the state has failed to deliver on promises of development), then resistance to adopting them is not surprising.

Before concluding this discussion of changing marital ideals and experiences, it is important to say something about marital violence among the Huli. Many Huli people speak of physical conflict as an inevitable dimension of marriage, and most of the participants, male and female, had exchanged blows with their spouse (Wardlow 2006b; for discussion of high rates of domestic violence more generally in Papua New Guinea, see Counts 1993; Toft 1985; Zimmer-Tamakoshi 1997). Marital fighting is a complex cultural and sociological issue, but rather than parse this behavior as solely an expression and means of male dominance (which it undeniably is—according to Barss 1991, the incidence of wife-murder among the Huli is extremely high), here I want to point out that it is also a manifestation of the prevailing Huli assumption that marriage is inevitably a battle of wills (Wardlow 2006b). Most participants in the study assumed that husbands and wives have competing desires and are unavoidably at odds over many things (e.g., domestic labor, money, sex, obligations to extended family). Moreover, Huli men and women share the idea that physical aggression is an important means for a person—male or female—to show self-respect during conflict and that a person who fails to defend himself or herself physically is a coward. Finally, many male participants (but no female participants) asserted that marital physical and emotional intimacy only exacerbate the ongoing struggle that is marriage, as illustrated in this quote from a middle-aged man:

> In my opinion, people used to be more free. . . . Nowadays husbands and wives live in the same house. It's not just me—all my friends and other men my age

also live with their wives. And I think this causes more fights and arguments. Before, men had their own houses and wives had their own houses, and they didn't fight as much. But now we live in one house and sleep in one room, and we get angry with each other over nothing. I think it's because we see each other all the time, see the same body all the time, hear the same talk all the time.

Although Huli men and women tend to share the idea that physical fighting is appropriate in some situations, including marital conflict, there are aspects of marital violence that indicate men's ability to use physical force to punish and intimidate in ways that women cannot. For example, men speak far more than women of physical aggression as a means of disciplining an unruly spouse (although some female participants also spoke of "whipping a husband with a stick" to chastise him for disrespectful behavior). In contrast, women speak of starting physical fights in public in order to make marital conflict visible. In other words, violent confrontation is a key female strategy for bringing marital conflict to community attention and for gaining community support (Wardlow 2006b).

Men's Extramarital Opportunity Structures

Almost all but the newly married and the very devout men interviewed had engaged in extramarital sex at some point during their marriages. Many had done so within the last month, and many spoke of it as a regular occurrence, particularly when they were away from home. Huli men described almost all of their liaisons as very brief in duration—not surprising since there are no brothels in Tari (and only two guest houses, both of which are religiously oriented), and thus most illicit sexual transactions occur outdoors, with couples quickly trying to complete the act before being caught (see also Hammar 1992, 1996).[7] Moreover, most of the men in the sample were of low socioeconomic status and could not afford to support a girlfriend or "outside wife" (a practice that seemed to be more common in both the Nigerian and Ugandan cases).

At first glance, there would seem to be many factors—both discursive and sociological—to discourage men's extramarital sexuality. In contrast with the other research sites, Huli people do not speak of men as "naturally" needing sexual variety or having avid sexual appetites. If anything, traditional discourses about masculinity emphasize abstemiousness, purity, and self-discipline, and Huli custom asserts the moral and hygienic importance of marital monogamy for *both* men and women (Glasse 1974; Goldman 1983; Wardlow 2006b). Both men and women claimed, for example, that they might be able to guess if a spouse had cheated because they or their children would experience weakness and malaise for no apparent reason. Further, as Haley (2007: 59) points out, "The peoples living in the western end of Southern Highlands Province . . . share the belief that they are part of a regional system deeply rooted in mythology and ritual, and that the fertility of their region is morally constituted. This means they must act and behave in certain ways for their world to be fertile." From this perspective, extramarital liaisons, in addition to whatever consequences they might have for the participants, do environmental and cosmological damage. According to Haley, "Even today, despite the almost complete absence of indigenous ritual practice, Duna [the ethnic group just to the west of the Huli] hold to the belief that moral behaviour conserves fertile substance, and that immoral behaviour sees it depleted and will ultimately bring about the world's end" (2007: 60). Perhaps because of greater exposure to schooling and a longer history of male out-migration, the Huli seem more dubious than the Duna about whether illicit sexual behavior actually drains the world of its fertile essence. Nevertheless, many male participants declared that they would never engage in extramarital sex on the eve of a tribal fight or an important political event for fear that it would endanger the success of the enterprise, suggesting at least some sense that individual sexual unruliness can negatively affect the sociopolitical body. Again, this would appear to contrast markedly with this book's other research sites, where men's extramarital liaisons were generally not seen as inherently destructive to the social (let alone the cosmological) fabric.

Finally, men are well aware of the potentially humiliating or even violent penalties of extramarital sex (Wardlow 2007). As one man said, "I used to have sex with lots of other women, but then I gave my wife gonorrhea, and it was very shameful. We had to go to the hospital together, and at the hospital they carefully checked over my penis and asked me all kinds of questions, and I felt completely humiliated. And my wife was very angry, and she made it public and took me to village court. I had to give her compensation pigs in front of everyone, and this was humiliating, so I stopped sleeping with other women." Village courts are basically outdoor gatherings where government-appointed mediators adjudicate local disputes. They are quite egalitarian in nature, and the whole community is welcome to attend and comment on the dispute in question, whether it involves theft, rape, adultery, or interpersonal violence. Perhaps it is not surprising, then, that when asked what the possible negative consequences were of extramarital sex, most men said "village court" or "paying compensation" (not illness or a damaged marriage). Moreover, if a man's extramarital partner is a married woman whose husband is living in Tari, having to pay compensation may be the least of his worries; being murdered by the woman's husband is also a real possibility.

That men's extramarital activity appears to be common despite these deterrents suggests that the social, cultural, and economic factors facilitating and propelling extramarital sexuality—what in this book we call "extramarital opportunity structures"—far outweigh those factors that hinder it. I now discuss these opportunity structures and the ways in which they shape men's extramarital sexuality into specific patterns and imbue it with particular personal and cultural meanings. The most important opportunity structures that emerged from the Papua

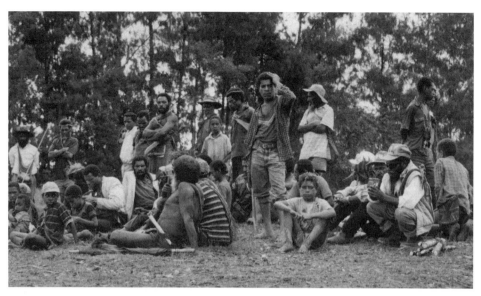

Village court cases are open-air, public events, and anyone may attend and comment on the proceedings. Huli men consider being taken to village court one of the serious risks of engaging in extramarital sex. Photograph by Holly Wardlow.

New Guinea research site were labor migration, compensatory masculinity in the context of economic disenfranchisement, and—despite this disenfranchisement—men's greater economic power relative to women.

Male Mobility and Labor Migration

Traveling outside of Tari, whether for work or some other purpose, seemed to all but guarantee that men would have extramarital relations, and men often described the process of becoming familiar with a new urban area as a ritualized event that involved going to bars with friends, meeting women, and taking them to low-cost guest houses for sex. Such activities were described as quintessentially modern and urban—simply what one did when one had the opportunity to go to a city—and thus almost a matter of course, regardless of a man's socioeconomic status. A wealthy businessman or a civil servant attending an in-service training workshop might go to a hotel bar, whereas a poorer man would be taken by *wantoks* to an unlicensed, makeshift bar under a tarp at the back of someone's house. Whatever the venue, drinking, laughing with one's male peers, and buying sex would be the evening entertainment.

In addition to their visits to urban areas, many men in our sample had worked at mine sites or on plantations. Colonial-period economic policies such as the Highland Labour Scheme, a labor recruitment program that lasted from 1959 to

1974, targeted men in the highlands to work on coffee, tea, and copra plantations located in other provinces; thus, there have been high rates of labor-related migration among the Huli since the Tari area came fully under the Australian colonial administration in 1961 (Ward 1990; Stewart 1992; Ballard 2002; Wardlow 2009). The extension of the Highlands Highway to Tari in 1981, and the recent development of resource extraction industries in and near the borders of Southern Highlands Province (particularly the PJV gold mine, the Hides gas fields, and the Kutubu oil project) have, not surprisingly, helped to maintain this enduring pattern of male migration out of the Tari area. Migration data from 1982, for example, shows that in some areas of the Tari Basin, approximately 45 percent of men between the ages of twenty and thirty-nine were absent (Lehmann 2002; Lehmann et al. 1997).[8]

In many men's interviews, labor migration was associated with what might be called a man's "extramarital sexual debut"—that is, his first experience of extramarital sex. As one man said:

> After I was married, I left my wife and children and went to Goroka for work, and it was there that I had sex with another woman. That was the first time. I went with another man. It was his idea—he was my boss and I was the driver. He said, "Let's go around and find some women. I'll pay for some food and I'll pay for the guest house." So I did this the first time because I was with him. We took a car and we went together. We impressed the women by riding around in a car. Lots of working men do this—they pressure each other to go drink and have sex with prostitutes. It was especially hard for me because I worked as the driver, so they expected me to drive them to hotels and other places and it was hard for me to say no.

Many men asserted that they had learned *pamuk pasin* (promiscuous behavior) through their experiences as either plantation or mine laborers, and many elements of men's stories about labor-migration-related sexuality were similar: they included predominantly male workplaces, heavy drinking at the end of an arduous week, and the fact that women tended to target employed men by gathering outside popular bars on men's paydays. Moreover, that labor migration was the context for many men's first forays into extramarital sex shaped the meaning that extramarital sex had for them: buying sex from sex workers or picking up women in bars was described as a kind of leisure activity men do together to relax, to escape the drudgery and anxiety associated with working for low pay, to experience the pleasures of having a paycheck, and to perform and participate in a more worldly masculinity.

Many men expressed some ambivalence about the ritual of buying alcohol and sex: on the one hand, they delighted in the male camaraderie, the sexual joking and teasing, and the attention of women; on the other, many also experienced the pressure to drink and buy sex as a kind of coercive peer pressure, and they felt guilty about wasting money on fleeting pleasures. As one man who had worked as a driver in a mining town said,

> Working for money is good, but only if you can stay with your family—if you have to go somewhere else to make money, it's only good if they can come with you. There is a lot of beer available in most places where you can find work, and that's not good. And spending the money you make instead of giving it to your family—like when you waste it on beer, or buy sex from women, or give it to workmates who aren't your blood, who aren't really your family, who aren't your children—none of that is good. And then you get a letter from your family, and it says, "Daddy," or it says, "My husband," or it says, "Honey." And then it says, "We really need money, we don't have cooking oil or soap." When I got a letter like this and I didn't have money to send them, I would worry. Worry would kill me.

Surplus Time: Compensatory Masculinity in the Context of Economic Disenfranchisement

Because I didn't have a rich sense of how men actually spent their time, I added some questions to our interview instrument that asked participants to describe what they had done the day before. The responses were illuminating: women most often reported doing agricultural work, taking care of pigs, taking sick family members to the hospital, preparing meals, and (for those who were not religiously devout) selling cigarettes. The men, in contrast, most often talked about strolling around town with male friends, cruising the marketplace, and gambling. The following male response was typical:

> Yesterday I got up, roasted some sweet potato on the fire, ate, and went to the market. I asked a friend if he had money, and he did, and so we played darts to try to win cans of Coca-Cola. We each won a can and we drank them, and then we went and walked around the market exchanging glances with various women. We talked with the women, and flirted and joked with them. Then, late in the afternoon, I walked back home. . . . I walked to our sweet potato field, I dug up some sweet potatoes, and I went to my house [he and his wife lived in separate houses]. . . . My sons and I made a fire and cooked some sweet potato and we ate. And then I went to sleep. [*Interviewer*: Do you do agricultural work or is that your wife's work?] That's my wife's work. I'm a man. I wander around. Wherever I want to go, I go. Staying at home to work in the fields, that's women's work.

Thus, an important factor that enables men's ability to engage in extramarital sex is the surplus time they have on their hands compared with women, who are typically kept busy with agricultural and domestic labor. However, men's "surplus time" is actually a complex phenomenon—one produced through social constructions of men as the primary providers of cash for the household, even though the grim lack of economic opportunity within Tari and the feminization of agricultural labor there means not only that women *do* most of the labor, but also that many men consider it shameful for a man to devote too much time to subsistence agriculture.

Procuring money is now the proper purpose of men, and although a paying job is probably the most prestigious means of doing so, women are well aware that there have never been many economic opportunities in Tari, and that the opportunities that once existed have evaporated as businesses and government services have shut down. Thus, other activities are also considered legitimate, particularly if a man is successful at them. When asked, for example, how their husband made money, a surprising number of women answered, "He gambles," and a few said, "He's a criminal." When describing how they spent the money they earned selling cigarettes or produce, women often said that they set aside a few dollars for their husband to play cards with, both because it made him happy and because every once in a while he would win big and the household would be able to buy a chicken or a new outfit for a child. That gambling (let alone robbery) is considered by so many women to be a legitimate form of "work" for their husbands is, I think, another indication of the profound lack of economic opportunity for men in Tari.

In the past, Huli men engaged in a range of activities: they did the heavy work of preparing fields for planting (which most still regularly do), dug deep moat-like trenches around household and clan territories (which most still regularly do), harvested their own sweet potato gardens and cooked for themselves and their sons (which a minority of men still regularly do), raised their own pigs (particularly premaritally, since a young man was expected to provide many of his own bridewealth pigs), engaged in warfare, patrolled clan boundaries, guarded women engaged in agricultural work, negotiated treaties and organized the huge feasts that marked the end of warfare, orchestrated complex and lengthy regional religious rituals, and went on extended trade-related journeys. In fact, many men still engage intermittently in all but the last two activities. However, warfare is now only sporadic, and when forewarned, the police prevent battles by arresting the key instigators. Further, most men now rely on their wives to provide food for them and assert that agricultural labor is women's work, unless it is for a cash crop such as coffee. Thus, many men are caught in the classic postcolonial bind in which many precolonial masculine activities either no longer exist or are now feminized (and thus devalued), while the most prestigious (and increasingly normative) postcolonial masculine activities—in particular, making money through waged or salaried work—are not available to most men. Many men, with "surplus time" on their hands and with few avenues open to them for achieving "hegemonic masculinity" (Connell 2003), therefore engage in what has variously been analyzed as compensatory or protest masculinity (for examples and critiques of these concepts, see Bourgois 1996; Chen 1999; Razack 2002; Tomsen 1997; Walker 2006). That is, in response to their powerlessness to realize hegemonic masculinity, they forge masculine identities by turning to other, often dangerous or destructive activities that are culturally coded as masculine, resulting in "selves distorted by their relations to the ideal type" (Walker 2006: 8).

It is important to note that compensatory and protest masculinity are not equivalent concepts, and that these terms come from quite different analytical and political locations, compensatory masculinity being more psychological in orientation and protest masculinity being more suggestive of resistance to structural—and most typically class—relations of inequality. Some scholars of masculinity have avoided these terms by instead talking about the "hegemonic bargains" (Chen 1999) that disempowered men strike, consciously or unconsciously trading on whatever social privileges they might have (in relation to women, for example, or through their physical looks or athletic prowess) in order to come closer to the hegemonic masculine ideal. Other scholars examine the ways that marginalized men "reconstruct their notions of masculine dignity" (Bourgois 1996: 414) through dangerous, violent, and dominating behaviors. My purpose here, however, is not to wade into this conceptual debate, but only to assert that Huli men experience strong social and internal pressure to perform potent masculinity, and that their conduct stems in part from the fact that they have little access to the avenues of real economic and political power.

Among the Huli, these compensatory or protest practices can be seen in a range of venues: the "gangsta" look and demeanor adopted by many young jobless men in Tari and elsewhere in Papua New Guinea (MacIntyre 2008), the extremely high levels of sexual violence in Tari, and young men's deliberately insouciant attitudes about rape, often dismissing their assaults against women by saying, "Chans, yia" (literally, "chance," but implying, "I saw an opportunity and all I did was take it"). However, like much of the literature on compensatory and protest masculinity, these examples focus on young men and violence. I am suggesting that older, married men also engage in compensatory or protest masculinity, but that their practices more often take a sexual form—specifically drinking, buying sex, and discussing their sexual escapades with male peers. Thus, while the man quoted earlier spoke only of flirting with women at the market, most men spoke of the Tari market as a primary location for finding women who were willing to sell sex. (Most of the women at the Tari market are not there to sell sex; however, the market is so big, bustling, and chaotic that it is easy for subtle sexual negotiations to take place without too many people noticing.) Interview after interview contained segments like this one:

> First, I take a good look at them and try to catch their eye. If they look back at me in the same way, then I'll edge a bit closer to them. And then I'll give her

some small thing like a Coke or some betel nut. And then, just from the way we look at each other, I know that she's willing, and we'll agree to meet somewhere later. We talk about which road to take, and who will go to the agreed-upon location first and who will come later, and where exactly we will meet in the bush off the road. When a woman agrees to meet a man like that, it only means sex—that's the only reason for it, even if it's never actually said. So if a woman agrees to follow me to a certain place or to meet me there later, then I know she's willing to have sex with me.

The ebullient tone in the men's voices, and the elaborate and often funny stories they told, suggested that buying sex is an important means for them to experience a sense of economic power and carefree bravado. Much like the Mexican case, their buying of sex "indicates that there is money to spend on discretionary pleasures, the refusal to be beaten down by poverty" (Hirsch, this volume), and the refusal to let one's life be reduced to the struggle to meet basic needs. Moreover, men often band together to look for women and frequently boast and joke about their liaisons in the company of male peers, suggesting that having an encouraging and appreciative male audience (after the fact) enhances the pleasures and sense of triumph that come from an illicit liaison. Indeed, having a ribald and riotous story to share seemed in many cases to be more pleasurable and meaningful than the sex itself, as seen in these quotes about "passenger women" (a widely used term for women who exchange sex for money; see Wardlow 2002c and 2004):

> I talk to my friends about the passenger women I have sex with, but not about the married women or students I have sex with. I worry that they might tell someone. Those women are my secret pleasures just for myself. I only tell my friends about the sex I have with passenger women—then they will know which woman to approach for sex. For example, I'll tell them, "Sex is better with big women. When I had sex with _____ it was the best. You should try her. Big thighs, big vagina, big everything!"

> I get very graphic when I talk about passenger women. I say, "This woman is willing to do this or that." Or, "Her genitals looked like this." Or, "That woman's genitals feel like that." My friends are the same—they boast about the different styles they've tried. They say, "She was in this position and I did this" or "I pushed her down and did it to her like that." We really talk about sex and passenger women in a very graphic way. And when one man does this, it gives the rest of us the idea to try a particular style or try a particular woman.

In the Nigerian case (Smith, this volume), wealthy men also engaged in humorous and boastful banter about their extramarital liaisons, suggesting that these practices are not solely a compensatory response to marginalized status or a "reconstitution and reclamation of indigenous masculinity" (MacIntyre 2008: 186). However, in contrast to the Nigerian case, drinking and buying sex in male groups in the Huli case is an important venue for crossing socioeconomic lines: men employed by PJV were often the ones who bought the alcohol, for example, treating their unemployed peers to a night of drunken fun. These trans-class get-togethers are significant in the Tari context in part because the PJV office is a gated and guarded compound, and the men who work as security guards must turn away almost all of the many petitioners—including male kin and peers—who are seeking employment or asking PJV to fund community projects. Orchestrating these evenings enabled PJV employees both to ameliorate the humiliations they had to inflict on rejected petitioners during the work day and to display their modern, employed, and generous masculinity. Moreover, when poorer men in the sample were trying to explain their extramarital liaisons, they often invoked their employed peers or their images of elite urban men, saying, for example, "Rich men in the cities have lots of women and girlfriends, and go drink at fancy hotels. We are just trying to do the same thing with less money." In other words, poorer men often seemed to see themselves through the eyes of urban, salaried masculinity, and they framed their extramarital liaisons (and bawdy stories about these liaisons) as a simulation of the practices and privileges of more powerful men.

Women's Dependence on Men for Money and Other Resources

Despite the general dearth of economic opportunity in Tari, it was nevertheless apparent from both men's and women's interviews that women's dependence on men for money and for access to other resources sometimes put them in sexually coercive situations. The clearest example of this was the easy availability of women selling sex in Tari in 2004. Although most men in the sample did not have waged or salaried jobs, they still often had enough money to buy sex since, as they described it, a sexual transaction could be obtained for as low as five kina (about US$2) plus a can of Coke (for the initial encounter in the marketplace). This low price represented a dramatic change from the past: interviews that I had conducted with passenger women in the mid-1990s showed that most had been paid at least ten kina and often more—at a time when the kina had been worth almost three times as much as it was in 2004—and that they had typically rejected men who had had the gall to offer them less. In other words, women in the mid-1990s could have expected about US$12 per sexual transaction, but the rate in 2004 easily went as low as US$2. This drastic reduction in price reflects the women's reduced asking power, which was likely due both to the women's knowledge that most men cannot afford to pay more and, by all accounts, to a significant increase in the number of women selling sex. As one man said, "We would have to blindfold ourselves not to see all the willing women here now." Moreover, women's motivations for selling sex seem to have changed somewhat. During the mid-1990s, very few women had asserted economic need as their primary motivation; instead, they had talked angrily about incidents in which they had felt betrayed by their husbands or natal families, and their desires to shame and punish those people through revenge promiscuity (Wardlow 2002a, 2002c, 2004, 2006b). In 2004, by contrast, female participants who had sold sex talked bluntly about needing money for children's school fees and other basic household goods.

Men's inability to act as providers, even when they leave home to find work, has exacerbated this dire predicament and has probably propelled some women into sex work who had never before considered the possibility. For example, my friend Roni had been relatively well-off in the mid-1990s: she herself had no formal education, but her husband had a job as a government driver, and although his salary was quite low, they and their two children had lived free of charge in a small government flat, and her sister worked as a schoolteacher and often gave them additional money. However, when I returned in 2004, Roni's husband had lost his job because of government downsizing and was looking for work with companies that had employed him before he married, all of which were located in other provinces. He had been away from Tari for most of the previous three years and had only been able to send money home once. In fact, I ran into him by chance in another town. He was distraught about his inability to obtain a secure job; at the same time, he admitted to spending money on beer and passenger women in part because the *wantoks* he stayed with in various towns and mine sites did so, and in part to experience at least a momentary freedom from the anxiety of being unable to find work.

Back in Tari, Roni was trying to care for their now six children, but could not manage both this and agricultural work. Her sister was still trying to work as a teacher, but she hadn't been paid for a year due to the collapse of the provincial government. In fact, most of the other teachers had left or stopped coming to work, effectively closing the school. Roni said that it finally had become a choice between trying to sell sex, a possibility that was clearly alien and abhorrent to her, or stealing from a neighbor's fields for food. She chose the latter, was caught, and was so embarrassed by the public denunciations and demands for recompense that she could barely talk about it. She hadn't left her house for days afterwards. Many women in comparable situations choose to sell sex, which, it must be said, is probably socially safer, at least in the short run, since it is easier to hide one's transient sexual dealings than one's pilfering of neighbors' sweet potatoes. Even if neighbors find out about the former, they aren't directly affected by it and are thus more likely to spread gossip than to create a humiliating public scene.

Finally, men are also able to exert sexual power through their control over some of the modern technologies that occasionally become necessities. A man who worked as a long-distance bus driver, for example, said that he regularly took sex in lieu of fares because so many women could not afford to pay. A woman who had not sold sex before or since told of the one occasion when she did: she had desperately needed to use a telephone to reach her brother who worked in another town. The phones were not working in Tari. She managed to make her way to Mendi, where the phones were working. She walked into a small government office, begged the man behind the desk to let her use the phone, and was allowed to do so once she agreed to have sex with him. Thus, men are sometimes able to use their positions as "gate keepers" over certain services and technologies to coerce women into using their sexuality as a kind of currency.

The Discomfort of "The Family House" and the Delights of the *Dawe Anda*: Gendered and Sexualized Geographies

The extramarital opportunity structures discussed above are buttressed by the homosociality of adult life, a facet of social organization that is readily apparent as one walks through Huli space. The sprawling main market is divided into two areas separated by a fence—the main area where women sell produce, and a smaller area where men, and only men, play darts. In church, regardless of denomination, men and women sit on opposite sides. Even spouses who live together in one house typically divide the house in half, so that the husband and any male visitors sit on one side of the central fire, and women sit on the other.

One survey I did in the mid-1990s showed that two-thirds of married couples were living in the same house, a significant departure from traditional practice in which men had their own houses or lived in clan men's houses. However, this mission-spurred change in living arrangements does not mean that men are completely comfortable inhabiting what Huli call (using the English phrase) "the family house." Tellingly, a man will sometimes refer to his "family house" as his "wife's house," suggesting that in adopting co-residency he feels not that he has created a new (modern and Christian) space, but instead has moved into a female space. While most men in the sample said they enjoyed the company of their wives, and some said that they preferred the company of their wives to other people, most men also expressed discomfort and irritation with having to stay for extended periods in "the family house," particularly as the number of children in the household grew and a wife became absorbed in the labor of being a mother.

Men also commented, often unhappily, on the changes they observed in wives once they had had three or more children. Specifically, wives were said to become more willful, demanding, and quarrelsome, as seen in the quote from this middle-aged man:

> When women have children, there are changes. Before, my wife was young and she never talked back. She just sat there and agreed with me and laughed at my jokes. But once she had children, she decided that she was a citizen—that she had the right to speak, the right to carry a stick and hit me when she was angry, the right to disagree with me. She really thought she was a citizen. And when we

had children, she got very busy with the children and only thought about them, and they were always around crying or demanding something, and this would get on my nerves, and I lost interest in being at home with my wife.

Setting aside what this man's use of citizenship discourse might tell us about how the State is conceptualized, it is clear from this and other interviews that men are sometimes discontented about the ways in which women transform from amenable wives into demanding mothers. Such changes are not surprising when understood in terms of how women's social power changes over the course of their life cycles: women gain authority not from being good emotional and erotic companions to their husbands but through bearing and raising children. Having children gives them the legitimate right to make demands of husbands and to complain when husbands are not fulfilling their obligations as fathers. Thus, women can be seen as patiently biding their time (and perhaps biting their tongues) until childbearing enables them to be more forthright. Huli men tended to "biologize" these changes, describing women as "naturally" docile when young and then "naturally" becoming more querulous because of biological changes associated with reproduction. The discomfort many men feel about spending time in "the family house" motivates them to spend their leisure time (of which, as I said earlier, there is a "surplus") with their male peers. Moreover, discreetly seeking out other sexual partners at this juncture in a marriage was described as normal, harmless, and even beneficial for a marriage—certainly wiser than attempting to demand sex from a tired and irritable wife.

The men's and women's interviews also powerfully showed how men's mobility is assumed while women's is highly constrained (particularly young women and married women who have fewer than three children). For example, one interview question asked what the interviewee usually did when he or she wanted to leave the household in order to go to market or to visit relatives. Men typically said either that they would inform their wife first or that they would just leave, and that they would only provide a wife with details about their whereabouts if they planned to be away from Tari for more than a couple of days (and some women's interviews confirmed that men were sometimes away from home overnight with no prior notice or later explanation). In contrast, most women said that they would ask permission to leave the household, and men universally said that they expected their wives to ask permission. Moreover, men often spoke of children as a kind of "fence" that kept wives within the domestic and agricultural sphere: a wife might want to stroll around town or visit kin, but once she had young children, the amount of labor she had to do would keep her housebound. Thus, although men worried that wives would find out about their extramarital dalliances through gossip, most were supremely confident that their wives were at home and would never actually witness them flirting or negotiating rendezvous with women in the marketplace.

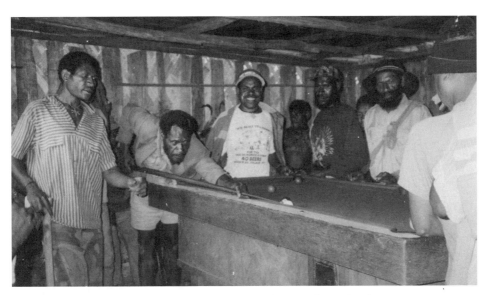

Huli men typically socialize in all-male spaces such as small snooker houses. Women rarely enter these all-male domains. Photograph by Holly Wardlow.

In addition to the Tari main market, the one other space that men frequently mentioned as a venue for finding extramarital partners was the *dawe anda* (literally, "courtship house"; see Wardlow 2006b for a detailed discussion). Traditionally, the *dawe anda* had been a cultural institution that enabled married men to find additional wives. Never-married and newly married men had not been allowed to attend, since just being in the overtly erotic atmosphere was thought to be dangerous to virgin male bodies and inappropriate to newly married men's proper goals of reproduction and establishing a secure household. Married women were and are strictly prohibited, and when spouses catch each other at a *dawe anda* (typically because a wife suspects her husband of going to one and follows him there; more rarely because a wife has decided to try to make some money selling food or cigarettes just outside the *dawe anda* fence), a violent altercation is virtually guaranteed.

Ritually, the *dawe anda* has not changed much from the past: men and women gather at night in a well-secluded house, where the men form competitive singing teams and vie for the women. The women sit together on one side of the house while the teams take turns serenading each woman with traditional courtship songs that employ erotic metaphors. Only after a woman has chosen a particular man are the teams supposed to move on to the next woman. What has changed is that *dawe anda* are now described by many people as *haus guap* (literally, "houses for going up"; that is, houses for sex). In other words, *dawe anda* now serve more as brothels than as venues for men to find additional wives. While some of the women who attend hope to find husbands, it is often because they have spent a year or more as passenger women, have tired of the stigma and violence associated with sex work, and are hoping to reintegrate themselves into their communities and reinvent themselves (to the extent possible) as respectable women. And although some men do develop enduring relationships with particular *dawe anda* women and end up taking them as third wives (the second wife role is usually considered too prestigious for a *dawe anda* woman), men generally consider *dawe anda* women unsuitable marriage partners. Most men who participate in *dawe anda* do so either for the male camaraderie of singing traditional Huli songs together or for sex.

Although the various Christian missions have tried to discourage *dawe anda*, and although the hospital (when it had more money) used to pay the police to burn down *dawe anda* sites and to arrest *dawe anda* women, the *dawe anda* remains a robust social institution. There are a number of reasons for this, but an important one is the way in which "the family house" and the *dawe anda* have become mutually constructing sexual geographies. While the Christian missions have successfully promoted the idea that God wants husbands and wives to live together and that the nuclear family house is therefore the morally preferable way to organize social space, they have not succeeded in ameliorating the discomfort men experience at having to spend prolonged periods of time in "the family house" (Wardlow 2008b). Ironically, some men say that the missions—and their promotion of spousal co-residence—have made *dawe anda* more necessary, since many men no longer have their own houses to escape to. After a long day spent gardening, cooking, eating, and talking with wives, many men spoke with relief of being able to spend their nights singing erotic songs, competing with other male teams, engaging in bawdy joking, and being chosen by *dawe anda* women who then were willing to have sex for not too much money. In a sense, men's participation in *dawe anda* can be seen as a kind of resistance to the modern, nation-making hegemony of the companionate marriage ideal in which masculinity is domesticated, tribal warfare is pacified, and men are expected to sacrifice their autonomy for the benefits of marital intimacy. As Stephen Tomsen comments, men's popular leisure activities (in the case he examines, Australian men's drunken fighting) can "often be understood as a form of symbolic protest against aspects of bourgeois morality (hard work, saving, self-discipline and useful leisure)" (1997: 91), and this social protest overlaps with "constructing a strong or tough male image" (1997: 96).

Social Risk: The "Safety" of "Women Who Don't Belong to Anyone"

The social risks of men's extramarital sex—particularly with whom to have it—pivot around the issue of bridewealth. The importance of bridewealth has both intensified in the contemporary context and become more problematic. On the one hand, marriage is defined as the transfer of bridewealth from a man's family to his bride's family, and only when bridewealth has been given is a marriage considered legitimate. Women who have sex with men outside of the system of bridewealth marriage are usually considered passenger women; thus, social respectability is tied to bridewealth. Moreover, as economic opportunities have evaporated and people are no longer able to pay for things like school fees, bridewealth has become an important means of acquiring cash. Indeed, people continually seek reasons for inflating bridewealth demands; some families, for example, now demand that a fiancé's family reimburse them for their daughter's education-related expenses (high school and tertiary tuition fees, transportation, uniforms, etc.). On the other hand, because bridewealth demands have increased dramatically, young, unemployed men now find it very difficult to get married, and once married, husbands often expect obedience from wives as a kind of recompense for the hardships they endured amassing the money for bridewealth.

Men also say that bridewealth distinguishes which women are sexually off-limits because they "belong" to their husbands. Once a man has given bridewealth to his wife's family, it is understood that he has sole claim to her sexual and reproductive body. Thus, bridewealth is as much a compact between men as it is a tie of obligation between husband and wife, and men's extramarital liaisons—at least with married women—were described by most men in the sample as transgressions against other men. This male compact is enforced by the threat of violence: adultery, which in the Huli language literally means stealing a man's wife, can lead not only to punitive violence against the wayward wife but also to retaliatory violence against her male partner and his clan. Thus, when asked what the possible consequences were if a man had extramarital sexual relations, the most common answers were "tribal warfare," "being taken to village court," and "having to pay compensation to a woman's husband." Anxieties about damaging one's marriage or hurting a wife's feelings were less common.

An important corollary of this conceptualization of marital infidelity is that as long as a man's extramarital sexual liaisons do not infringe upon other men, little moral disgrace and few social or economic penalties are attached to the liaisons. A man's sexual itinerancies are only consequential to his community—and thus count as infidelity—if he foolishly and selfishly ignores their interests by having sex with an already married woman or a young woman whose bridewealth he cannot afford to pay. Thus, as many men said, it is only common sense for a man to avoid marital discord through secrecy about his extramarital liaisons, but he has a moral obligation to protect his kin from tribal fighting and compensation claims by choosing "safe" partners—traditionally, widows and divorced women. "Safe" in this context means sex that is less likely to result in retaliatory violence or in adverse economic consequences for one's self and one's clan.

Traditionally, the only safe extramarital female partners were widows and divorced women—i.e., women who occupied a liminal social position because their earlier marriages had removed them from the custody of their fathers but their divorces or spouses' deaths meant that they were no longer in the custody of husbands. However, passenger women (who are sometimes divorced or widowed, but more often abandoned by husbands or on the run from them) now comprise an important category of "safe" women. The following quote was typical of what men had to say about their safe extramarital partners: "I have been careful not to have sex with married women. I wanted to avoid any trouble with other men, and so I've had sex with divorced women or widows. I've also avoided young women who had reputations for being well-controlled by their parents or brothers. Usually, I just try to find passenger women. You know—women who don't belong to anyone." Many of the factors discussed here make *dawe anda* appealing places for men: the passenger women there are "safe," it is a venue for some men to display and share their wealth with their less fortunate peers, men can be fairly sure that their wives will not find them there, and although women are present, the atmosphere is reminiscent of the way bars and pepper-soup joints are described in the Nigerian case: the singing is male singing, the boisterous banter is male banter, and the drama is male drama.

Married Women's Strategies: Colluding with "the Secret" or Violent Confrontation?

Before the "Love, Marriage, and HIV" research team as a whole began this research, we had two rough, competing formulations of the possible relationship between increasingly pervasive ideologies of companionate marriage and married women's risk for HIV. On the one hand, it was possible that ideologies of marital intimacy, trust, and companionship might be a sort of safeguard—making it *less* likely that men would engage in extramarital sexuality (whether that was because of guilt, fear of social censure, or satisfaction at home). Certainly this would seem to be the underlying premise or hope of some "be faithful" HIV prevention campaigns (Wardlow 2007). Alternatively, we thought it was possible that ideologies of companionate marriage (in tandem with other factors, such as male migration or women's economic dependency) might make women *more* vulnerable to HIV because of a woman's need to ignore a husband's infidelity and to maintain the appearance of a union based on love and trust (Hirsch et al. 2002).

We found evidence of both of these dynamics, but the latter pattern seemed to stand out more conspicuously in most of the field sites. In Nigeria, for example,

> women have multiple reasons to remain silent about suspicions or evidence of their husbands' extramarital affairs. In more modern marriages . . . women risk undermining whatever leverage they have because their influence is directly

tied to the presumption of an intimate and trusting relationship. . . . Women are less willing to call on their kin and in-laws for support in such cases, not only because these marriages are more independent from extended families but also because of the ideology that in such marriages a man's happiness (and thus his proclivity to seek outside women) is directly related to the capacity of his wife to please him. (Smith 2007: 1002)

Thus, there would appear to be a number of factors that motivate women to keep "the secret" of their husband's infidelities. There is, of course, women's economic dependency, which may make a husband's sexual fidelity a secondary concern as long as economic fidelity is maintained. Further, as Smith's observations suggest, in some contexts—in this study, most notably Vietnam and Nigeria, but also Mexico and Uganda to some extent—women bear the emotional and erotic onus for maintaining the companionate marriage: if a husband strays, the wife may be blamed for failing to be a good companion. Finally, it is important to remember that an important dimension of the ideology of companionate marriage is the "privatization" of the couple. That is, the ideology of companionate marriage emphasizes the primacy—and privacy—of the emotional intimacy between spouses: the marital relationship is meant to be the couple's own business, extended family should not feel entitled to interfere, and neither husband nor wife should seek out others' intervention, except perhaps in cases of domestic violence. In other words, the intimacy of companionate marriage is often expressed through neolocal residence (rather than living with extended family) and through a conviction that it is the right and responsibility of the couple to monitor, manage, and repair their own relationship (including conflicts over infidelity). This conviction is often accompanied by a sense that because the couple is supposed to find pleasure and satisfaction primarily in each other, the failure to do so is shameful and should be kept hidden. It is often women who maintain their own respectability as good wives by managing the appearance of their marriages as harmonious and loving, which may include ignoring a husband's sexual itinerancies.

The Huli field site was conspicuous, then, in comparison with the other field sites, for women's resistance to this "privatization" of the marital relationship, particularly when it came to men's infidelities. First, unlike the researchers in the other project sites, I encountered almost no discourse suggesting that a man's adultery is somehow the fault of his wife; not once, for example, have I heard a Huli person, male or female, say that because a wife didn't satisfy her husband sexually she was to blame for his going to a *dawe anda*. Indeed, both men and women expressed ambivalence about the eroticization of marital sexuality. As I noted at the beginning of this chapter, Miriam's marriage had been an exception in terms of mutual sexual pleasure being an explicit and candidly articulated goal; recall that Miriam's delight about her marriage was in part due to her sense that their sexual practices were transgressive, distinctively un-Huli, and thus symbolic of a unique intimacy. In contrast, most of the Huli male and female research participants expressed strong reservations about prioritizing sexual pleasure within marriage. They asserted that marital sex is dangerous as well as pleasurable; that sexual substances have potent physical properties and should be carefully managed; that sex should be limited to reproductive purposes; that nontraditional, unregulated sex makes husbands and wives *overly* intimate and thus more likely to quarrel; that openly expressing desire and pleasure can destabilize marital relations of power, potentially positioning one spouse as the vulnerable desirer and the other as the powerful desired; and that while marital sexuality is, of course, private, it is also public in the sense that a couple's excessive sex, or their failure to confine sex to its proper meaning and purpose, can affect the health of society and the cosmos (Wardlow 2008).[9] Thus, the idea that a wife could be erotically inadequate, and therefore to blame for her husband's infidelity, was alien to most participants.

Since women did not attribute their husband's infidelities to some inadequacy of their own, most did not feel that airing such "dirty laundry" might be embarrassing to themselves. Rather than worrying over whether other people might find out and trying to preserve the appearance of domestic harmony, they were often quick to make such knowledge public, to insist on having a hearing in village court, and to demand compensation from husbands. Very few women spoke of colluding with "the secret" of men's extramarital sexuality, and as mentioned above, most had no compunction about creating loud, confrontational, and sometimes violent public scenes when a husband's infidelities were discovered. For example, much like Miriam, when Helen suspected her husband of cheating, she hunted him down at his favorite drinking club and stabbed him and the woman he was with. As she put it,

> He initially told me that she was a relative of his on his mother's side, but it turned out he was sleeping with her. There were two incidents when I cut that woman with a knife, and three times that I cut him with a knife. Once he had to go to the hospital and get eight stitches, and another time he had to get four stitches. . . . Finally I said, "I might end up killing you, and then I would be causing a lot of trouble for my clan. So you tell the company to transfer you to some other hotel. [Both Helen and her husband worked for the same tourism company, he as a driver and she as a maid.] We shouldn't live in the same place—I might end up dead, or you might end up dead, or she might end up dead. And then we are causing trouble for all of our clans. So get a transfer and take that woman with you."

When another woman's husband came home late and drunk, she accused him of cheating and threw boiling water in his face while all their neighbors looked on.

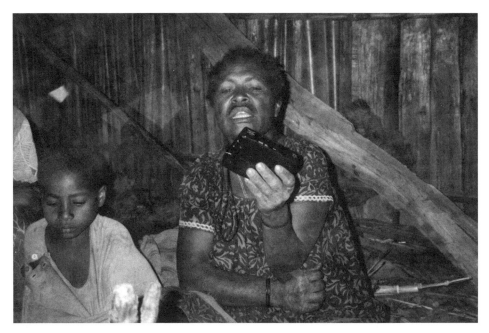

Most Huli female participants were not reluctant to share their stories of romance, marriage, and marital conflict. Photograph by Holly Wardlow.

Another woman's husband worked as a high school teacher and was unexpectedly transferred to a boarding school a day's journey from where they were living. When she learned he was being "too friendly" with one of the female students, she took a bus to the school and "beat him in the head with a stick." Finally, another woman who was reluctant to beat her husband because she "loved him and wanted to be a good Christian" was angrily confronted by her three sisters who told her that she was "indulging his bad behavior as if he were a child," and that if she "wasn't willing to show her self-respect by whipping him in the head, then, of course, he would not respect her either."

It would seem, then, that to the extent that ideologies of companionate marriage smuggle in Christian bourgeois expectations about female respectability and forbearance, and thus require women to suffer men's sexual and other infractions in silence, Huli women—despite their stated desires for love-based marriages and more marital intimacy—reject companionate marriage and its attendant pressure to keep "the secret" of male infidelity. If men can be said to resist the aspects of companionate marriage that would literally domesticate them and reduce their autonomy, women resist the aspects that would transform female physical and verbal assertion from practices that demonstrate a woman's self-respect and that enable her to secure public support to behaviors seen as undignified, unseemly, and backwards.

Conclusion

Although the descriptors "traditional" and "untraditional" are problematic and are typically avoided by anthropologists, I think it is fair to say that Huli men's extramarital sexuality is in fact untraditional, and in the precolonial context was strongly discouraged. The dramatic change in men's extramarital sexual behavior and in what it means to them is largely driven by structural factors, such as an organization of economic opportunity that requires men to leave home to make money. Indeed, the colonial and postcolonial history of Tari is a history in which men's extramarital sexuality has increasingly become the norm, suggesting that men's extramarital sexuality is intimately interwoven with processes of development. In particular, it would seem that economic policies that interpellate and recruit men as moveable bodies for labor are simultaneously policies that produce extramarital sexuality, a conclusion also supported by the Mexican case. In addition, men's extramarital sexuality is also shaped by their resistance to the domesticating ideologies of companionate marriage and by their "surplus time," which again is largely a consequence of their marginalization in the changing national and global economies.

The rare exceptions to Huli women's typically confrontational responses to male infidelity reveal the important ways in which the companionate marriage ideal is tied to class status and patterns of consumption (Illouz 1997). There were two women in the sample who, fully aware of their husbands' philanderings, either said nothing or privately appealed to them to stop. Both of these women were married to civil servants, and both said that they worried that an aggressive response would jeopardize their children's future. Having risen into the middle class through marriage, they were not about to risk divorce and the possibility that their children might descend into the rural poor. Moreover, both women ruefully admitted that they weren't sure that they could rehabituate themselves to the life of subsistence agricultural labor. They had become used to living in government houses, cooking over kerosene stoves instead of wood fires, and spending their extra time selling used clothing (one way that a civil servant can enable his wife to have an independent income is by giving her enough start-up capital to buy a bale of secondhand clothing). Both said that trying to appeal to a husband's love and sense of responsibility was a better strategy than public confrontation (though perhaps not entirely effective, since one had been repeatedly infected with STIs by her husband). Moreover, both felt that public confrontation would be considered inappropriate, "bus kanaka" (backwards, rural, and uncivilized) behavior for a civil servant's wife.

In both cases, then, an investment in the ideologies, strategies, and proper deportment of companionate marriage went hand-in-hand with an economic investment in it. As mentioned at the outset of this chapter, companionate marriage is perceived and experienced as a unified package among the Huli: it is at once an emotional orientation toward one's spouse and a set of deportments appropriate to, or even expected of, the Christian middle class. Thus, the question of how best to exert influence over a wayward husband—through private moralizing language about the obligations of love, or alternatively, through publicly hitting him with a stick—depends both on what a woman is willing to risk economically and on how she thinks her behavior will be interpreted. These interpretations, in turn, depend on emerging class distinctions (e.g., depending on one's class identifications, female silent suffering can be perceived as either dignified or cowardly, and female aggression can be seen as either righteously defiant or embarrassingly uncouth). Thus, while the companionate ideal may offer the pleasures of marital intimacy and the promise of more egalitarian decision-making, in the Huli context it also seems to be associated with a particular Christian and middle-class construction of female propriety that "privatizes" marriage, constrains a woman's ability to make conflict public and visible, and limits her means for seeking social support. In addition to the extramarital opportunity structures discussed above, these latter aspects of companionate marriage also contribute to married women's HIV vulnerability.

6

Going Public

Modern Wives, Men's Infidelity, and Marriage

in East-Central Uganda

Shanti Parikh

It was Isabella's usually calm demeanor that made her public rampage against her husband and his lover compelling gossip.[1] After hearing news that her husband would be taking his lover to Kasokoso (the outdoor drinking area in Iganga Town), Isabella had decided it would be a perfect opportunity to catch the couple "red-handed," a phrase popularized by Uganda's tabloid media to refer to catching someone in an illicit sexual act. As the rumor went: Isabella had sat in the bushes surrounding the drinking area for almost an hour, waiting for the couple's arrival. Once her husband and his mistress had been seated outside one of the grass-thatched drinking huts, an enraged Isabella had darted from her hiding place and violently attacked the mistress with a long-handled cooking spoon while screaming profanities and accusations at the startled couple. The chaotic scene had drawn quite a crowd as the husband and other evening drinkers tried to pull the incensed wife off the mistress who was subsequently rushed to the hospital with blood dripping down her face. The sheepish husband had returned home after several days in hopes that Isabella's temper had cooled. The story quickly spread through town.

Since Charles's return from military duty on the Uganda-Zaire border about a year earlier, rumors had been circulating about his sexual trysts with women in town. I, however, had not heard of the rumors when I began my interviews with Charles.[2] During our interviews, he repeatedly declared his love and appreciation for his wife, which I had no reason to doubt. When I asked him what he does to show his wife love, he included the English phrase "being faithful," which is part of Uganda's well-known "ABC" HIV prevention mantra ("Abstinence, Be faithful, and Condom use") and a central vow in Christian marriages. His answers about love and fidelity demonstrate the flexible meanings and demonstrations of love, and how in some situations love for a wife can co-exist with extramarital relationships with little conflict. Similar to findings in Smith's chapter in this book, many residents in Iganga are tolerant about men's extramarital sexuality as long as it is conducted within acceptable parameters and in ways that do not threaten their economic and emotional bond with wives and their own social reputation.

Isabella had surely suspected her husband of having dalliances since returning from the military, I was told by several mutual friends. During an interview earlier in the month, Isabella had spoken hesitantly when asked if she had ever suspected her husband of having an extramarital lover. "It's possible," she had responded quietly, after a thoughtful pause, "for I don't know everything Charles does or everywhere he goes." But like many respectable wives, Isabella had not taken public action or spoken easily about his affairs to her friends, deciding instead to preserve her reputation as a respectable middle-class woman as well as the reputation of her marriage.[3]

Over time, however, Isabella could no longer willfully ignore her husband's brazen indiscretions without risking that her public silence would be taken as an endorsement of his behaviors or as her own weakness. If taken too far, such non-response would have eventually raised questions about her own self-respect and desire to protect herself, both of which are promoted as constructions of modern selves in development discourse and public health campaigns in Uganda. When Charles's philandering exceeded acceptable parameters for men's extramarital sexuality and became too blatant to ignore, the normally reserved and restrained Isabella was forced to react.

Had Isabella been a poorer woman in the village or simply an *ababulidho* (common woman)—who, it is assumed, have less social prestige or respectability to lose—or a woman with an already sullied social reputation, her public outrage against her husband and his lover would not have been such a tantalizing piece of gossip. But, as explored in this chapter, public demonstrations are now considered less and less socially improper, even for middle-class women, and are becoming a useful and sometimes necessary strategy for them to maintain their own reputations as modern women.

While it might be tempting to wonder if this research project prompted Isabella to become more vigilant about her husband's infidelity, I doubt that it had such a powerful effect. Rather, as I demonstrate, the timing of my research converged with discourses already circulating in Uganda that have challenged the hegemonic male sexual privilege that had undergirded men's misbehaving while simultaneously encouraging women's public inaction. I am not suggesting that these recent challenges in popular discourses—such as HIV prevention campaigns that stress fidelity, media coverage of the revised adultery laws, and the Pentecostal movement's emphasis on monogamy—have radically changed gender inequalities or marital practices. Rather, I argue that these recent discourses have provided residents of Iganga with newer moral templates and ways of thinking about and discussing older practices. They also have led to new motivations and arenas for

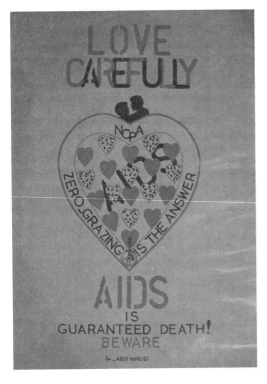
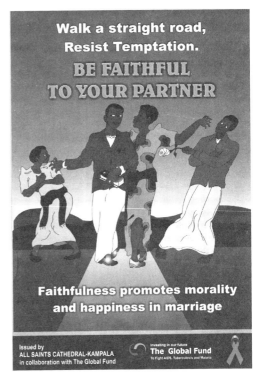

Monogamy has been a central aspect of Uganda's internationally recognized HIV public health campaign, a strategy commonly referred to as the "ABC" approach—"Abstinence, Be faithful and Condom use." From the popular "Zero Grazing" slogan during the late 1980s to more recent morality-based and Christian-influenced campaigns, everyone in Uganda is well aware of and often anxious about the connection between multiple partnerships and HIV transmission. Photographs by Shanti Parikh.

sexual secrecy as men and women seek to construct certain types of public reputations within a shifting moral landscape in which men's concurrent multiple partnerships presents a paradox for both men and women.

The Kasokoso scandal begs these questions: What does Isabella's decision to confront Charles and his mistress publicly tell us about changes in marriage, extramarital liaisons, and the wider moral and social contexts that shape both? What are the social risks and rewards associated with a wife going public or choosing to remain willfully silent about her husband's extramarital sexuality? Why would a man such as Charles so intentionally and blatantly flaunt his extramarital affairs in ways that defied prevailing conventions of respectable infidelity and risk becoming the target of his wife's anger and of wider community critique? Finally, what roles do local and popular conceptions of infidelity that blame the mistress play in the maintenance of modern marriage, and particularly in the construction of a modern woman?

The practices, conceptions, and meanings of men's concurrent partnering and wives' reactions have shifted over time and emerge within historically specific moments. In order to locate contemporary practices within Iganga's historical trajectory, in this chapter I use marital histories from three different age cohorts to chronicle how wider changes have shaped expectations and experiences of marriage, and how they have enabled historically specific forms and meanings of men's concurrent partnerships. The three historical moments I consider are colonial (1930s to 1960s), postcolonial (mid-1960s to mid-1980s) and contemporary (mid-1980s to current-day). In examining the historical shifts, I am interested in how the wives' responses and strategies make sense given the wider political and moral economies of the particular time. I provide this temporal overview in order to demonstrate two points: The first is how gender and marital propriety and strategies intersect in specific ways at different historical moments. My second aim is to highlight how men's and women's locations in Uganda's socioeconomic landscape shape the way they engage with the range of options for marriage in response or resistance to particular forms of moral regulation. Borrowing from Michel Foucault, I use the term "regulation" to mean not only judicial judgments in the form of laws or physical surveillance, but also to indicate the broader social processes of normalization through which people are disciplined through the (often very subtle) deployment and reinforcement of norms. In the process of normalization, certain marital and sexual practices are constructed as ideal or normal and others as immoral or deviant through "the deployment of force and the establishment of truth" (Foucault 1978: 184). I show here how those constructions of gendered propriety are highly gendered and classed.

Research Setting

This chapter is based on six months of ethnographic research in 2004 and two months of follow-up research in 2005 in the agrarian-based, east-central town of Iganga and its network of outlying villages, a region in which I have conducted research since 1996. Iganga Town is the rapidly growing administrative and commercial center for Iganga District (the population of the district was roughly 600,000 in 2004). The town sits along the Trans-Africa Highway, which is the major international road that runs from the coast of Kenya through Rwanda and into the Democratic Republic of the Congo. The Bantu-based, patrilineal Basoga is the main ethnic group in Iganga, though other Ugandan and East African ethnic groups have easily integrated into the community. Over the last few decades, many East Indians have opened shops and businesses in town.[4]

Historically, residents of Iganga relied on subsistence agricultural and livestock activities, and Basoga living closer to Lake Victoria also engaged in small-scale fishing. To meet their needs in an increasingly monetized economy, today households must supplement farming with other income-generating activities such as small trading, shopkeeping, manual labor, driving bicycle or motorcycle taxis, repair work, selling cooked food, and working in service industries. Having a salaried position in a school, government office, bank, or a local branch of a development agency elevates a person's socioeconomic status, but such positions are few and more readily available to men, exacerbating gender inequalities.

When this research was conducted in 2004, Iganga Town had no formal manufacturing industry; however, given the pace of economic development in the region, it is possible that a major industry or manufacturing plant may emerge in the near future. While Iganga has no large industry, there is an active and visible informal artisan economy that sits along Iganga's portion of the Trans-Africa Highway. Its cottage industries consist of metal fabricators, carpenters, tailors, casket makers, and other craftsmen who provide residents with many of their household wares and furniture. Iganga is commonly known as "the iron-roofed town" because its landscape is dominated by hurriedly constructed buildings with patched-together iron roofs. The landscape and name call attention to the town's relatively slow formal infrastructure development and town planning as compared to its more bustling neighboring towns, Jinja and Mbale.

Like other urban settings in Uganda, Iganga Town has experienced rapid population growth over the last few decades. The population of Iganga Town, excluding the outlying rural areas, has grown from twenty thousand in 1990 to fifty thousand in 2003 (Iganga Municipality Profile 2004). This rapid growth reflects a general rural to urban migration in Uganda as people look for wage labor and better schools for their children. Residents commonly note how recent developments in town have led to an expansion of Iganga Town borders into outlying villages. Iganga's growth has been further facilitated by its location along the Trans-Africa Highway, as entrepreneurs from other regions have opened shops in town.

Over the past ten years of conducting research in Iganga, I have seen tremendous changes in Iganga's economy. It has gone from a sleepy, dusty town in 1996 to a small but bustling commercial and social center for residents of nearby villages in 2004. Main Street (a.k.a. the Trans-Africa Highway) has gotten so crowded with pedestrians, bicycle and motorcycle taxis, and public minivans that crossing the busy highway has become a task of dodging people, vehicles, and the occasional herd of cows or goats. There is also a growing group of middle-class professionals formed in part by the wave of young college-educated people who have moved to Iganga, either returning home after graduation or relocating for an existing or recently opened office in town. Whereas residents used to travel to the capital, Kampala, or other neighboring cities for electronic goods, the latest fashions, and other luxuries and services, now they can obtain these in Iganga. From the construction of new shops selling foreign items to the wide variety of goods and services available, Iganga's marketplace is active. A common Saturday activity is browsing through the rows of Indian- and African-owned storefronts along the main street and the maze of side streets while socializing and looking at the trendy clothes and shoes, cell phones, and other electronics brought to Iganga from the capital, neighboring Kenya, or Dubai.

Residents view the availability of modern sources of prestige and forms of consumption (such as formal education, allopathic medicine and services, and commercial leisure) and luxury goods (such as televisions, mobile phones, refrigerators, and cars) as desirable indicators of progress and modernity. But for most residents in Iganga, access to cash has not kept pace with changes in the consumer marketplace and people's desires, leading to increased socioeconomic stratification among households and tensions between husbands and wives. While there has been an influx of young professionals and a growing middle-class, un- and under-employment remain rampant in Iganga. Households are in a constant state of searching for money to afford the new luxuries and to pay for the increasing costs of everyday living, including health care, school fees, food, clothes, taxes, and the unexpected upkeep of orphans left by deceased relatives. During our research, both husbands and wives said that one of their greatest marital disappointments or sources of conflict has been not achieving the material success they had imagined for themselves; wives commonly complained that they have not seen the level of wealth their husbands had promised them during courtship. Many older residents told me that they feel they and their younger kin are poorer today than twenty years ago precisely because they cannot afford the basic essentials needed to survive in the monetized economy, much less luxury items and services. Life and marriage in Iganga can be characterized as existing in economic uncertainty, and this uncertainty has implications for marital happiness and for men's extramarital behaviors, as explored in the next section.

HIV and AIDS in Uganda: Gender, Marriage, and HIV Status Anxiety

Uganda is cited as the HIV success story in Africa. Despite the country's poor social and public health infrastructures, which had virtually collapsed during the post-independence unrest from the late 1960s to the early 1980s, President Yoweri Museveni was able to spearhead an aggressive HIV awareness campaign shortly after his regime gained power in 1986.[5] His swift and bold response has been widely credited for the 30 percent decline in HIV prevalence rates in two urban antenatal sites in the early 1990s (13 percent in eighteen sites outside of urban areas) to an estimated 10.1 percent in urban sites in 2007 (5.7 percent in rural sites) (UNAIDS/WHO 2008).[6] Most observers agree that Uganda began experiencing a decline in HIV prevalence in prenatal sentinel sites starting around 1992 in the southwestern regions of the country (Rakai and Masaka Districts and Kampala); however, considerable debate exists concerning the extent of the decline (Parkhurst 2002), how to interpret the numbers (Zaba et al. 2000), and reasons for the decline (Brody 2004; Gray et al. 2006; Green et al. 2006; Halperin and Epstein 2004; Wawer et al. 2005). During the years of President George W. Bush's PEPFAR (President's Emergency Plan for AIDS Relief) program, disagreement about the causes of declining HIV prevalence in Uganda took on new political meaning and motivations. The contention focused on whether Uganda's success was driven by the abstinence-until-marriage and fidelity messages (key components of Bush's global prevention strategy) or by structural conditions such as post-civil-war social stabilization, gender equality, protection of girl children, and the natural evolution of the epidemic (HIV mortality exceeding incidence). Most anthropologists and other observers of Uganda's situation argue that the explanations that emphasize individual behavior change models—specifically Uganda's "ABC" model—are short-sighted and fail to recognize the major role that the country's changing social, economic, and political contexts played in Uganda's HIV reduction.

Uganda's HIV prevalence decline is further complicated when one examines the trends more closely. First, there are notable gender differences in the trends. During the years of Uganda's declining HIV rates, women aged 30–34 and 35–39 (the age groups whose members are most likely to be married or ever-married and are thus the main subject of this project) comprised the only age-sex groups to experience increases in HIV rates (Mbulaiteye et al. 2002). Second, Uganda's HIV prevalence rates appear to have risen during the early 2000s. According to the World Health Organization, HIV prevalence rates rose in sentinel sites outside major urban areas from 5.1 percent in 2002 to 11 percent in 2003, and to 11.9 percent in 2004 (UNAIDS/WHO 2008). These recent increases in HIV prevalence have been used to call into question the effectiveness of abstinence-until-marriage programs and fidelity messages pursued by Bush's PEPFAR policies, as well as the limited attention paid to promoting condom use.

Uganda's HIV epidemic has had a tremendous impact on people's lives. Like other sub-Saharan countries hard hit by HIV, the twenty-five-year epidemic has exacerbated social and economic hardships for all families in Iganga (even wealthier ones) particularly because the illness tends to afflict the most productive segments of the population—young and middle-aged adults—leaving older people to care for children. Most households in Iganga have had to care for ill or dying kin, absorb orphaned relatives, and provide economic and social assistance to extended families affected by HIV. Uganda's first AIDS orphans, whose parents passed away during the mid-1980s and early 1990s, are now young adults who are trying to navigate through Uganda's difficult economic climate without the traditional security of parents and their property. The devastating impact of the country's long HIV epidemic at the individual, household, and national levels cannot be overstated.

The participants of this study were well aware that they might contract HIV from their spouses, and my research assistants and I noted how some participants were visibly anxious about the possibility. Women frequently made comments about how they did not know if their husbands were coming home with HIV, and all participants said that "remaining faithful" to one's spouse was the main way to avoid HIV transmission within marriage. Nonetheless, most wives and some husbands suspected that their spouses had had extramarital relationships at some point during their marriages. Very few participants felt they had had a productive discussion (as opposed to threats, yelling, arguments, or accusations) with their spouse about premarital or extramarital sexual behaviors, preventing illness, or getting tested for HIV. When asked if he and his wife had ever discussed HIV, one man stated, "Yes, I tell my wife that she will get HIV if she goes outside our marriage and acts like a prostitute." His comment and others like it reflect Basoga gender ideologies in which advice on propriety and reputation tends to flow from husbands to wives, and less commonly the other way. But, as I argue in this chapter, these gender ideologies that constrain and enable the marital and extramarital behaviors of husbands and wives are historically situated. I now turn to these wider historical changes.

The British Colonial Era: Economic and Legal Influences on Marriage, Polygyny, and Adultery in Iganga

Beginning in the early 1900s, British colonial policies and ideologies interacted with the precolonial Basoga agrarian economy and patrilineal kinship system in ways that provide important historical trajectories from which to understand contemporary marriage and men's extramarital sexuality in Iganga. Marriage in Iganga was and remains an important marker of adulthood. As anthropologists have long argued, marriage is not only a relationship between two people but, at least historically, it establishes a relationship between two kin groups. This relationship between two groups is solidified through a series of bridewealth payments from the groom and his family to the bride's family (Radcliffe-Brown and Forde 1950). In the academic literature on bridewealth, as well as in residents' discussions, there are competing explanations about the purpose of bridewealth: one side suggests that bridewealth payments remunerate the bride's family for their past investments in raising and educating the young woman, and another side argues that bridewealth payments compensate the bride's family for the loss of her future labor. Although the exchange of bridewealth does not represent the buying and selling of women per se, in practice bridewealth exchange does establish a gender hierarchy within marriage in which a wife is beholden to her in-laws and to her husband. Furthermore, the patrilocal residential system, in which the couple resides near or on the land of the husband's family, can lead to the isolation of the new bride from her natal family and social networks; the insertion into a new kin network leaves her dependent on and subordinate within her husband's clan.

During precolonial times, men owned land and crops through their patriclans, and wives both provided and oversaw the labor on farms, managed the production of foodstuffs, and controlled home gardens. As historians have shown about various parts of sub-Saharan Africa, the colonial introduction of cash crops and other capitalist enterprises exacerbated gender inequalities.[7] In Uganda, the British colonial government encouraged and in some cases coerced small farmers to enter into commercial agriculture enterprises as the basis for its capitalist endeavors. In Iganga, these new crops consisted of coffee, sugar, cotton, and tea. This economic shift led to two major changes in marital gender relations. First, informed by prevailing British gender ideologies regarding property rights, colonial officials gave men greater control over economic resources, further distancing women from new forms of capitalist wealth. The workload of ordinary women increased as they were expected to work on their households' subsistence gardens as well as their husbands' cash crop farms, yet women controlled the profits from neither (see also Allman and Tashjian 2000: 3–18).

Second, more wives and children translated into greater wealth for men in the form of crop production, social prestige, and subjects (Kalema Commission 1965). Hence, polygyny became a way for men to secure labor for cash farming: both headmen whose status was inherited and enterprising capitalist farmers had incentive to marry more wives. As documented by anthropologist Lloyd Fallers, who conducted research in Iganga in the early 1950s, some women adapted to their subordinate position in the cash economy by employing creative marital strategies that gave them more control and autonomy (1969: 101–99). The interviews my research team and I conducted in Iganga echo Fallers's findings, and also illustrate many cases in which women went around the colonial system by deciding to separate from their spouses and migrate closer to town, where they could engage in income-generating activities. For instance, we interviewed an elderly man in Iganga whose father had been a prominent local chief during colonial times. He recalls his mother moving off the family compound, and attributes his own lack of economic mobility to having been raised by stepmothers who had been more interested in educating their own children. When asked why his mother had moved away, he says that while he does not know, he speculates that she had preferred to live on her own rather than as a neglected older wife of a man with many wives.

A set of contradictory marriage laws (and when and to whom to apply them) caused much contention during colonial times, creating what Allman and Tashjian described as "gender chaos" (2000: 169–210).[8] Initially, British colonial administrators did not seem concerned about polygyny, partly because the multiple wives benefited the colonial rural economic system by guaranteeing a labor supply on farms. However, Christian missionaries disagreed with what they considered the colonial administrators' complacency, for the missionaries believed that polygyny was backwards and sinful (Kalema Commission 1965; Morris 1967). Through schools and churches, the missionaries implemented a civilizing campaign in which they aggressively promoted monogamy and discouraged polygyny. They directed the campaign mainly at Uganda's small but growing number of educated Christians, believing that their targets' new middle-class sensibilities would eventually trickle down to rural peasants (see also Allman and Tashjian 2000). Local appropriation of the ideological agendas of the missionaries' civilizing and domesticating projects were slow and uneven. As will be seen, the attempt to abolish polygyny and construct it as morally and socially backwards was met with resistance and had mixed results locally.

British administrators may have been less concerned about polygyny than the missionaries were, but the high rate of divorce and separation among the Basoga—as compared to other Bantu groups—did draw their attention (Fallers 1957). Convinced that marital instability was the result of Basoga women's autonomy, British officials collaborated with local male leaders to institute laws and policies to increase rural crop production by giving husbands greater control over their unruly wives (Fallers 1969). In an effort to stabilize and regulate marriage, the 1904 Divorce Law required a full refund of bridewealth (either by the woman's father or new husband) upon the dissolution of a union, effectively making divorce more difficult for women to initiate. Fallers found that half of the domestic court cases tried in the native courts involved a man suing his wife's father for "harboring his wife" without the consent of the husband. In such cases, the husband could demand her return as well as compensation for the temporary loss of her labor (1969).

Another common offense that Fallers found was that of a man suing his wife's lover. Following British law and as outlined in the Divorce Law, adultery was defined differently for husbands and wives. For a married woman, adultery was having an affair or running off with another man. For a man, adultery was defined as sexual relations with a married woman, with the offense committed against the "owner" of the woman, such as her husband (see also Wardlow, this volume). Sexual relations with an unmarried woman was not considered adultery. The law codified a gender double standard: a man could *safely* have an extramarital liaison without any legal ramification or wider social consequence as long as it was with a woman over whom a male did not claim rights, such as a prostitute, divorcée, widow, or orphan. In other words, while a man could divorce a wife if she had extramarital sex, his own extramarital sexuality was neither legally nor socially considered grounds for divorce.

In my discussions with Iganga residents about their parents' marriages, the double standard regarding the definition and consequences of adultery clearly emerges. When asked to reflect on their parents' marriages, the oldest participants (and some younger ones) recounted stories about how their fathers' flagrant extramarital liaisons and children born of these liaisons had been at the root of their parents' marital problems and of their mothers' social and economic suffering. For instance, Tapenesi, an older woman in her late sixties whose mother had come of age during the colonial period, explained that her mother had protested her husband's repeated bringing of other women into their bedroom by eventually refusing to sleep in her matrimonial bed. She chose, instead, to sleep on the floor of their bedroom. When I asked Tapenesi how this affected her behavior within her own marriage, she responded that she had been determined to never "surrender control over my bedroom as my mother did." After she had borne five children, her husband had brought a younger woman into the home as a second wife to bear more children, without Tapenesi's prior knowledge. Remembering the fate of her mother, she had remained steadfast about giving up neither her bedroom nor her senior position in the household. She describes how this had occurred twice, with both co-wives eventually leaving when Tapenesi's stubbornness and oversight became too much for them. After two failed attempts at polygyny, her husband did not bring another woman into the house, keeping his extramarital lovers outside the home and their marriage.

Tapenesi's reflections about her mother's and her own marital strategies bring to the surface at least two points relevant to this chapter—the complicated relationship between formal polygyny and extramarital liaisons, and historical roots of women's agency in the face of their husbands' multiple partnering. First, although Tapenesi had been unable to stop her husband's relationships with other women during his younger days (he claims he is now "too old" to have mistresses), she considers it a success that she was able to prevent his attempts at polygyny and to partly control where and how he conducted his subsequent affairs. Second, while in theory polygyny and infidelity are two different phenomena in Basoga ideology, in some cases they emerge from the same social forces—men's personal motivations (be they reproduction, social prestige, or companionship) and the availability of young women. In sum, colonial policies interacted with precolonial Basoga kinship and economic systems in ways that facilitated and encouraged different types of men's multi-partnering. While the dependence of Igangan wives on their husbands was structurally bolstered through adultery and divorce laws, and they had limited resources from which to assert their marital desires, women did employ strategies of resistance, including divorce, silent protest, and managing domestic interactions.

The Postcolonial Era: The Emergence of the Middle Class and the Myth of Monogamy

The marital histories of three generations reveal a pattern in which the hegemonic notion of wealth in the form of wives and children gradually was challenged—

although it did not completely vanish—as capitalist desires and Christian ideologies were further absorbed into the local landscape. In Uganda's increasingly monetized economy, wives and children not only meant more labor for farming but also more household dependents to feed, clothe, educate, and the like. The notion of "wealth in people" as a motivator for a man to marry multiple wives was displaced—in ideology if not in practice—by the ideal of marital monogamy, particularly among Uganda's emerging elite. In some cases, in order to manage multiple partnerships while not officially participating in polygyny, wealthy men took on informal "outside wives," a term used by Wambui Wa Karanja (1987) to describe the elite Yoruba men in Lagos setting up secondary households with young professional women. These transformations in polygyny and extramarital sexuality as well as men's management of multiple partnerships are clearly demonstrated in marital histories of Iganga's first postcolonial educated adult men, for whom professional mobility and success depended on depicting a certain type of marital image to European patrons and other elite Africans (see also Obbo 1987; Mann 1994). In the literature on postcolonial elite marriages, the role that the wives played in determining and managing the desired marital configuration has been underemphasized.

Take, for example, Joshua Waigona, who had been a top civil servant in Uganda's first postcolonial government. He had married Mary in 1965; he was twenty-five and she was sixteen. He described how monogamy and big church weddings were expected at that time within his social network. While he had had several lovers before marriage who were, according to him, "ababulidho" (common women), he had selected Mary as his wife because she was "a conservative, educated girl" from one of the female boarding schools in the area. She seemed to be "well-disciplined, respectful, and gentle," and compared to his premarital lovers, he had thought that Mary would fit in nicely in his peer network and would represent him well. In addition to the pragmatics behind his selection, he elaborated on the affective basis of his choice: according to him, love and communication were essential for marital harmony, and he had demonstrated his belief in this by taking his wife with him on social outings with their group of European, African, and Indian friends and their wives. He noted how activities such as attending movies in the city, eating at fancy restaurants, and taking weekend trips were inaccessible to most Ugandans but had formed an important aspect of their middle-class identity. As he reflected on the prestige and the social worlds associated with Christian, monogamous marriage, he simultaneously talked about the various lovers he had maintained while away in England for training and in the Ugandan towns he had frequented for work. His European and African co-workers and bosses had indirectly encouraged such behavior as a form of male bonding, camaraderie, and status-building.

In the late 1970s, Joshua, Mary, and their children relocated to the capital, Kampala, so that he could to take a management position at a British company. While the family stayed in Kampala, Joshua had made frequent trips to Iganga for work and to visit his natal family. He had met and become "familiar with" the daughter of the owner of a popular pub, impregnating and eventually marrying her. The story has an interesting twist, which he discussed during one of my interviews with him. As we sat in the lovely gazebo inside his compound in Iganga Town, he explained how he had unintentionally become a polygynist:

> *Joshua:* I met her in 1980 or 1979, I think. She was born of this place, Iganga, and I used to pass through Iganga to go to my home village, where I was born. And you know every time you pass through your hometown, you are bound to go to a pub or some place like that. So I used to branch [stop off] at a pub here in Iganga. And in fact that is how I met her. She was born to the owner of the bar. And she looked attractive and you know you get there, you drink a beer and then you pass a joke one or two, but when you come once twice and then you become intimate and then, you know. And then the friendship starts there and then the relationship. That is how I think I met her.
>
> *Interviewer:* How old was she at the time?
>
> *Joshua:* She was much younger than myself. She was as old as my first son, I think. [*a quick glance at the interviewer, and slight laughter*]
>
> *Interviewer:* Did you know when you had just met that you were going to marry her?
>
> *Joshua:* Oh, no, I thought it was casual relationship, then things developed and sometimes you get reckless and somebody gets pregnant and so on. After she got pregnant, she said, "I want to go back to school. You must give me a house to stay." Then her parents came to know, and they said you must come and introduce yourself. And then my wife got involved. [*a long sigh and pause*]
>
> *Interviewer:* If she had not gotten pregnant, would your wife have known?
>
> *Joshua:* My wife knew only afterwards. She wanted me to marry the girl but keep it as a secret, but eventually it came to be known to others.
>
> *Interviewer:* Would you have married her if she had not gotten pregnant?
>
> *Joshua:* Well, I say these things are not really well planned and calculated. Very few people in my circle really plan to say, "I want to get a second wife." These come as accidents of life and you look at the girl: you have more or less spoilt her future, and then she says, "Now what do I do?" Then you say, "Okay, what do we do?" She says, "Okay, now you have to put me in some home." So I bought her a house in Wanyange and she started giving birth to children.

Ironically, it was an angry and disappointed Mary who insisted that he take his pregnant lover as a second wife, so that she could keep a watchful eye on the younger woman's behavior, and in hopes of having greater surveillance over the rumors about the affair and her marriage. Joshua initially opposed turning the extramarital liaison into formal polygyny for fear that his reputation among European patrons and other African elites would be tarnished, but in the end, he gave in to the pressure from his wife, his mother, and the mother of his pregnant lover. His second wife, however, never gained the full social status of a wife of a wealthy man. This was partly because Mary's clever planning and her position as an educated woman left no room for another wife in their social networks, and because their Christian community only recognized one formal wife. The second wife passed away in 1989, to which Mary commented, "My marriage was able to return to normal—the way it was supposed to be."

Mary's interview also revealed a more private act of rebellion: revenge sex. She stated that after discovering Joshua's infidelities, she had run away to her stepsister's house in a nearby town and had an affair with one of her neighbors. The man had tried to persuade her to leave Joshua and marry him, but Mary had said she was still in love with her husband. Mary explained that her revenge affair had allowed her to more easily forgive her husband.

Joshua and Mary's case offers insight into how marital practices and men's management of multiple partnerships became important class markers and indexes of modernity during Uganda's recent history. Although the public appearance of marital monogamy was expected by their social networks, the wealth and mobility of many middle-class professional men gave them great access to a large pool of women—who, in turn, found them highly desirable. Furthermore, while formal polygyny was frowned upon in elite circles, the maintenance of girlfriends was quietly accepted and facilitated by men's peer groups. Although Joshua formalized his marriage with his second wife, it was and still is not uncommon for a long-term girlfriend relationship to turn merely into an informal secondary household, particularly after the birth of a child. Joshua and Mary's story also reveals the way in which a wife can participate in presenting a certain type of public appearance of her marriage in order to maintain her public reputation as well as to exert some influence over her husband's actions.

Poorer men's marital histories show class differences in the men's management of multiple partnerships and the strategies employed by the wives of cheating husbands. For instance, a contemporary of Joshua, Mugoya, was a peasant farmer outside Iganga Town during this same period. Unable to pay the costs associated with formally marrying a second wife, including the bridewealth, he opted to maintain a series of lovers outside of his marriage, one of whom was a premarital girlfriend. According to him, his jealous wife had confronted him about his infidelities, and when she did not get the response she desired, she had eventually begun "running around the village," spreading rumors and complaining about his behaviors to neighbors. Frustrated and embarrassed by her public outbursts, Mugoya had decided to "chase her away" (a common phrase meaning to divorce or force a woman to leave, often against her will) and later married a "more respectable woman" who kept their marital issues more private. As in the past, the first wife had had limited legal or social recourse, and she had most likely left the marriage with no matrimonial property and with limited claim over the children if Mugoya had demanded custody. Hence, going public meant she had risked not only the reputation of her marriage but also the economic support of her husband. Since women did not inherit or legally own property, remaining silent would have been a more prudent strategy, and in some cases still is.

The Contemporary Era: Modern Marriage and the Project of "Developing the Home"

Scholars have noted that over the last fifty years, changing consumer markets, the monetization of daily needs, and global influences regarding the significance of individuality (as opposed to kin obligations) in the expression of modern love have had a tremendous impact on people's notions of modern marriage (see also Ahearn 2001; Bailey 1988; Collier 1997; Wardlow and Hirsch 2006; Illouz 1997; Rebhun 1999). The same can be said of marriage in Iganga. In our study, both men and women described marriage today in terms of "developing the home," in which the primary goal is to acquire consumer goods, formal education for offspring, and social and economic status within the community. According to both wealthy and poor people in Iganga, this goal requires mutual economic and emotional commitment from husbands and wives to the marital project, the cornerstone of which is communication and cooperation.

When discussing modern marriage with us, people in Iganga conceptualized it as intricately intertwined with and shaped by the wider demands of the economy, and talked about how selecting a marriage partner is motivated by individual desires, kin obligations, and economic considerations. As they reflected on their fathers' multiple wives and numerous children, they stated how the large number of dependents hindered their own ability for economic and social advancement, since their fathers' resources were distributed among many. Both the men and women in our study saw multiple wives and many children as obstacles to and the antithesis of modern and successful marriages. Men were very critical of what they believed to be their fathers' irresponsible use of income on women other than their own mothers, although this did not necessarily stop them from engaging in similar behaviors. Women commented on their mothers' passivity and seeming complacence regarding their fathers' philandering. As a result, when asked how they wanted their marriages to be different from those of their parents, most men and women said that they wanted fewer children and more equal participation in decision-making and income-generation. The joint economic and social investments in developing a modern household were regularly contrasted to the past in which husbands were seen as autocratic leaders who made decisions without input from or consent of their wives. Today wives can and do express their anger to hus-

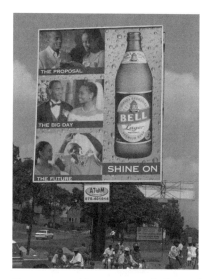 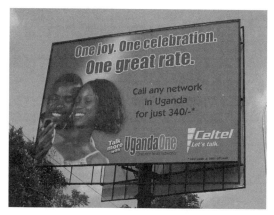

Romance and love are regularly used to sell modern goods and lifestyles in Uganda, building on and fueling residents' ideas of modern relationships based on intimacy and togetherness. Photographs by Shanti Parikh.

bands who misuse household funds for their own pleasures, including inquiries about suspected extramarital liaisons.

Recent global ideologies have also placed importance on the display of emotional and intimate bonds in marriage. These have been absorbed in Iganga's local landscape in ways that have influenced the moral economy of marriage. Uganda's economic and social liberalization policies under President Yoweri Museveni have contributed to the proliferation of global ideas, media, and goods in Uganda. The commercialization of romance is reflected in Uganda's vibrant marketplace, where images of romance and love are regularly used in advertising. They not only sell consumer goods and services but they also promote a certain image and ideal of a modern relationship. Stories and advice programs about love, pleasurable sex, and how to keep one's mate monogamous are in-demand features in Uganda's daily newspapers, glossy lifestyle magazines, and radio shows, and such concerns also drive a thriving commercial counseling industry.

While the commercialization of love has allowed people to achieve modern marriages through consumption and public representations of affection, Uganda's aggressive HIV prevention campaigns have served to further reinforce public discourses of monogamous relationships and fidelity. The omnipresent public health campaigns have provided medical reasons and scientific support for avoiding certain types of sexual behaviors in favor of marital fidelity and partner reduction. The Igangan residents in this study recited earlier HIV prevention slogans such as "Zero Grazing" and "Love Carefully" when discussing reasons for monogamy

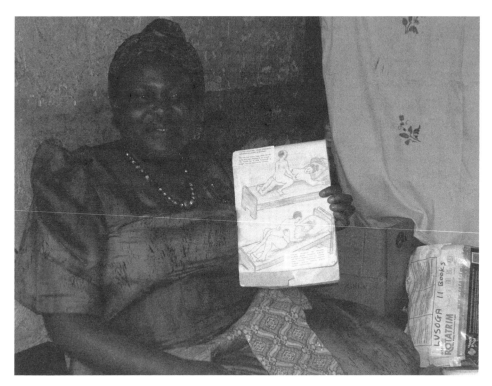

Ugandans are surrounded by messages on how to improve their sex and love lives. The *ssenga* (paternal aunt) has evolved from the kin-based "traditional" sex educator of unmarried adolescent girls to a profitable commercial icon. Today *ssenga* is used as a label for a variety of sex advice services such as newspaper columns, radio shows, television programs, and even this sex counselor's shop near Iganga Town. She holds a sex manual that she drew and is surrounded by the local medicines she uses to treat sexual problems such as impotence, jealousy, and unrequited love. Photograph by Shanti Parikh.

and partner reduction. Simultaneously, within the last couple of decades, the quickly growing Evangelical Pentecostal (or, "born again") movement has had a tremendous impact on residents' ideas about the connections among marriage, monogamy, and capitalist consumption. Many residents, particularly younger and university educated ones, have left the churches established during the British colonial period (Anglican, Protestant, and Catholic) and are flocking to the Pentecostal and other charismatic churches that have sprung up around Iganga and Uganda in general.[9] Many of these churches feature local or traveling preachers who are surrounded by material wealth, further reinforcing the connections between Christian ideals and capitalist accumulation. In sermons, weekend conferences, and seminars, these churches have put marriage, sexual restraint, and abstinence at the center of their agendas and activities, turning marital practices into

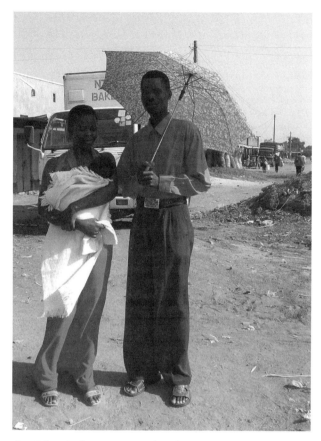
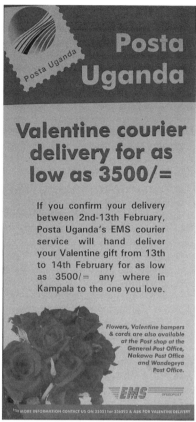

On Valentine's Day, married and unmarried young couples proudly parade around town dressed in red, publicly declaring their love. Photographs by Shanti Parikh.

moral (versus kinship) issues. Several leaders of the Pentecostal churches in Iganga told me that they suspect that the HIV epidemic and people's fear of the virus have attracted to their churches people who are looking for hope, a moral compass, and safe (both morally and disease-free) mates.

Both men and women in our study thought that monogamy was economically and socially more desirable than polygyny. Although the ideal of monogamy was pervasive, actual practice was different. In a baseline study I conducted in 1998, about a third of all household heads ($N = 423$ households) in my sample village were at that time in a polygynous union (Parikh 2001). People in Iganga hold conflicting thoughts about today's constructions of ideal marriage: On one hand, older people and some younger ones regularly lament the decay of marriage as an institution, which they see demonstrated by the decline of family involvement and the frequency with which young people enter into informal marriages without the consent (or sometimes the knowledge) of senior kin.[10] As one participant said,

"Marriage today is the result of pregnancy." Some argue that this is a strategy to ensure the reproductive capabilities of a potential spouse (most often that of a potential wife). Christine Obbo wrote of elite Ugandan women's double constraints: unmarried women "must try to prove that their chastity is beyond reproach . . . while they must also demonstrate their fertility" (1987: 265).

On the other hand, most residents feel that today's emphasis on monogamy represents a positive shift, as it allows people to invest their emotional, economic, and labor resources more effectively into a smaller family unit. While it may seem contradictory on the surface, the belief that monogamy is an achievable ideal is held simultaneously with the belief that men's infidelity is virtually inevitable and sometimes expected. But as my data suggests, moral discourses against men's poly-partnering and the threat of HIV infection have enabled more women, elite and poor, to make their grievances public. If the practice of men's concurrent sexual liaisons is under increasing public attack, what opportunity structures exist and how does Iganga's sexual geography continue to enable and facilitate extramarital sexuality?

Opportunity Structures and the Sexual Geography of Men's Extramarital Liaisons

Notions of modern marriage—in which marital success is defined by monogamy and the capitalist endeavor of developing the home—have been gradually, partially, and contradictorily absorbed into everyday realities in Iganga. Residents in Iganga recognize that wider social and economic forces have set an ideal stage for male extramarital sexuality, making it almost impossible for couples to achieve marital monogamy throughout their entire marriage. Three main opportunity structures facilitating men's extramarital liaisons in Iganga emerged in our research, namely (1) gendered patterns of mobility within Iganga's sexual geography, (2) unmet marital expectations, and (3) a distorted economic and demographic structure that had resulted in a perceived abundance of *nakyewombekeire* (free young women who are unattached to a father or husband). Socially respectable husbands are expected to manage their extramarital affairs in ways that keep them safely hidden from certain social groups, kin groups, religious communities, and the like.

In order to illustrate how these opportunity structures are interconnected and play themselves out on the ground, I will return to this chapter's opening vignette involving Charles, Isabella, and the schoolteacher. I do so in order to highlight where he transgressed social convention and why his wife could no longer comfortably ignore his actions, which I argue were scandalous not because he took advantage of the opportunity structures and had an extramarital liaison, but precisely because he decided to transgress the social conventions of secrecy. I also discuss what types of behaviors can be done in which spaces in Iganga's sexual geography.

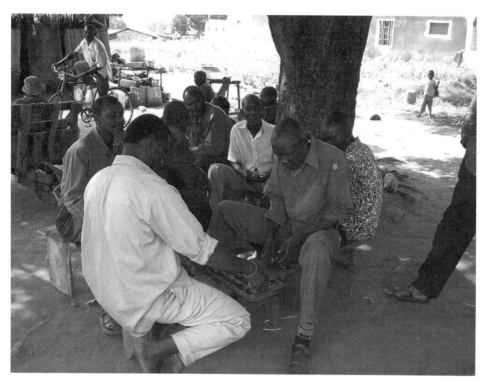

Men's leisure spaces in Iganga Town offer places away from home and the village where men can joke with each other about relationships or meet up with extramarital lovers. Photograph by Shanti Parikh.

Gendered Mobility and Infidelity: "He Wanders All Day and Night"

While research on sexuality and HIV infection in sub-Saharan Africa has drawn attention to the role that labor-related migration plays in men's extramarital sexuality and the spread of HIV (Anarfi 1993; Campbell 1997; Jochelson et al. 1991; Romero-Daza and Himmelgreen 1998; Schoepf 1988), this chapter highlights two aspects that are often neglected in discussions of men's extramarital sex—the gendered nature of daily mobility patterns and how daily mobility patterns shape men's and women's experiences with extramarital sexuality. Temporary migration for work or education is no doubt a common feature of people's lives in Iganga, but a more salient characteristic is daily, prosaic mobility within the Iganga region.[11] These daily patterns of mobility are highly gendered and an integral part of performing gender prestige and identity. As the chapters on Mexico and Vietnam in this book nicely demonstrate, differences in men's and women's economic opportunities interact with gendered patterns of mobility and structure men's access to extramarital sex. The gendered daily mobility patterns of Iganga's residents interact with its sexual geography in ways that allow men to engage in a variety of recreational and extramarital activities outside the purview and scrutiny of their wives, neighbors, kin, and other critical observers.

The anonymity of Iganga Town is partly the result of population growth and rural-urban mobility connections. In 2003, the estimated residential population of Iganga Town was fifty thousand, while the day population was estimated to be close to eighty thousand. This population swell of about 60 percent reflects the increasing rural-urban circulation found throughout Uganda as rural residents access urban services, employment, social networks, and transportation hubs. Younger and adult males account for the majority of daily commuter traffic; many remain in town each evening as Iganga transforms from its structure of daytime businesses and formal markets into a lively nighttime outdoor bazaar with a wide variety of drinking and eating places peppering the landscape. An irony emerges: although husbands are considered the "rulers" of their households, many men feel they have a limited place in the home. According to a middle-class public servant, "If you go home, what is there for you? Your wife quarrels with you about this and that; wonders why you are not looking for money. Or, she and children have their chores so you sit alone. Nothing to do."

The semi-anonymity of town and its social distance from overseeing wives and kin serve to facilitate men's sexual networking (see also Pickering 1997). Married women with young children tend to have particularly limited mobility (because of breastfeeding and other childraising obligations) and often encounter a shrinking in their social networks, leaving them more dependent on husbands and nearby in-laws and less able to keep an eye on their husbands' recreational activities. For instance, Mariam, a young woman in her early twenties, was newly married with one young infant and pregnant with another. Her responsibilities of caring, cooking, and cleaning for her own child, her aging parents-in-law, and the orphans from her husbands' relatives meant that she had very little time to leave the family compound, let alone the village. At most, she ventured to town once a week to shop at the municipal market on a bicycle taxi that her husband had arranged. The bicycle taxi waited while she shopped and sometimes carried her goods through the market, limiting Mariam's opportunity to make small talk with other women.

During an interview, Mariam proudly told me of a recent time when she had gone to town to meet a cousin who was in town for a wedding—that is, for a reason other than to shop at the market or run an errand arranged by her husband. Being new to the region, she had not explored the town or made friends with anyone other than her neighbors in the village. However, her husband, who had been raised in the area, had an elaborate social—and, it turned out, sexual—network, which was ever-expanding given his growing business of buying and selling fish to markets outside Iganga Town. When asked what her husband did that made her sad, disappointed, or upset, Mariam responded, "He wanders all day and night." She said she would like to ask about his whereabouts and daily activities, but she felt he would not tell her and seemed to fear the consequences of seeming too inquisitive. That he was a good economic provider and returned home most nights was how Mariam said he was a good husband. While the contrast between Mariam's highly supervised and limited mobility and her husband's great daily mobility was more extreme than for most of the couples I met in Iganga, it demonstrated how gendered mobility structures husbands' extramarital sexuality and impedes wives' knowledge of their husbands' actions and whereabouts.

In his ethnographic study of sexuality in Guadalajara, Héctor Carrillo argues that the city's radical transformations from daytime activities to nightlife are marked by a shift in sexual propriety; the evening allows for behaviors and personal comportment that would not be acceptable during the day (2001). Similarly, in Iganga, the evening sexual landscape allows an outlet for behaviors that on a wider social level have been rejected as reprobate and morally inexcusable. In other words, although recent moral ideology has dictated that certain behaviors and places are immoral and scandalous, the historical and social forces from which they emerged still exist, pointing to an ambivalence about the expectations of modern morality. More than once, I witnessed an unspoken code of silence being upheld when I saw people I knew from more professional or morally upright settings in places considered morally questionable such as bars, pool halls, discos, and even once a video hall showing porn movies.

Charles's scandal shows how things can go wrong when a husband does not adequately (whether intentionally or not) hide his affairs from his wife or their mutually shared social networks. As a professional woman, Isabella's social and physical mobility extended to Iganga Town, where she came in regular contact with Charles's evening drinking buddies. Moreover, like many wives of absent husbands, she had become more familiar with various networks and more mobile around Iganga Town while Charles was away for military service, in order to obtain basic necessities for their household and keep up with local happenings. Given Isabella's unusually expansive social world in Iganga, Charles would have needed to conduct his extramarital liaison much more secretly or in another town, as some middle-class men tended to do. In short, Charles had not adequately kept the evidence and rumors of his affairs contained to the spaces that existed away from his wife and their shared social network, subsequently calling into question his respect for his wife, himself, and the expectations of their friends and family.

Unmet Expectations of Modern Marriage
Consumer goods and modern lifestyles have become markers of successful modern marriages. Yet given fluctuations in individual income and expenses, they are often unobtainable or unsustainable for many residents in Iganga, and in Uganda as a whole. We asked the wives in our study why they had decided to marry their spouses (as opposed to other men who might have been courting them). A common answer was that they had been attracted to the economic promises and statements about upward mobility that their husbands had made. When a husband

could not meet his premarital promises of wealth and luxuries, it frequently led to frustrations and disagreements within the marriage. In order to avoid conflict and questions about their failed economic pursuits, a strategy that men employed was to stay away from home, finding solace in mistresses who seldom required the same financial investment as wives and households. While lovers frequently demanded some material reward such as rent, money, gifts, or assistance with children, they did not require the same amount of emotional attention as wives, and the men had freedom to use their money as they wished without being subject to criticism.

While marital discord caused by unmet economic expectations leads some men into extramarital liaisons, discourses that have challenged gender inequalities within modern marriage cause a different set of problems. Although women generally believe that the social campaigns surrounding gender reform and women's rights are positive, some husbands see them as threatening to their status. A man in his late sixties explains the effects of Uganda's gender equality campaigns on marriage:

> Women [in the past] had good discipline. They were not behaving like today's young wives. There was a lot of respect given to the husband. If the man said, "I want to find such a thing done," that will be final and by the time he came back, the thing will have been done. The wife would not have any complaint or anything to add. Marriage then was good, although there was a lot of wife beating.

Throughout this research project and the ones I previously conducted in Iganga, men repeatedly expressed the feeling that their masculine authority—once seen as both natural and a cultural given—was constantly under attack on multiple fronts, including development discourses, HIV prevention messages, women's rights campaigns and legislation, and popular songs, plays, and radio shows. Charles's actions can be read as a "protest" against the new gender regime in his marriage and perhaps in Uganda in general.[12] While he was away, Isabella's work as a secretary for an international development agency had basically supported the household and many extended family members. Thus, Charles had returned from the military feeling as if Isabella had usurped his position of authority and that of being the primary breadwinner. Being between assignments, he had had no flow of steady money, yet he had desired to maintain the masculine prestige he had earned in the community from his deployment on secret missions and to violent regions. Importantly, by selecting a woman from the professional class, a schoolteacher, instead of the more usual barmaid or unemployed young woman, he had asserted that he had the financial and romantic ability to win over even middle-class women.

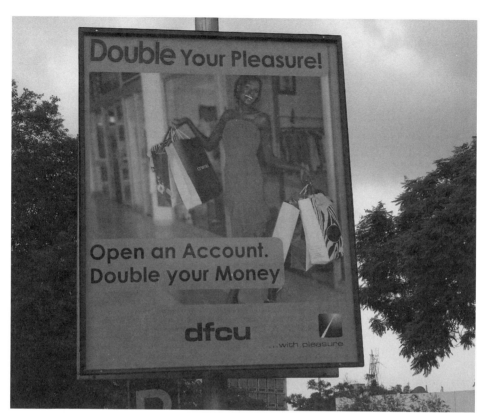

According to popular discourse, young women's desire for luxury goods leads them into relationships with married men who are willing to give them money and gifts. This common interpretation of men's infidelity renders married men as innocent victims to young women's material desires. The mistress is frequently blamed for the affair, not the married man, allowing some wives the rationalization they need in order to forgive their husbands. Photograph by Shanti Parikh.

Unmarried Young Women: Nakyewombekeire

Residents of Iganga recognize how poverty drives young women into transactional (or sex-for-money) relationships with older men and sugar daddies, as commonly noted in the literature on HIV and women in Africa (see, for example, Schoepf 1997; Susser 2002). The connections between women's poverty and HIV in Uganda are reinforced by media stories and public health campaigns. The discourse about young women's vulnerability to sugar daddies, however, is often overshadowed in Iganga by moral discourses about *nakyewombekeire* (literally, "a young woman who lives on her own," which can also be understood to mean "lacking steady employment").[13] According to talk in Iganga, the growing supply of unmarried young women poses the most immediate threat to the stability of marriages. Local interpretations of the problem can be understood as a reversal of general scholarly analysis, which portrays young and adolescent women as vulnerable victims of wealthier men's sexual advances. Conversely, residents as well as the media often construct a narrative in which unmarried women are intentionally pursuing married men; particularly "vulnerable" are wealthy men and men of social power. Within this men-as-victims trope, male infidelity is depicted by men and women as less the result of men searching for women and more as a function of too many single women chasing after the few men with money. As men get more money, they are in greater demand by more women.

The anxiety surrounding young women's sexual agency has been heightened by people's awareness of the HIV epidemic and Uganda's sizable population of young people who have come of age as orphans. This pool has contributed to the growing number of young men who find themselves searching for income opportunities, suspended in menial work, or in between jobs, and consequently delaying marriage. As younger men postpone marriage for economic reasons, relationships with older and wealthier married men provide young women with opportunities for economic support and social networks. Residents of Iganga echoed messages in popular culture when they depicted attractive, nicely dressed, leisure-seeking women as preying on married men, a construction that stood in stark contrast to public health and feminist analyses. When asked why men cheat, one man remarked, "There are just too many unmarried beautiful young women without money and they simply tempt us [*light laughter*]." Both men and women in our study often blamed young women—not married men—for men's infidelities, rendering men partly innocent and absolving them from blame.

Modern Husbands: HIV Prevention Campaigns, Morality, and Managing Social Risk

In this chapter, I have chronicled how global forces—colonial economic and legal systems, the emergence of a postcolonial middle class, and today's notions of modern marriage—have interacted with marriage and gender inequalities in Iganga in ways that have transformed the practices and meanings of married men's concurrent sexual partnerships. I have argued that the formal polygyny and men's indiscreet infidelities found in Iganga residents' narratives about the past have not disappeared; rather, there have been shifts in how men's poly-partnering relates to their public reputations and status, and thus how they manage their multiple partnering. In today's shifting moral economy, dominated by religious, public health, and popular culture discourses, a new demand for discretion has emerged—an image of discretion that privileges the appearance of sexually safe and monogamous couples. Managing social reputation requires conflicting actions from men: appearing to have sexual prowess and vitality remains an important aspect of masculine status within many male peer groups, but uncontained public knowledge of his sexual exploits can ruin a man's reputation in the wider community. Hence, a man's friends or co-workers might serve as accomplices or encouragers for his dalliances, but he may also go to great lengths to keep knowledge of his extramarital relations away from people in his home and his family's social networks. Having liaisons with women not in his wife's socioeconomic group is the socially safest type of affair from the perspective of not getting caught.

Given that Uganda is held up as the global HIV success story for reducing its prevalence rates, it might be useful to look more closely at how its campaigns fit into local moral landscapes. The evidence from this project suggests that while the "ABC" message and other campaigns may have contributed to risk reduction, certain forms of morality propagated by the "ABC" approach—and more generally by the enormous presence and impact of institutional public health responses to HIV and AIDS—have created perceptions of social risk that have led to new strategies that may be counterproductive from the point of view of HIV prevention. Recent HIV prevention campaigns equating infidelity and condoms with immorality have meant that some men and women choose not to use condoms and deny their risk of HIV infection in order to maintain the appearance of being moral and monogamous; hiding their liaisons and convincing themselves that extramarital sexual encounters are not immoral are higher, more immediate priorities than the biological consequences (for a fuller discussion, see Parikh 2007).

For husbands and wives in the small town of Iganga, it is also important to keep marital problems from neighbors who might revel in the couple's misfortune or whose jealousy might have caused the marital strife in the first place. Middle-class couples are often more guarded, for they have more to lose in terms of public reputation and the effects of neighbors' jealousy.

Modern Wives: Love, Geographies of Blame, and the Other Woman

During the research period for this project, the album *Spare Tyre* was wildly popular. Beloved Ugandan wife-and-husband musicians Sophie and Sam Gombya appear on the album's cover, smiling and affectionate, with Sophie embracing her husband from behind. She appears to be vigilantly protecting him from an "other woman"—a "spare tyre," as she demeaningly refers to mistresses. The album's title song is a contemptuous rant against "ignorant" spare tyres. Singing in the language of Luganda, Sophie asserts that official wives have the real power and that mistresses are simple fools who are just being (ab)used and discarded like spare tires.[14]

The music video depicts a doting Sophie hugging and intimately touching her "husband" (portrayed by an actor). Interspersed throughout the video as dramatic asides, Sophie speaks to and points her finger at the other woman, and looking directly at the camera, she reminds all spare tyres of their subordinate and temporary position. The video ends with a defiantly bold Sophie pulling the wig off the head of the other woman in front of a crowd of onlookers, at what appears to be an intimate party at someone's house, symbolically and publicly baring the inauthenticity of her husband's lover.[15] In response to what Sophie and other wives see as such women's unapologetic and boastful flaunting of their affairs with married men, the delightfully feisty singer reminds them, "You are my helper[16] . . . / I am his real wife."

By the end of our initial research period, and during my follow-up visit the next year, "Spare Tyre" had became almost a sort of theme song for married (and many unmarried) women in Uganda, invoking delighted screams and rhythmic swaying from them whenever they heard it. The song easily resonated with women in Iganga rebelling against its history of philandering husbands. These acts of rebellion have been gaining further validation and moral support through a variety of public movements in Uganda that forcefully denounce the historical norms that have allowed men to have multiple partners without major consequences.

In addition to Sophie Gombya's popular lyrical vituperation, another highly publicized challenge to male infidelity during our research was the amendment of the adultery law that sought to make grounds for divorce the same for husbands and wives, hence allowing women to file for divorce on grounds of their husbands' infidelities. The day after the legislation passed, the front page of the daily newspaper *The Monitor* ran the headline "Wives Can Divorce Cheating Husbands."[17] Women activists with whom I spoke doubted the law would greatly alter Uganda's deeply entrenched social ideologies and marital practices anytime soon, but thought it would give women of all socioeconomic statuses legal ammunition against "cheating" husbands, as well as simply exposing the double standard surrounding expectations of infidelity. Furthermore, sex scandals involving Uganda's political and social elite have been constantly featured in the country's many lucrative social media. These public scandals can be read as counter-narratives, representing resistance and ambivalence toward the rigid moral ideology surrounding modern marriage, its uncritical emphasis on monogamy, and its expectation of wives' obedience.

I am not trying to suggest that Sophie's song, the ratified adultery laws, or interest in the sex scandals of public figures will transform or liberate women from straying husbands or even keep men from straying. However, the popularity of these moral discourses reflects a wider social anxiety that surrounds the contradictions inherent in conceptions of modern marriage and persistent expectations, opportunity structures, and gender inequality that facilitate male infidelity.

Christine Obbo observed that in the early 1980s in Uganda, "high status women, while striving to make their homes as comfortable as possible for the husband, [would] turn a blind eye and deaf ear to his extramarital activities" in part to spare their reputations and maintain marital harmony (1987). As I have shown, I found similar patterns. However, twenty years after Obbo's study, my data suggests that among women in Iganga, men's infidelity is becoming increasingly intolerable, even for middle-class women who might have more at stake in terms of public reputation. In fact, during our interviews with women in Iganga, most spoke easily about their husbands' misbehaving (most commonly womanizing or overdrinking) as the source of their marital discontent.[18] Public outcries by women were not uncommon during the research period, and like Isabella's investigation into her husband's affairs, there were cases in which a wife or an assigned intermediary secretly followed an adulterous husband to "catch him red-handed" with his mistress.

Wives are presented with a paradox that seems unique to the Uganda case: while the search for prestige—the appearance of modern monogamous marriage—largely motivates women's silences around their husbands' infidelities, the desire for another kind of prestige—the status of being "rational" modern women who have the knowledge and desire to protect their bodies and rights—leads some wives to go public with their complaints about their husbands' infidelities. Feigning indifference or being willfully ignorant, if done too long, can prove detrimental to a woman's reputation, particularly in a context in which women's rights agencies, public health campaigns, and global discourses of modernity promote notions of personhood based on rational choice, individual agency, and self-efficacy. While the consequences of going public can in some cases be dire, if executed well such displays can prove to be a productive and almost necessary reaction. In airing their grievances to the wider community, women can hope to prompt three effects—to shame the husband in hopes of securing greater community surveillance, to gain sympathy from her neighbors, and finally to present herself as a modern woman, which as conceived by rights and public health discourses is based on a model of rational choice in which a woman has the will to protect her self-interest and well-being.

Yet rarely did wives' outcries or public acts of rebellion lead them to initiate a divorce. As in the case of Isabella and in Sophie's song, a wife's anger is often not directed at the husband, but at the other woman, who is often referred to by what has turned into the derogatory term *nakyewombekeire*. No longer publicly tied to fathers, brothers, or uncles, and not yet tied to husbands, *nakyewombekeire* have been set free to compete with each other and, importantly, with older or married women. The conflict between wives and mistresses is not simply about generational tensions, but also reveals class conflicts among women. While an elite man might befriend a driver or subordinate and have him collaborate in his secrets, people in Iganga speak about relationships among women in different age groups and socioeconomic classes as being fraught with distrust and animosity. This vertical class animosity among women provides another opportunity structure that facilitates men's extramarital liaisons. For mistresses, relationships with the husbands of older women or women from a higher class can be read as a form of social revenge against women who look down on them.

By breaking their silence and going public with their knowledge of their husbands' infidelities, women such as Isabella rebel against the (not so) secret contradictions that exist between what has come to be expected of modern monogamous marriage and the realities of marriage in contemporary Uganda. More important, going public reveals what an older man called "sexual hypocrisy" in contemporary Uganda. But like the song "Spare Tyre," in local geographies of blame, the mistress (not the husband) is constructed as the perpetrator of men's infidelity. Blaming the other woman for a husband's behaviors is not only a way of articulating awareness of wider opportunity structures that propel men into extramarital liaisons, it is also a way in which a wife can make her husband's infidelities a bit more tolerable, and a way for her to protect her own reputation as a modern rational woman when she forgives him and attempts to maintain her modern marriage.

Conclusion

"World Enough and Time": Navigating Opportunities
and Risks in the Landscape of Desire

As we discussed in Chapter 1, sociocultural anthropology has been deeply ambivalent about the project of comparison for at least twenty years.[1] On the one hand, most anthropologists engage in informal comparative discourse all the time—juxtaposing case studies from different regions in order to illustrate analytical points to students, reading deeply into other regional literatures in order to seek inspiration for one's own research, and exchanging knowledge about ritual, marriage, or forms of leadership as a mainstay of collegial conversation. On the other hand, many of these same anthropologists would likely assert that actually doing multisited comparative research is intellectually untenable (because of any or all of the problems discussed in Chapter 1) and thus to be avoided as an explicit or formal objective. While we would certainly agree that comparative research is challenging, and perhaps problematic from some standpoints, we have demonstrated here that it can be a methodologically powerful means both for analyzing the local materializations and consequences of globalizing processes and ideologies, and for mounting a more formidable and persuasive voice when approaching the institutions that are able to implement policy change.

The methodological and rhetorical power of our particular mode of critical comparative ethnography derives from three specific characteristics of the approach. First, a recognition of diverse and unequal resources and social conditions was built into the research design through the deliberate sampling of couples with variable socioeconomic status and migration patterns. Thus, for example, we were able to compare not only women's interpretations of and responses to men's extramarital sexuality across different field sites, but more specifically, the interpretations and responses of poorer and richer women both within each field site and across the five field sites. This attention to social class and migration was also incorporated into our strategies for participant observation, so that, for example, we all made a point of spending time in the homes of both richer and poorer families to investigate how the division of material and emotional labor differed, again both within sites and between sites.

Second, at the outset we all shared a conviction that the best ethnography is rich in particularity and historical specificity, and so we all harbored some misgivings about having to sacrifice some of that specificity and richness for the purposes of carrying out comparison. Thus, we all experienced what might be described as competing centrifugal and centripetal impulses, with the former pushing each of us away from the shared project and toward the particulars of our own field sites, and the latter pushing us away from specificity and toward the emerging resonances among our research sites. Similarly, our detailed yet open-ended interview protocol allowed us to elicit expansive accounts about individuals' experiences and opinions, but it also forced us to collect life-history data on the particular topics of interest to the project as a whole. Our grounding in a shared theoretical framework meant that when we diverged from the specifics of the research protocol, we could do so with confidence, since we had a clear sense of—and commitment to—shared intellectual goals. We are still unsure about how to know when local meanings and histories are so significant that they create incommensurability or make comparison the less compelling question, or when, alternatively, such context-specific details can comfortably and legitimately be set aside. However, we are sure that the ongoing tension between our desires for contextual richness and our desires for systematic comparison improved the validity of our results. This is in part because of the third distinctive dimension of our methodology: our constant communication before, during, and after fieldwork, so that we were able not only to adjust our shared interview protocol as needed, but also analyze together why the methods or interview questions needed to be adapted to account for site-specific social relations or nuances of meaning.

Perhaps the greatest value of critical comparative ethnography is the way in which it can catalyze abstraction and theory-building by creating an intense and focused intellectual community. The extent to which ethnographic research can and does lead eventually to a deeper understanding of regularities in social processes through the use of comparisons has generally been haphazard and variable, depending both on the individual agency exerted by always overcommitted individual academic actors as well as the structures available to them, such as conferences, small working meetings, organized panels, edited volumes, and the like. By availing ourselves of generous funding from the NIH, we created an intensive study group to consider and explore new ways of thinking about love, marriage, and intimacy. Most scholars, even those with the most generous colleagues, only have access to the benefits of peer review when they submit articles to journals or book manuscripts to presses. In contrast, we have enjoyed nearly a decade of collaboration on this project, and within that crucible produced work that has far exceeded in analytic depth that which any of us could have conducted on our own.

We pointed out in Chapter 1 that "polygyny is not polygyny is not polygyny"—and this volume could be read as arguing also that homosociality is not homosociality is not homosociality—but our goal (and thus our analytic strategy) extends far beyond collecting materials on the same topic in order to highlight the variations in what they look like ethnographically (as is quite common in edited volumes). In choosing to emphasize the cross-cutting analytic themes presented in the Introduction and developed in the ethnographic case studies, we have also chosen not to focus on other striking correspondences—and equally notable differences—across the sites, particularly in relation to the roles of religious institutions and the State in regulating everyday life and in terms of the organization of same-sex sexual behavior. Although much more could have been said about the state of play of all of these topics at each field site, we have deliberately de-emphasized that sort of comparative description; focusing on cross-site variation in the ways in which particular categories play out seems to us a sort of analytical dead end, one that would have led only to the conclusion that different things are different in different places. Instead, we have striven for an analytic approach in which raising the level of abstraction throws broader social regularities into relief. Our readers, of course, are the best judges of the novelty and importance of the findings generated through comparison. The first substantive section of this Conclusion returns to the core notions of opportunity structures, the navigation of risk, and the social construction of sexuality. In the second section, we explore the public health policy implications of our work on love, marriage, and HIV.

Intellectual Contributions

Theorizing the Structure of Extramarital Opportunities

The concept of "opportunity structure" in sociology has been developed within two distinct substantive arenas. The first, and the one that we draw on primarily, was pioneered by Peter Blau (1994) and further elaborated within the context of research on probabilities of marriage and (more recently) divorce (South and Lloyd 1995; South, Trent, and Shen 2001). The second comes out of research on social movements and calls attention to aspects of political contexts (e.g., characteristics of nation-states, alignment of political elites, transient events) that facilitate or hinder movement organization and action (Kitschelt 1986; Meyer and Staggenborg 1996; Tarrow 1998). Critically, the latter school of thought places particular emphasis on the notion that opportunities must be grasped. Opportunities alone are insufficient. Movement entrepreneurs and the groups they lead must be positioned and motivated to take advantage of the opportunities with which they are presented.

The aesthetic appeal of this concept to any dyed-in-the-wool sociologist lies in the fact that it is "quintessentially macrosociological" (South, Trent, and Shen 2001: 745). Investigating the probability of marital dissolution, Scott South, Katherine Trent, and Yang Shen propose that "the real or perceived opportunities to form postmarital relationships are largely a product of the social structure," operationalized for purposes of their research as "the numerical distribution of men and women in the population" (745). In other words, the probability of marital dissolution increases as a function of the "relative number of attractive marital partners who might serve as alternatives to one's current spouse," and not (or not as much) with the social, economic, and psychological characteristics of couples and individual spouses. Opportunity structure theory (or at least this branch of it) is grounded on the simple assumption that "the probability of social relations depends on opportunities for contact" (Blau 1994: 29).

There is a substantial body of sociological literature testing inferences drawn from this premise, not only in the domain of marital dissolution but also with respect to the probabilities of marriage, social mobility, intergroup relations, and timing of sexual debut (Lichter, LeClerc, and McLaughlin 1991; Nathanson and Schoen 1993; Blau 1994). In light of the complexities described in the preceding chapters, this literature is extraordinarily narrow in its conceptualization of opportunities, limited for the most part (due no doubt to sociologists' privileging of quantitative analysis) to the relative *numbers* of individuals with given characteristics in a given population (e.g., the number of attractive alternative partners). The rich data provided by these five case studies offers an opportunity (if we may say so) to greatly extend the scope and reach of opportunity structure theory. Although our focus has been on extramarital opportunity structures, these extensions have the potential for much wider application.

As elaborated in the sociological literature, opportunity structure theory has two dimensions, corresponding roughly to the anthropological concepts of structure and agency: the "macrosociological" dimension (e.g., the distribution in a population of "opportunities for contact") and what might be called the "demand" dimension (articulated most clearly by social movement theorists)—the presence of incentives and rewards for taking advantage of those opportunities. Empirically, of course, these two dimensions overlap: if you want something badly enough, you will be very creative about finding opportunities to have it. We propose, nevertheless, to maintain the conceptual distinction because it helps show how the case studies contribute to our understanding of opportunity structures, and it enables us to consider what they tell us about when, why, and for whom those opportunities are irresistible.

Structures of Opportunity

As the use of the plural is intended to suggest—and as all five case studies make clear—opportunities are multidimensional. The probability of extramarital dalliance is a function not only of the *number* of attractive partners available in a given population, but also of the availability of *space* and *time* to access those partners. At the risk of vast oversimplification (which we promise to complicate below), the resulting probabilities are displayed in the accompanying table. The lower right-hand box—no partners, no space, no time—presents few problems of prediction (and closely corresponds to the opportunity structures confronted by married women in each of the five settings we describe). The probability of extramarital

Table 1. Probabilities of Extramarital Sex

Is there space?	Is there time?	Are there available partners?	
		Yes	No
Yes	Yes	++++	–
	No	+++	––
No	Yes	++	––
	No	+	–––

Note: The likelihood of an extramarital affair is represented here by a scale wherein ++++ equals "extremely likely" and ––– equals "extremely unlikely."

sex under such circumstances is extremely low (indicated by –––). Similarly, given an abundance of available partners, space to meet those partners, and time not accountable to family and kin, the probability of an extramarital affair is very high (++++). The other cells are harder to predict, although we have taken a stab at it (e.g., even assuming the availability of space and time, if no suitable partners can be found, the probability of extramarital sex is surely quite low, hence the minus signs in all the cells in the last column). Material from the case studies complicates (in a useful way) each of these three variables. Since almost all of the action is among men, our analysis focuses on their opportunities (and constraints).[2]

PARTNERS

Men's opportunities for contact with sexual partners other than their wives are legion, facilitated both by the organization of family, social, and economic life and, in each of the five settings, by the widespread and increasing availability of unattached and economically dependent women—a reality confirmed by men's remarkably consistent perceptions about the availability of young women. The social, economic, and demographic conditions underlying this reality vary somewhat across settings—delayed marriage, men's labor migration, young women's rural-urban migration, absence of economic alternatives for women—but the outcome is the same: a "surfeit of tempting young beauties" (Hirsch, this volume). Men's opportunities depend, however, not only on the sheer number of available partners, but also on the relative "attractiveness" of those partners. Youth and beauty aside, the criteria for attractiveness are variable and require, among other things, a careful weighing of the balance between the prospect of pleasure and the danger of exposure. Men in Papua New Guinea, for example, avoided women who "belonged" to a particular man. Ugandan men were careful to choose women of lower social status and younger ages than—and therefore unlikely to socialize with—their wives. In Nigeria, age differences between married men and their younger, unmarried partners served a similar purpose. Vietnamese men preferred sex workers, because contact with them was reliably short-term and did not require substantial commitments of time or money. Mexican men emphasized the safety of certain spaces—the cantina, the rodeo ring in a distant town, or almost anywhere far from Degollado's main street and central plaza—for their extramarital dalliances. While opportunities to find a partner are legion, married men's choice among available partners is constrained by considerations that stem from these men's positions in valued networks of family and kin.

SPACE

Absent altogether from the demographic analysis of marital dissolution cited earlier—but elaborated in these five case studies—is the seemingly obvious point that (at least for most men) the existence of social spaces beyond the reach of the wifely gaze is a necessary condition for extramarital dalliance.[3] Indeed, the implication of an exclusive focus on the relative *numbers* of available partners in a population would be that sex-segregation is inimical to the formation of extramarital partnerships, a proposition wholly contradicted by the findings reported in this book. Socially created sex-segregated spaces where men can bring—or encounter—women other than their wives are a critical dimension of contemporary social structure in every one of the five ethnographic sites. These spaces may vary in their amenities and in their degree of institutionalization—from the sports clubs of Nigeria and cantinas of Mexico to the bushes of Huliland—but they are nonetheless omnipresent. Not only are wives (and often other unwanted observers as well) segregated *out* of these male spaces, wives are segregated *in* to domestic spaces where their involvement with chores and children severely restricts their ability to survey their husbands' extracurricular activities.

TIME

In addition to available partners and unobserved spaces, engagement in extramarital sex requires time that does not have to be accounted for to legitimate stakeholders—spouses, in particular, but often other relatives, friends, and employers as well. Surplus time may be created by poverty, such as with underemployed Huli men, or by affluence, as is the case for men zipping around Hanoi's increasingly crowded streets on their new motorbikes. Irrespective of whether it was the result of economic affluence or economic decline, surplus time accrued to the men in these settings and not to their wives.

MOBILITY

Mobility—whether it is across town or across the continent—at one and the same time expands the range of potential partners and increases access both to private space and to private time, arguably in proportion to the distance traveled. For a man with a motorbike and a cell phone, as in Hanoi, even barriers of time and distance meant little. In all of the five countries included in this project, social, economic, and kinship organization facilitated and often demanded men's mobility for work (and often for leisure as well) and severely constrained the mobility of women; in Vietnam, political organization contributed to this as well, and in Iganga colonial economic structures facilitated this gender difference. Gendered patterns of mobility are critical to understanding the probability of extramarital sex because these patterns impact all three dimensions of extramarital opportunity structure: partners, space, and time. They facilitate these opportunities for men by at one and the same time removing husbands from "the wifely gaze" and severely limiting wives' opportunities for gazing. By the same token, these patterns limit the likelihood of women engaging in extramarital sex by confining wives to home and hearth, thereby depriving them of time, space, and access to partners.

Irresistible Opportunities

Opportunities for extramarital dalliance may be legion, but there is no law that says these opportunities must be grasped. The second piece of this analytical puzzle is to unpack the circumstances that lead men (and, again, it is more often men than women) to take advantage of these opportunities. At least three kinds of answers to this question emerge from the five case studies: First, in the context of many masculine social networks, men are both prompted to play around with women other than their wives and rewarded for doing so (we use the phrase "playing around" advisedly, since not every flirtation leads to sexual intercourse, it just increases its probability). Second, apart from the not inconsiderable risk of exposure, as long as the man is fulfilling his role as economic provider, there are relatively few sanctions against this behavior. Third—and elaboration of this point is a major contribution of this project—the spaces that men seek out and the time they have on their hands are not simply neutral "opportunities." They have meanings that incite and even legitimize extramarital sexual behavior. Let us briefly illustrate each of these propositions.

Men's performance of extramarital sexuality was often—not always, of course, but often—a show put on for the benefit of their buddies, and the better the performance, the greater the applause. Two remarkably similar extracts—the first from Papua New Guinea, the second from Mexico (echoed as well by the Nigeria and to some extent Uganda findings)—exemplify this point:

> Men often band together to look for women and frequently boast and joke about their liaisons in the company of male peers, suggesting that having an encouraging and appreciative male audience (after the fact) enhances the pleasures and sense of triumph that come from an illicit liaison. Indeed, having a ribald and riotous story to share seemed in many cases to be more pleasurable and meaningful than the sex itself. (Wardlow, this volume)

A great deal of men's emotional focus is actually on their relationships with their male companions. These long boozy evenings can be about the pleasure of affect, of *cariño*, of the touch of a true friend and the ear of someone who cares deeply—but this *cariño* is shared not between men and their hired girlfriends but among the men themselves. The sex is, in a way, incidental. (Hirsch, this volume)

The opportunities represented in the probabilities table are, then, far more than just opportunities to have sex—as noted about the Mexican example, "the sex is, in a way, incidental." They are opportunities to act before an audience of one's male peers, where successful performance may symbolize economic capability and class status (such as in Nigeria and Vietnam) or, as Wardlow puts it, "resistance to the domesticating ideologies of companionate marriage" (as in Papua New Guinea, Mexico, and Uganda). Or, it may simply be the oil that lubricates the bonds of masculine friendship. In any case, it's not entirely about the sex. No doubt, the sex is sometimes rewarding in and of itself, but if the ethnographic research presented in this book makes anything crystal clear, it is that men gain rewards from this behavior that go far beyond any physical pleasure they may experience from the act itself.

Clearly male peers egg each other on, and indeed they may be sanctioned for non- or reluctant participation. At the same time, as long as men abide by the unspoken rules of the game—that is, as long as they fulfill their economic responsibilities to their wives and children, and do not flaunt their extramarital affairs in inappropriate places and at inappropriate times—they are unlikely to be censured by their peers, their communities, or even their wives. Where the boundaries of respectability lie is best demonstrated by their violation: the Ugandan husband who flagrantly treated his schoolteacher girlfriend to drinks in the local bar; the Mexican husband who took his girlfriend to a wedding also attended by neighbors from his hometown; the Nigerian man who was threatened with expulsion from his tennis club if he didn't cease both his public displays of affection for his girlfriend and his social and economic neglect of his wife. Men who were careful to stay within the boundaries of acceptable behavior—however "acceptable" was locally defined—could grasp the opportunities presented to them with relatively little to fear in the way of negative consequences.

Our final point about extramarital opportunity structures, illustrated to a greater or lesser degree in all of the case studies, is that geographical spaces—the home, the church, the cantina, the tennis club—have subtle and sometimes not so subtle meanings that go well beyond their physical properties. Spaces that are known to privilege sexually explicit conversations and cues do more than merely *facilitate* extramarital sex by offering a private place to meet; extramarital sex (at the very least extramarital flirtation) is *incited* by the aura of expectation these spaces create. This point holds true even in spaces not populated by enthusiastic *compadres*—any hotel bar will do.

Beyond Extramarital Sex

The conceptual framework we have proposed is applicable in many circumstances where the question at hand is to estimate the probability of other forms of behavior that might also be described as "public secrets"—that is, practices that are known to occur but whose existence can only with difficulty be publicly acknowledged. This framework has two underlying dimensions: "supply"—the distribution in a population of opportunities to engage in said behavior—and "demand"—the presence of incentives or rewards to take advantage of those opportunities. As we argued earlier, a major contribution of this work is to call attention to the multidimensionality of opportunities: which dimensions are relevant will depend on the behavior in question. To take just one example, we might want to predict variation in the probability of corruption in (let's say) US state government across the fifty states. Under the heading of "supply," we would want to know, first, what are the relevant opportunities in these settings—the equivalents of partners, space, and time—and, second, the distribution of these opportunities within and across states. Clearly, we would pay close attention to each state's regulatory system—to what extent is venality in office beyond the reach of the regulatory gaze? Under the heading of "demand"—the irresistibility of opportunities to be "on the take," we might look at such things as the payscale for government officials, the extent to which financial double-dealing is regarded as normal business practice (i.e., one is typed as "weird" if one abstains), and so on. Analyses along these lines—and in a variety of settings—would very likely suggest substantial modifications and additions to the framework we have proposed. We do not suggest that this framework is complete, only that it has the potential for application well beyond the confines of understanding intimacy in Mexico, Nigeria, Papua New Guinea, Uganda, and Vietnam.

Navigating Risks

With opportunities come risks.[4] Actions have costs as well as benefits, and these cases are particularly eloquent in articulating not only the nature and complexity of those costs but the extent to which they are embedded in and inextricable from the web of relationships that surrounds each actor in the marital (and nonmarital) dramas portrayed. Costs do not inhere in the actions of individuals but in the social context within which those actions occur and in the social meanings attributed to them.

In one of her illuminating essays on "risk and blame," Mary Douglas articulated the socially constructed nature of risk: "The thesis here to be proposed is that the self is risk-taking or risk-averse according to a predictable pattern of dealings between the person and others in the community. Both emerge, the community and the person's self, as ready for particular risks or as averse to them, in the course of their interactions. The person who never thought of himself as a risk-taker, in the unfolding of the drama of his personal life, and under the threat of the community's censure, finds himself declaring a commitment to high risk" (2002: 102). Going beyond the point that risks are socially embedded, Douglas would argue that dangers are defined so as to preserve and reinforce existing social structures: thus, in an exceptionally sharp illustration of this point, "even men who themselves cheat on their wives can be mobilized to scorn and sanction another man who allows his extramarital affairs to interfere with his economic obligations to his family . . . [or] who flaunts his infidelity too publicly" (Smith, this volume).

Less dramatically, men consistently evaluated potential partners and possible spaces not only with reference to the opportunities they presented but also with reference to their level of threat to the fulfillment of family-centered obligations for discretion (uniformly), economic support (usually), and companionship (occasionally). In Vietnam, a sex worker poses less risk to a family's economic and emotional stability than a man's lover. In Papua New Guinea, sex with a woman "not belonging" to anyone brings few penalties to husbands. Finally, the Mexican example emphasizes the spatial dimension as well; as Hirsch writes, "He should have known better than to bring his secretary into his home; as the saying goes, 'Hay que saber dónde y con quién' (You have to know where and with whom)" (Hirsch, this volume).

It is perhaps all too obvious that seizing opportunities for extramarital pleasure endangers the web of conventional domestic relationships. Less obvious is that *not* seizing those opportunities may also entail risks—to a different but often equally significant set of relationships. Douglas observes that "danger . . . is defined to protect the public good"; the "public good," of course, is in the eye of the beholder (2002: 6). Consider Smith's description of the rich and generous patron of his tennis club nicknamed "One Man Show." Suppose this jovial fellow, "always buying food and drinks to go around, and contribut[ing] heavily every time the club tried to raise money for an event, an outing, or a building project," should suddenly decide to turn off the tap. The ensuing outcry from his fellow members is not hard to imagine. Earlier, we called attention to the rewards men gain from their peers for "playing around" with women who are not their wives. Equally important are the sanctions in place—risks or costs we can call them—for not playing around. In several of these cases, male-centered social structures that essentially paralleled the structures of family and kin played an important role not just in social bonding but in the economic life of the community as well: just as men mobilized to sanction the pal who was playing around too publicly, they sometimes did the same to the pal who did not want to play at all.

In the cases described, among the most powerful forces in structuring the costs associated with affairs outside of marriage—whomever the partner and however short- or long-lasting the relationship—was gender. Although conditions varied somewhat across settings, women's opportunities for dalliance were limited and the risks they faced—of marital disruption and eventual poverty, loss of children, loss of personal and familial reputation—were uniformly greater than the risks for men. If danger is, indeed, defined to "protect the public good," then women's transgressions were clearly perceived as more threatening to the public good than those of men. With the partial exception of Papua New Guinea (and Uganda, where it is becoming more common), the danger for a woman of confronting a husband with his extramarital affairs was much the same as the danger of engaging in an affair herself: disruption to the web of social relationships on which she depended not only economically, but—in these settings—for status and reputation and for the power commanded by a network of supportive kin.

Occasionally, of course, women do assume the risks of going public with accusations of infidelity but only as a last resort (Papua New Guinea again an exception) and only when the costs of inaction appear to outweigh the costs of action—and by costs we refer not so much to personal costs (e.g., humiliation) but to the costs to a woman's position among her family and friends. In this volume, Smith describes married women in Nigeria as much more likely to seek confrontation—and also more likely to find the desired supportive public response—if the infidelity-related neglect they perceive is economic, rather than emotional: "Indeed, a woman who seeks assistance in the face of a man's infidelity will find a much more sympathetic audience if she can show that her husband is failing to provide for his family than if she merely complains that he has failed in his promise of love and fidelity." Parikh describes how "a normally reserved and restrained" married woman in Iganga was driven into a state of public fury when the secret about her husband's affair became too blatant to ignore. These authors suggest that women acted when they felt disgraced or when their self-respect was threatened. Somewhat similarly, Huli women tied their ready physical aggression against cheating husbands to their own dignity and self-respect. When men went too far in endangering the web of domestic relationships on which women depended (and clearly what constituted "too far" was highly variable), women invoked those same relationships to restore (or occasionally to legitimize breaking) the conjugal bonds.

Contributions to Sexuality Studies

Our foremost contribution to the social science of sexuality is the notion that in these five diverse contexts, social organization facilitates extramarital sex. In addition to being produced by social structure—rather than just occurring because men can't help themselves and their wives are not powerful enough to stop them— these "publicly secret" practices in many ways themselves produce critical social bonds. This expands upon anthropological work on sexuality published during the 1980s and 1990s, in particular Gayle Rubin's distinction between those practices that fall within the "charmed circle" of socially valued practices and those socially despised practices that fall outside it. The cross-cultural variability of this charmed circle—in which, to draw the sharpest contrast, intergenerational same-sex practices are in one context grounds for public shaming and in another context a critical step on the road to developing adult personhood (Herdt 1981, 1984, 1987)—has been well established. Our work calls attention to the fact that societies do not have a single shared "charmed circle"—for example, men's extramarital sexuality is outside the charmed circle from the perspective of wives, the Church, and so on but well within the charmed circle from many men's perspectives as long as it abides by certain rules.[5]

Rubin did not emphasize the culturally productive nature of "stigmatized sexual behavior," and certainly practices outside the charmed circle are more frequently referred to by US right-wing politicians and social activists as proof of the breakdown of society, if not the actual cause. Our research, however, has led us to recognize the salience of extramarital sexual relations and the associated homosocial behavior as central to the production of culture and masculinity. Bringing marital and extramarital sex together under one critical optic does more than just show how the contrast between socially valued and illicit sexual intimacy creates "the normal" through the articulation of "the abject." We show how extramarital sexuality is itself productive of diverse social bonds, both heterosocial and homosocial. Raewyn Connell and Gary Dowsett articulated the notion of "the sexual organization of society" to mean the way in which heteronormativity, the unequal relationship between homosexuality and heterosexuality, forms an element of social stratification equal in importance to class, ethnicity, or gender (1999). Here, we extend that notion of the sexual organization of society, showing that across the spectrum of moral valuation, a wide range of practices of intimacy contribute to the development of social bonds.

Second, in addition to demonstrating the mutually constitutive and socially productive nature of marital and extramarital sexuality, we underline the need for a reintegration of work on hetero- and homosexualities. The insight that the category of heterosexual only came to exist through the articulation of homosexuality as a deviant identity is not a new one (Weeks 1986, 1989; Foucault 1985; D'Emilio 1997, 1998), but ethnographic work on sexuality has persisted in a sort of either/or approach—revealing, perhaps more than anything, a sort of overspecialization on the part of social scientists themselves, who go to the field focused on a set of problems and a population, and limit their inquiry accordingly. The chapter on Mexico further suggests the potential of ethnographic research that acknowledges the malleability and instability of categories of sexual identity and integrates spaces and informants from across the local spectrum. Our exploration of married men's sexuality in Degollado gained nuance and complexity from hearing from those men's partners across the spectrum, ranging from the married woman who told us "you have to be willing to be a little bit of a whore for your husband" to an older man, a frequent purchaser of transactional sex with other men, who asserted that ultimately, pleasure is pleasure—"cualquier agujero, aunque sea caballero" (any hole, even if it's a man's). Moreover, the prominence throughout this volume of reputational aspects of identity might serve to de-center object choice as the sole relevant axis of sexual identity; across all five field sites, the relative respectability of sexual practices and relationships was a far more critical aspect of what those practices or relationships meant locally than object choice, transactionality, or even the affective nature of the relationship within which particular practices took place. The overemphasis on identity in sexuality studies recalls the ethnocentrism of early kinship theory, with its overemphasis on studying kinship forms in relation to normative Western categories—underlining, more broadly, the culture-bound nature of all social theory.

Third, our discussions of the spatial aspects of sexuality have helped us understand, and will perhaps serve to illustrate for others, what it means to talk about desire as "incited." Social constructionist work on sexuality has made it clear that desire is to a great extent taught by media, language, and example, rather than innate. The history of fashion similarly has demonstrated that various body parts rise and fall in their erotic appeal. The idea that what people desire can change, however, does not necessarily move us conclusively away from the idea that sexuality is, as Carol Vance famously noted, "a kind of universal Play Doh . . . on which culture works, a naturalized category which remains closed to investigation and analysis" (1991: 878). Our explication of sexuality as a quality of spaces, and not just of individuals in those spaces, presents concrete examples of desire as produced by particular sets of circumstances and social relations, rather than as a naturalized sort of lust that is produced by individual bodies and just waiting for a chance at release—what is frequently referred to as the "hydraulic model" of sexuality.

Fourth, exploring the geography of desire also creates new possibilities for thinking about the political economy of sexuality. Spaces of sexual risk and desire can be seen as material manifestations of gendered economic organization; the men spending time in bars, whether Igbo or Huli, are there because they have greater access to wage labor, greater mobility, and fewer responsibilities for the caretaking aspects of social reproduction. In and of themselves, these diverse forms of watering-holes represent in some instances important sectors of local economies, but above and beyond that they are products of specific political economies. The best example in that regard is probably the intensely rapid growth of Hanoi's pleasure industries after Doi Moi.

Many have written about poverty as a risk factor for HIV, describing how limited opportunities drive men and women into transactional sex (Brennan 2004; Padilla 2007; Kelly 2008; Fox 2009), and our spatial analyses show concretely how political and economic organization intersect to create sexual opportunity structures. Our take on the political economy of sexuality goes beyond that, though, as we show sexual risk to be produced by economic organization at all levels: by businessmen networking with each other, by workers whose jobs draw them away from home, and by young women for whom the riskiest form of desire may be not for men but for cell phones or fashionable clothes. In each of these cases, it is neoliberal capitalism working as it is intended to that produces sexual risk, rather than some breakdown or malfunction of the system. As we discuss later in this chapter in the section on the policy implications, this analysis of sexual risk as expressed in historically specific ways by modern capitalism presents a much greater challenge for policy than does an analysis which focuses only on economic inequality. Also, while it is commonplace to show that participation in wage labor provides men with the cash to spend on commercial sex, we trace out more nuanced connections between the men's experiences as workers and their sexuality. The ethnographic chapters describe how the alienation and loneliness of working as migrant wage laborers, and economic transformations that frustrate men's desires to succeed as providers, help pave the way for men's extramarital sexual liaisons.

Policy Implications

In closing, we wish to address our work's policy implications. We do this both to answer the inevitable (and reasonable) "so what?" questions on the part of our public health readers, and because even those whose expertise lies in social rather than policy science might be interested in how our findings fit into the broader picture of HIV prevention programs. Moreover, the divergence between what should be and what is—that is, between what our work suggests might be effective, and the most common prevention approaches we saw during the years in which this research was carried out—provides an excellent example of public health as one of the terrains through which the secret is itself both constituted and contested.

In the first decade of the twenty-first century, in response to citizen and scientific activism, the United States government significantly increased its commitment to funding both HIV prevention and treatment, becoming the largest single-country donor. PEPFAR represented a historic commitment (on the order of US$15 billion between 2003 and 2008, with an additional $48 billion in spending authorized in 2008) to expanding access to the almost miraculously effective, highly active antiretroviral therapy (ART). Through the funding for prevention activities, however, PEPFAR also exported American debates about public health and morality, in ways that extended even beyond sexuality to other areas of controversy. For example, despite the significant body of evidence demonstrating the efficacy of needle exchange programs, under the Bush administration PEPFAR funds could not be spent on needle exchange as a means of HIV prevention. This reflected the US federal government's longstanding refusal to support these programs—a refusal that stems from a concern that working to mitigate some of the detrimental health effects of intravenous drug use might be mistaken for condoning the drug use itself.[6] Other notable areas of debate included the requirement that agencies receiving funding from the United States Agency for International Development (USAID) must sign the "anti-prostitution pledge," through which they agree not to "promote, support or advocate the legalization or practice of prostitution"; PEPFAR's emphasis on the "ABC" approach to prevention (Abstinence, Be faithful, Condoms) (Halperin et al. 2004; Green et al. 2006; Green and Witte 2006; Thornton 2008), and the argument made by some that US-funding priorities had the effect of discouraging condom promotion, resulting in what was essentially an "AB" approach.[7] These prevention programs form part of the cultural framework within which HIV comes to have specific local meanings. Particularly in Nigeria, Uganda, and Vietnam, the three of our five countries with substantial US-funded HIV prevention and AIDS care and treatment programs, the meaning of HIV has been shaped substantially by the export of American moral projects of public health.

To the extent that marital HIV risk has been acknowledged as an issue that ought to be addressed through prevention efforts, US-funded or otherwise, a predominant approach has been to emphasize the value of mutual monogamy as an HIV prevention strategy. Even aside from the intense debates about the historical and potential efficacy of fidelity promotion (Epstein 2008), our findings suggest a number of ways in which the very notion is problematic.[8] We found significant cross-cultural variability in ideas about the meaning and value of fidelity, as we did in the extent to which monogamy was even relevant as a cultural ideal. Further, our findings about extramarital opportunity structures point to the limits of individuals' agency to live up to this ideal, to the extent that they desire to do so. Our work also calls into question the justice (not to mention the efficacy) of encouraging women to adopt what amounts to unilateral monogamy.

The prominence of individual-level approaches within US-funded HIV prevention programs provides an excellent example of public health policy as a cultural production—that is, an ideological assertion of how the world is rather than a road map for how to make it the way it should be. By seeking to improve public health through changing the behavior of individuals, these programs reflect a neoliberal approach to public health, overemphasizing the agency and responsibility of individuals to produce their own health and downplaying the responsibility and potential for governments and institutions to create the conditions that facilitate health. The history of public health depicts a tradition of improving the health of populations through policy and infrastructural interventions such as clean water and the enforcement of workplace safety regulation. The enthusiasm for behavioral interventions represents a lack of faith in the appropriateness or efficacy of government-level solutions to social problems. The roadside billboards in Uganda urging passersby to "Love Carefully," then, signal not just an export of the moral value of monogamy, but also of the Horatio Alger–esque belief that people should choose health as they choose toothpaste.[9]

Our work builds on the substantial and growing body of literature (Blankenship et al. 2006; Friedman and O' Reilly 1997; Friedman and Reid 2002; Parker, Easton, and Klein 2000) calling for structural interventions to reduce the risk of sexual transmission of HIV.[10] "Structural" denotes a diverse range of interventions at community, institutional, and policy levels; what they share, as a group, is a focus on changing the conditions that facilitate or discourage the individual-level practices that lead to transmission, rather than trying to reduce transmission by affecting individual practices directly. The notion of extramarital opportunity structures is particularly important in this regard, as it provides a road map through which researchers in other contexts could assess the specific elements of social inequalities that create differential vulnerability. Despite the growing literature on structural violence and HIV vulnerability, there are still all too few concrete explanations of the specific processes through which structural inequality becomes embodied as suffering—and it is vital to articulate structure in a way that makes it recognizable by someone who is not a professional social scientist. Specifically, our work leads us to recommend a wide variety of structural interventions focused on the migration-HIV nexus, as well as more specific intervention approaches building on what we have learned about men's leisure-time activities, possibilities for working with faith communities, and the relevance of sexual minority rights to heterosexual risk.

HIV and Migration

It has become commonplace in HIV prevention to hear migrant workers listed as a "vulnerable population" toward whom special HIV prevention programs ought to be directed, and it is equally commonplace to see prevention programs both exhorting migrant workers to adopt safer sexual practices and attempting to facilitate this behavior change by enhancing access to condoms. Our point here, however, is somewhat distinct. Drawing on the economic notion of "externalities," our work emphasizes how the global reliance on migrant labor itself facilitates HIV risk. Externalities are an unmeasured cost of the production of a good—one that is borne neither by the producer nor the consumer; the classic example of an externality is the pollution created by a factory. Sexual risk, we believe, could be considered "an externality" of a global economic system that demands a mobile and flexible labor force. Whether the case is one of a middle-class Nigerian whose participation in short-term training to do international development work provides opportunities for casual sexual liaisons, that of a motorbike taxi driver in Hanoi who takes advantage of his daily mobility to discreetly maintain multiple partners, or that of a Mexican migrant whose longer-term patterns of circular migration keep him far from his wife for months at time, across all five sites we saw countless ways in which mobility has been a fundamental element of extramarital opportunity structures. Hidden in the artificially low price of the products created by these migrant laborers is the cost of HIV risk for their primary partners.

In all five sites, work-related mobility was at times virtually compulsory as people tried to provide for their families in the face of severe economic hardship. This same mobility facilitated access to extramarital sex in diverse ways. In Nigeria, approximately half of all the cases of extramarital relationships described in the marital case studies occurred in situations where work-related mobility was a factor. Men whose work took them away from their wives and families appeared more likely to have extramarital relationships, and men frequently attributed their behavior to the opportunities and hardships produced by these absences. Men who were migrants sought partners not just out of lust but also out of loneliness, a need for social support, and a desire to find women to replicate the gendered division of labor to which they were accustomed in their residence of origin. Sex filled a need for solace—a need that was especially acute because of the meager options for diversion in the communities in which labor migrants are concentrated. As other research we have done in both Atlanta and New York has shown (Hirsch et al. 2009; Muñoz-Laboy, Hirsch, and Quispe-Lazaro 2009), those Mexican migrants in the United States who are not interested in spending their free time either at church or playing soccer have little to choose from other than cantinas, dollar dance halls, or brothels. Facing loneliness and alienation that makes them hungry for human warmth and confronted by a social geography that provides few health-enhancing ways of finding that warmth, new migrants learn the tricks of survival from those with more experience. As an informant from the Papua New Guinea site recounted, reflecting on labor-related migration and what might be called men's "extramarital sexual debut": "After I was married, I left my wife and children and went to Goroka for work, and it was there that I had sex with another woman. That was the first time." He emphasized that it was another man's idea: "I did this the first time because I was with [my boss]." In Papua New Guinea, as in the other four locations, men's narratives of the extramarital relationships they'd had during the course of labor-related migration typically emphasized acutely missing one's family; a simultaneous feeling of exuberant freedom from community scrutiny; predominantly male workplaces where drinking and buying sex was the norm at the end of a long and arduous workweek; and the fact that women tended to gather outside popular bars on men's paydays.

The relation between migration and sexual risk may be a structural determinant of sexual risk, but these social structures are produced—and can be changed—by organized social action; *modifiable* political and economic factors amplify the correlation between migration and sexual risk. In Vietnam, men negotiate for success in the emerging market economy in contexts in which providing colleagues with alcohol and purchased sexual pleasure is frequently a key part of the game—and Hanoi's engagement with the market economy has nodded at, or even exacerbated, men's reliance on purchased sex as the cost of doing business. The unspoken goal of US migration policy is to guarantee a flow of low-cost laborers, but an unintended result is to intensify migration's sexual risk; denied a path to legalization and thus family reunification, undocumented laborers are separated from their spouses for months or even years at a time. Military conflict provides a parallel example of government-directed mobility placing men in contexts of sexual risk: in Uganda, a soldier returning from the war recounted his liaisons over the course of his long-term conscription. He framed them as a product both of his extended separation from his wife and of his feeling that the risk of sexual infection with HIV meant little in the face of his very real risk of dying in battle before the year was out.

Housing policy is another domain through which migration relates to sexual risk. In Papua New Guinea, mining companies' refusal to provide family housing guarantees that men and women are separated for long periods of time. In essence, the companies' decision to economize by housing only the workers is passed along to the workers' families in the form of HIV risk (as well as other health risks). Policies regarding migrant labor figure prominently not just in terms of housing but more broadly in terms of the extent to which minimum benefits are guaranteed to workers: when, as with Mexican workers in the United States, migrants are seen as disposable bodies—cannon-fodder in the global wars of capitalism—many opportunities for primary prevention, for HIV testing, and for access to care are missed because the jobs at which migrants work provide no health care. Similarly, when migrants are shunted off into trailers, crammed into company shacks, or crowded into neighborhoods with little in the way of public services, the absence of any explicit policy to create opportunities to build human capital amounts to a de facto community development policy of deliberate underdevelopment. In none of these situations is there an explicit policy goal of creating HIV risk for migrants. However, by not acknowledging that the labor is rendered by humans with complex needs, the result is essentially an implicit policy that permits this situation. In all of these situations, the relatively low price of goods and services provided through migrant labor is predicated upon a hidden cost—the cost of sexual and HIV risk, borne not by the company that takes the profit, nor by the consumer who enjoys the product, but by the laborer who produced it.

The analytic purchase afforded by being able to look at this problem broadly across five very different contexts also leads us to see some specific policy solutions. The first step is a more accurate social diagnosis—that is, to raise awareness of HIV as a hidden cost of goods and services produced with migrant labor or by mobile populations, and to make consumers aware of the role that we play as avid beneficiaries of a global system of production that relies heavily on migrant labor. The economic sectors that benefit from this low-cost labor must be part of the solution, which could lie in social entrepreneurship to brand and promote products generated in healthy workplaces. Producers increasingly see a marketing advantage in differentiating commodities on the basis of the moral superiority of the social conditions under which they were produced (conflict-free diamonds, fair trade coffee, etc.). The fact that consumers already make use of a product's moral qualities, in addition to aesthetic and sensory ones, as they seek to act out social values through purchasing practices suggests that there might be a niche for food produced in health-promoting workplaces; the populations who already willingly pay more for cruelty-free eggs and meat would at least potentially demonstrate the same caring toward their own species, if afforded the opportunity. (An example of this is the nascent movement in the American Conservative Jewish community toward a seal for kosher foods that "reflect . . . production benchmarks consistent with Jewish ethical standards, including how companies treat their employees.")[11] HIV risk needs to figure in discussions of labor policy; labor regulations that require multinational corporations to provide family housing, basic medical care, workplace HIV education, and structured recreational activities could all serve to disentangle the migration-HIV nexus. The migration-HIV nexus also needs to be included in conversations about migration policy, because the long separations of workers from their families play such a prominent role in shaping migration-related risk.

Local Geographies of Risk

Our work on the social geography of sexual risk and on men's homosocial leisure-time activities, similarly, points to ways in which rethinking the physical organization of communities might mitigate the risk of sexual transmission. This might help public health program designers move beyond an almost compulsive reliance on interventions targeted at identity-oriented risk groups. Faced with the continuing disproportionate impact of the HIV pandemic on men who have sex with men (MSM), as well as growing awareness of the lack of concordance between sexual identity and sexual practices (Carrier 1984, 1985, 1994, 1995; Parker 1985, 1991; Parker and Caceres 1999; Young and Meyer 2005), programs have defaulted into using MSM as a sort of generic placeholder for a culturally meaningful sexual identity, rather than remembering that the category "MSM" was not initially intended to denote a meaningful social category. Thinking about the spaces that produce risk, rather than approaching risk as a category inherent to individuals, might be a way out of the dead-end of identity. Indeed, given the ways in which cantinas, tennis clubs, *bia hoi*, bars, and beer gardens facilitate men's access to extramarital sex, mitigating HIV risk in these spaces seems like the low-hanging fruit of HIV prevention. (We focus on the potential value of expanding men's recreational options not because women do not engage in extramarital sex, but because in none of the locations in which we worked do women do so in quite the same public, institutionally facilitated way that men do.)

Whether men are migrants or not, one of the privileges of masculinity is access to spaces hidden from the wifely gaze, and it is in these homosocial contexts that men most easily engage in liaisons with women other than their wives. With the exception of institutions such as the *dawe anda* in rural Huliland, most of the leisure-time spaces that create such propitious settings for casual sex are private-sector profit-making ventures. Interventions could either work with the proprietors of these institutions (as has happened with public health interventions at bathhouses in the United States and elsewhere) to enhance the likelihood that sex transacted as a result of interactions on the premises will be safer sex, or else promote the development of new forms of leisure-time activities that would be profitable, more widely open to the public, and provide fewer opportunities for extramarital sex.[12] Alcohol consumption is the other shared characteristic of most of these all-male spaces, and channeling alcohol taxes to HIV interventions or involving alcohol producers in HIV prevention campaigns would help offset costs of interventions and might lead to other creative strategies. Although the production of HIV risk due to alcohol consumption is not quite equivalent to the production of lung cancer and heart disease due to cigarette consumption, it is certainly possible to see a parallel. Building on this analogy, companies that profit from alcohol sales (not just the owners of the venues in which it is sold, but the national and sometimes even multinational corporations that produce it) might reasonably be held responsible for addressing (through additional taxes) some of the social damage created by the use of their products. Finally, raising the awareness of private sector decision-makers about the costs of HIV that they are already bearing, as well as the role of their businesses in the spread of HIV, could potentially lead to innovative and contextually sensitive approaches to HIV prevention and testing.

Sexual Rights

A third line of intervention suggested by our work would be to promote respect for the human rights of sexual minorities, both by advocating for the passage of laws protecting those rights and by demanding that existing laws be enforced. In communities with significant epidemics linked to men's sexual behavior with other men, homophobia increases HIV risk for men and women. In many of our field sites, men who experience same-sex desire do not have the option, as they do in much more cosmopolitan urban settings, of assuming an openly gay social role and building a life as a respected adult member of their community. For instance, in Degollado, acknowledging one's same-sex desire during the day, in the street—as opposed to at night, or behind closed doors—closes down a whole set of life options, both personal and professional. Indeed, Brazil, Mexico, and a number of other countries in Latin America have recognized the connection between sexual inequality and HIV transmission, and have sought to break this link by articulating and protecting the rights of sexual minorities. In Hanoi, and throughout Vietnam, homosexuality has become a topic of public discussion, particularly on the Internet. This is also becoming relevant for the field sites in Nigeria, Uganda, and

Papua New Guinea as new evidence is emerging, at least in the African context, that sexual relations between men may in fact account for a greater proportion of the sexual transmission than has been generally thought (Epprecht 2008; Beyrer 2008; Sandfort et al. 2008; Sharma et al. 2008; van Griensven and Sanders 2008; van Griensven 2007).

Partner with Faith Communities in New Ways

In each of our field sites except Vietnam, where the role of religion in public life remains sharply curtailed even after Doi Moi, religious leaders have played a central role in shaping the moral terrain of HIV, AIDS, and sexuality. Although in many contexts religious leaders have spoken out courageously about the need to care for individuals with AIDS, messages from the pulpit about the evils of promiscuity have—as was made clear quite sharply in the chapters on Uganda and Nigeria—complicated HIV prevention efforts by encouraging men to reframe what they are doing (both to themselves and others) so as not to appear debauched. By reinforcing a moral hierarchy of sexuality in which mutual monogamy is the ideal, these religious messages underline the importance of keeping "the secret," making it harder to mitigate the risks of these hidden practices.

Despite the growing power of the media, the marketplace, and public institutions to shape shared notions about sexuality, religious leaders are likely to continue contributing in powerful ways to the cacophony of messages about what sex is and what it should be, and so it is important to consider potential areas in which the public health commitment to healthy bodies and the religious commitment to saving souls might intersect. Our work generated four ideas in that regard: First, for both regional and international migrants, religious institutions are frequently the only ones that bridge the multiple locations across which they live their lives. There could be potential for faith-based initiatives that acknowledge the challenge to fidelity posed by labor migration. In the Mexican context, for example, it might be possible to use the omnipresence and power of the Catholic Church—coupled with Mexican Catholicism's embrace of embodied suffering as an expression of religious devotion—to develop a new sort of invented tradition, in which Mexican men commit to abstinence—or at least managed infidelities—in a parallel to that paradigmatic moment of embodied suffering and the deliberate abstention from pleasure, Jesus' encounter with the devil in the wilderness. The Church is, after all, led by men who commit themselves to a lifetime of controlling their own desires for the good of the greater community. Second, faith-based organizations could provide other forms of community and social support for migrant laborers—not just helping them deal with the challenges of temptation, but working with them to build up stronger communities that provide more options for diversion and more avenues to build up a sense of successful social personhood. Third, religious leaders could speak even more broadly (and realistically) about fidelity, providing pastoral guidance for married couples that candidly acknowledges the many challenges to fidelity in resource-poor settings and provides these couples not just with ideological frameworks within which to resist those challenges but also with alternative social spaces that could help mitigate some of those challenges. Fourth, and in some ways most important, we have shown here some of the damage that has been done by framing HIV as a disease of immorality. Religious leaders could do more than almost anyone else to undo that damage.

Prevention Opportunities: Stop Keeping "The Secret"?

Although mass media communication programs are by themselves insufficient as HIV prevention, there is no question that providing people with access to medically correct information and strategically shaping the way people think about HIV are important components of a comprehensive strategy. Our fieldwork and analysis lead us to believe that it is important to break the silence about the risk of marital sex and the likelihood of extramarital sex, but that it is crucial to do so in a way that avoids scare tactics. It is certainly necessary to disseminate information about the risk of marital HIV transmission, but the health risks of sex are, as we have shown, not always the most critical determinant of actual practices, and so it is equally imperative to think about how this information will be circulated, and by whom. Promoting community-based dialogues about sexual risk might be one approach for encouraging communities to generate their own strategies to address this issue, rather than trying to impose externally generated (and unsustainable) solutions. Men, as we have striven to show, are not the enemies of public health, and prevention interventions might consider drawing on existing constructions of masculinity—associating condom use with ideal masculinity and building on men's sense of responsibility to their families—rather than emphasizing, as is common in programs targeting men, the need to change indigenous masculinities.[13] Most important, our work underlines the importance of avoiding moralistic approaches to talking about extramarital sex, which just exacerbate the stigma of HIV and encourage people to be more secretive about infidelity—thereby making honest conversations about HIV risk in marriage even less likely.

A Final Word

We close by articulating briefly the points we have *not* made—indeed, the points on which we have particularly striven for clarity are also those areas in which we most fear being misunderstood. We have not argued that infidelity is inevitable at the individual level; our point, rather, is that it is inevitable at the social level, or at least nearly so, given current circumstances and social organization in the locations where we worked. Nor have we said that extramarital sex is bad, or good—indeed, we have endeavored (sometimes with great difficulty) to pull back from moral judgments. Instead, we have focused our attention on analyzing actual practices and on understanding how the tension between those practices and the quite distinct shared notions of what people should do—the push and pull between the "is" and the "ought"—serves as a fundamental element of social organization. We have tried not to reproduce xenophobic, ethnocentric, or simplistic characterizations of women as silently suffering victims or of men as unable to control their bodies. We have demonstrated instead that women are sometimes complicit in keeping "the secret," that women do sometimes resort to harsh words, unexpected actions, and even physical violence when evidence of a man's liaisons becomes impossible to ignore, and that some men feel considerable ambivalence about extramarital sex, while others seem to experience little internal conflict about where their penises go, as long as enough of the money goes where it ought to.

We have written not just about one secret, but about multiple secrets. The first one—the one which initially spurred us on—was the secret danger of marital sex: the shivers-inducing fact that for most women around the world, their greatest risk of HIV infection comes from having sex with their husbands. We began with the goal of exploring the social production of this risk, investigating how the notion of risk as well as the actual possibility of transmission are not just biologically produced, but culturally and socially embedded, meaningful and variable. Our pursuit of these objectives led us to the unexpected conclusion that the conflation of epidemiologically risky sex with morally devalued sex (and thus the implied equivalence of proper sex and safe sex) has contributed in fundamental, and erroneous, ways to making marital risk seem inconceivable and even oxymoronic. Our concern, however, that love and marriage are sometimes followed by HIV rather than (or in addition to) the more comforting and expected "baby in the baby carriage," was complemented by our attention to another secret: not just that many people, men in particular, participate in extramarital sexual intimacy, but that there are broad social regularities across very diverse contexts that facilitate those intimate encounters.

Finally, we have not said—in the inimitable words of one blogger, responding to a 2007 press release discussing our findings—that "men are, in fact, dogs."[14] Through this emphasis on the social, cultural, and structural, rather than the individual or biological, we have pointed to the gendered opportunity structures, sexual geographies, and concerns about social risk that make extramarital sex in many instances the behavioral default option. In doing so, our work provides a novel way of thinking about the social factors that promote HIV transmission—in addition, of course, to providing an analysis of men's multiple partnerships that extends far beyond the notion that men do it because their bodies demand it and their wives are powerless to stop them.

Discourses and policies that veil the complex relation between moral and viral risk have obscured the dangers of marital sex. Our analysis foregrounds an additional set of secret-keeping efforts, in which the socially produced nature of extramarital sex is concealed by the deliberate efforts of policy-makers for whom marriage remains the only moral place for sex, as well as by married men and women as they strive to build good lives. In doing so, they refrain from acknowledging that which must not be spoken. Social scientists have themselves been party to keeping these secrets, as the limits of social theory have created analyses of sex that artificially separate marital from extramarital, heterosexual from homosexual, and transactional from affective, rather than analyzing them all within a single common rubric: the gendered sexual organization of society.

Appendix I. Table of Methodologies

Specific data elicited and relationship to project objectives

Participant observation

We conducted six months of data collected on domestic life and communal social life. These observations were critical for the study of courtship, marriage, family life, and men's patterns of socializing and participation in nightlife. They provided a vital source of knowledge of the contexts within which men engage in extramarital sex.

Marital case studies

In the marital case histories, we collected data on marriage and extramarital relationships from men and women. Most of the men and women, with the exception of those in Papua New Guinea, were married couples. Over the course of three interviews, the men and women talked about childhood and family life, courtship norms and experiences, and premarital, marital, and extramarital sexuality, and they provided detailed descriptive information on the social organization of gender (particularly around the key categories of labor, power, and emotion) within their marriages. These stories, together with the stories of couples we became acquainted with through participant observations, were the "outcome" data we sought to explain.

Key informant interviews

Interviews of people with special, privileged knowledge of the reasons for and consequences of men's (and women's) extramarital relationships, as well as greater understanding of circumstances within which such relationships are most likely to occur

Archival research

Analysis of current and historical popular media, review of regional demographic data, and collection of locally important religious texts on marriage, sexuality, and the family; the goal was to locate the data on individual experiences within economic, social, and cultural contexts

Mexico: Fieldwork specifics

Participant observation
- Families and domestic life: Sunday lunches, afternoon visits, birthday parties, casual socializing, and weddings
- Social spaces where nice women do not go (e.g., cantinas, commercial sex venues)
- Adolescent social life and courtship: indoor soccer leagues, discos, and terrazas (open-air bars), as well as domestic spaces
- Public spaces: the plaza, church, the Sunday market

Marital case studies

Axis of diversity: Generation	Axis of diversity: Migration status	Axis of diversity: Socioeconomic status (SES)	
		Lower assets and resources	Higher assets and resources
Newlyweds to couples with first young child	Neither mobile nor migrant	2 couples	1 couple, 1 man
	Mobile or migrant	1 woman	1 man
Couples with two or more children, not yet grandparents	Neither mobile nor migrant	1 couple	1 couple, 1 woman
	Mobile or migrant	3 couples	2 couples
Grandparents and people with adult children	Neither mobile nor migrant	3 couples	1 woman
	Mobile or migrant	2 couples	2 couples

Key informant interviews
- 2 priests
- 3 health professionals
- 2 lesbians
- 15 adolescent girls
- 6 feminine-appearing men who have sex with men
- 9 women with local reputations for "sexual behavior"

Archival research
- Current media contexts, including newspaper articles on gender, sexuality, migration, and HIV; locally popular magazines and telenovelas; and movies
- Changing demographic and epidemiological contexts

Nigeria: Fieldwork specifics

Participant observation

- Life course rituals: weddings, burial ceremonies, child naming rituals, baptisms, birthday parties
- Marriage/family settings: household activities such as cooking, washing clothes, and farming; childrearing practices; marital communications; visits to and from migrant family members
- Community groups and events: community development associations, chieftancy installation ceremonies, village council meetings, community courts
- Social geography of men's extramarital sex: brothels, bars, discos, hotels, eateries, car parks at university campuses, social clubs, sports clubs, other settings dominated by male peer groups
- Religion: church services, fellowship meetings, crusades, premarital counseling sessions
- Health services: maternal and child clinics, family planning services, HIV testing and counseling, HIV anti-retroviral treatment program, private contraceptive vendors
- Popular culture and media: Nigerian videos, radio, and TV programming; Internet cafes; bookshops

Marital case studies

Axis of diversity: Marital duration	Axis of diversity: Socioeconomic status			
	Low education/SES		High education/SES	
	Rural	Urban	Rural	Urban
Less than 5 years	2	0	1	2
5–20 years	3	1	4	1
More than 20 years	2	1	2	1

Key informant interviews

- 4 health professionals
- 5 NGO program officers
- 12 people receiving antiretroviral therapy
- 4 pastors/priests
- 4 commercial sex workers
- 3 traditional chiefs
- 3 women's group leaders

Archival research

- Newspaper articles and columns about sexuality, relationships, and marriage; popular magazines about love, sex, gender, and marriage; Nigerian drama videos; and radio and TV programs with relevant themes
- Government demographic data and reports and statistics on HIV/AIDS

Vietnam: Fieldwork specifics

Participant observation

- Social geography of men's extramarital relations: dancehalls and nightclubs, *nha nghi, nha tam*, garden cafés, fishing huts, hotels, karaoke bars, *cafés om*, cruising for street-side and park-based sex workers
- Public spaces: parks, lakes, swimming pools, ice cream shops, cafés, tea shops, restaurants, street-side stalls, *bia hoi*, sidewalk street vendors (corner fruit stand, alley noodle soup and tea stands), and other locations among street-side socializing for families, courting couples, and youths
- Family spaces (household doorsteps, weddings, bridal gown shops, birthday parties, stores that cater to children)
- Women's Union monthly neighborhood meetings

Marital case studies

Axis of diversity: Generation	Axis of Diversity: Mobility	Axis of Diversity: Economic Status	
		Lower assets/ education level	Higher assets/ education level
Newlyweds and couples with first young child (up to 5 years of marriage)	Neither mobile nor migrant	2 couples	3 couples, 1 woman
	Mobile or migrant	0 couples	3 couples
Couples with children in the house (not yet grandparents)	Neither mobile nor migrant	2 couples, 2 women	2 couples, 2 women
	Mobile or migrant	1 couple	4 couples
Grandparents and people with adult children	Neither mobile nor migrant	3 couples	0 couples, 1 man
	Mobile or migrant	1 couple	2 couples, 1 man

Key informant interviews

- 1 economist (female)
- 1 Women's Union official (female)
- 1 lawyer for the Women's Union (female)
- 1 district commune official (female)
- 2 sociologists (one male, one female)
- 1 Vietnamese nongovernmental HIV/AIDS organization project officer (male)
- 1 hotel manager and *xe om* driver (male)
- 1 Vietnamese gay man who lives overseas
- 1 native Hanoi gay man (writer)
- 1 overseas Vietnamese man working in Hanoi
- 1 cook/housekeeper (female)
- 1 journalist (female)
- 3 health professionals (2 female, 1 male)

Archival research

Newspapers and magazine articles on marriage, love, HIV/AIDS, gender, and sexual relationships; educational material on HIV/AIDS; TV programs related to love and marital relationships; popular songs on love and romance (both contemporary and pre–Doi Moi); and government and international reports on HIV/AIDS

Papua New Guinea: Fieldwork specifics

Participant observation
* Families and domestic life: Casual socializing in the households of married couples
* Social spaces from which married women are generally excluded: snooker houses, *dawe anda* (local brothels)
* Public spaces: Tari market, local churches, small-trade stores, Tari District Women's Center, Tari District Hospital

Marital case studies

Axis of diversity: Generation	Axis of diversity: Migration status	Axis of diversity: Economic status	
		Low assets and resources	High assets and resources
Newlyweds (married less than 5 years, young children)	Neither mobile nor migrant	3 men, 2 women	
	Mobile or migrant	2 men, 4 women[a]	1 man, 2 women
Adults (married 5–20 years; young adult children; no grandchildren)	Neither mobile nor migrant	5 men, 1 woman	
	Mobile or migrant	11 men, 11 women	4 men, 2 women
Elders (married more than 20 years; grandchildren)	Neither mobile nor migrant	4 men, 1 woman	
	Mobile or migrant	7 men, 0 women	3 men, 2 women

[a] The Papua New Guinea research team interviewed men and women who were married, but not to each other.

Key informant interviews
* 1 priest
* 3 health professionals
* 1 women's center staff member

Archival research

Newspaper articles about HIV/AIDS, marriage, bridewealth, and the mining industry; educational videos about HIV/AIDS distributed by the Papua New Guinea National AIDS Council; reports based on the demographic data collected for 25 years by the Tari Research Unit; religious instructional texts on marriage, sexuality, and the family

Uganda: Fieldwork Specifics

Participant observation

- Households and domestic life: daily routines, meals, household chores, communication, interactions, comportment, use of space, and mobility
- Neighborhoods: public socializing, meetings, ceremonies, weddings and other life cycle events, tasks, markets, shops, paths and walkways, and private gathering spaces
- Men's homosocial spaces: evening commercial leisure places such as restaurants, bars, hotel bars, local drinking areas, pool halls, video and movie halls, outdoor eating places, dancehalls, live entertainment spaces for plays, concerts, traveling evangelical sermons, and other performances
- Health and HIV VCT (voluntary counseling and testing) and treatment centers
- Places where HIV+ groups meet: meeting content, presentations, and awareness performances in communities

Marital case studies

Axis of diversity: Generation	Axis of diversity: Mobility	Axis of diversity: Economic status		
		Lower	Middle	High
Newlyweds (married less than 5 years; young children)	Neither mobile nor migrant	3 unions	1 union (2 wives interviewed)	Could not find any
	Mobile or migrant	1 union	2 unions	3 unions
Adult (married 5–20 years; young adult children; no grandchildren)	Neither mobile nor migrant	3 unions (1 with 2 wives interviewed)	2 unions (1 with 2 wives interviewed)	1 union
	Mobile or migrant	1 union	3 unions	2 unions
Elders (married more than 20 years; grand-children)	Neither mobile nor migrant	3 unions	2 unions	2 unions (1 with 2 wives interviewed)
	Mobile migrants	2 unions	2 unions (1 with 2 wives interviewed)	1 union

Key informant interviews

- 3 mistresses
- 1 sex worker
- 1 male "pimp"
- 2 sex education teachers
- 1 commercial sex educator
- 1 district health officer
- 1 local healer
- 3 HIV healthcare workers
- 2 workers at an AIDS agency
- 6 HIV+ people
- 6 village-based HIV support groups (20–25 members in each group)
- 1 judge
- 1 officer from the Family Affairs (Probate) Office
- 1 head of a women's rights agency
- 1 Basoga cultural expert
- 3 hotel/bar managers
- 1 chairman of the Uganda Taxi Operator and Driver Association (UTODA)
- 4 religious leaders
- 1 bridal shop owner
- 1 editor of a gossip newspaper
- 1 journalist

Archival research

- Print, video, song, radio, billboards, advertisements, and plays; representations of sexuality, marriage, infidelity, HIV, and gender
- Public health information, campaigns, and billboards on HIV/AIDS
- Official reports on HIV sentinel data, demographics, marriage, women's issues
- Religious and other instructional materials on marriage, sexuality, and the family

Appendix II. Marital Case Study Interview Field Guides

Interviews 1–3

The marital case study guides and participant observation guides included here as Appendices II and III were part of a set of thirteen documents developed by the team over the course of several very intense planning meetings during the year before we carried out our fieldwork. We used these shared instruments to ensure the comparability of data both in terms of topics covered and underlying theoretical constructs explored. The marital case studies consisted of three interviews (conducted separately) with each member of a couple, and so each of the three sections of the guide below corresponds to one of those three interviews. Once in the field, each of us translated and adapted the guide to incorporate concepts and concerns of local relevance; in some cases, as discussed in Chapter 1, we also modified the overall approach to exploring the questions included below.

Because these guides and the other instruments were to be used only by team members and our field assistants (all of whom we would train ourselves), the guides were all characterized by a certain informality in formatting. For some of the questions, we spent a great deal of time working through specific wording for probes that were intended either to clarify the question or to ask follow-up questions, but in other cases the probes were just lists of topics. Most questions as written out included an explicit articulation of their purpose. As we developed them, we were acutely aware that as the guides were translated and adapted, the wording would change, making it all the more important to be explicit (and to remind ourselves) of the underlying goals of each question. For some questions, however, the relevance of the material to our work was so obvious that we did not find it necessary to articulate the purpose. Our original field guides as developed as a group are reproduced here without significant editing.

Interview 1: Coming of Age and the Early Years of Marriage

Relationships, Sexual Practices, and Individual Sexual Coming of Age

1. Tell me about how you met your spouse.

Purpose: To focus on courtship ideals as a way of uncovering marital ideals, gender ideals, and the rise of individualism; to elicit information about courtship practices/rituals, and reasons for choosing a spouse/this spouse.

Probes:
Tell me about the first time you saw your spouse.
How did you meet?
What did you like about him or her?
Were there any things you didn't like?
What were you looking for in a spouse?
What had your parents told you to look for in a spouse?

2. What was your relationship like before you were actually married?

Purpose: To elicit information about the social context and organization of courtship; quality of relationship; importance of various dimensions of the relationship (e.g., emotional, material, and sexual).

Probes:
How did you become a couple?
Who pursued whom and how?
What types of activities did you to together?
What feelings did you have for this person?
How did you show them?
How did he/she show his/her feelings? (Probes: gifts, kisses, sex.)
Did you ever give each other gifts?
Can you give me examples?
When and how did your family find out about the relationship?
How did they react?

3. Why did you marry this person?

Purpose: To explore marital ideals, and individual vs. family choice of spouse.
Probes:
What did you think were the important aspects of a good marriage?

4. Tell me about other times before you met your spouse when you had a boyfriend/girlfriend.

Alternative phrasing:
    Tell me about your first relationship with someone of the opposite sex?
Purpose: To elicit information about sexual coming of age, early learning about sexuality, sense of sexual self/identity, premarital behavior patterns, and differences between premarital and marital relationships.
Probes:
    How did you become a couple?
    Who pursued whom and how?
    What types of activities did you do together?
    What feelings did you have for this person?
    How did you show them?
    How did he/she show his/her feelings? (Probes: gifts, kisses, sex.)
    Did you ever give each other gifts?
    Can you give me examples?
    When and how did your family find out about the relationship?
    How did they react?
    Why did the relationship end?
    Why didn't this relationship lead to marriage?
    What is your relationship with this person like now?

Symbolic and Material Aspects of Wedding Ritual and Household Formation

5. Can you describe the engagement period and the preparations for marriage?

Purpose: To elicit information about courtship practices and marriage preparation, especially issues about individual/couple vs. family/community/social aspects of the process.
Probes:
    What were the steps in getting married?
    Who initiated the formal marriage proposal?
    Who had to consent for the marriage to happen?
    Was there ever any family conflict about the proposed marriage?
    Was anybody upset at the idea of you getting married?
    Was there any training or counseling you went through before you got married?
    What were the things you needed to learn to do before you got married?

6. Tell me about your marriage ceremony(ies).

Purpose: To elicit information about the process and meaning of marriage ceremony(ies), especially how ceremonies mark or signal different things about gender, who "owns" a marriage (i.e., couples or families/communities), how important love is/is not; how important parenthood is, etc.

Probes:
What type of ceremony(ies) did you have?
Why did you have it this way?
Who participated in the wedding, and what did they do?
What was said during the ceremony?
What was done?
Who was invited to the wedding?
What did people wear?
What kinds of gifts were given?
Who paid for which parts of the wedding?

7. What was the relationship/your life with your spouse like right after you got married?

Purpose: To elicit information about the nature and quality of the respondent's relationship (including affect and power) as well as its organizational context and structure in the first year or two after marriage.

Probes:
With whom did you live right after you got married?
With whom did you spend your time after you got married?
Did you have obligations to your in-laws after marriage?
Did this change your relationship with your spouse? How?
Did you and your spouse have your own bedroom/house?
    (possible—ask about first sexual intercourse with spouse)
How did you get along with your spouse?

8. Describe happy and unhappy experiences you had when you were first married.

Purpose: To elicit information about the role of affect in marriage.

Probes:
Tell me about your first big fight.
What were the things you did to show your spouse your feelings?

9. How did your marriage compare with what you thought it was going to be like?

Purpose: To explore the lived experience vs. ideals for married life.

Interview 2: The Lived Experiences of Marriage and Family Life

1. Tell me about what your marriage is like now.

Purpose: To elicit information about how elements of affect, work, and power play out in marital relationships; the idea is to get respondent to talk naturally/extemporaneously, using subsequent questions to guide conversation.

Probes:

How has it changed over time?

How have your ideas about what is important in marriage changed over time?

2. Describe your feelings for your spouse.

Purpose: The underlying question here is how important is emotion/love as an element of a successful relationship—and then the bigger question under that, of course, is the relative role of emotion (whether expressed verbally, sexually, or otherwise) in building the bonds of marriage.

Probes:

Tell me more about what those feelings mean.

If love is mentioned: what is love?

If not mentioned, ask them to define the feelings they list.

Within the last year, describe an event that made you feel particularly happy/good about your spouse.

Within the last year, describe an event that made you feel particularly unhappy about your spouse.

What do you think your spouse feels about you?

How important is love now in the marriage? Is it different now?

3. What are the times of day when you two talk? What do you talk about?

Purpose: To elicit information about what couples talk about and whether/how talking is part of creating an emotional bond.

Probes:

Ask about:

Family members

Children

The relationship

Worries/problems

Work

Money

Community

Gossip

Do you ever talk privately with your spouse?

How is that?

4. When you go out, do you always tell your spouse or the other people you live with where you are going?

Purpose: To elicit information about independence/autonomy and extent of
communication.

Probes:
Do you need to ask for permission? Under what circumstances?
Do you have to inform family members where you have been?
Does your spouse tell you where he or she is going?
Does he or she ask for permission?
Did you ever go someplace without telling?

5. What are the things that you do to be a good wife/husband?

Purpose: To elicit some sense of what the obligations of a good spouse are, especially as
these illuminate gender roles and the extent to which emotional quality of relationship
matters or doesn't.

Probes:
Cooking/cleaning
Gifting
Providing for the family
Care for children and elderly
Sexual performance
Fidelity
Intimacy
Social respect
Of these things, which ones are really important to your spouse?
Can you tell me about a time when your spouse got
    angry at you about one of these things?

6. What are the things that your husband/wife does to be a good husband/wife?

Purpose: To elicit some sense of what the obligations of a good spouse are, especially as
these illuminate gender roles and the extent to which emotional quality of relationship
matters or doesn't.

Probes:
Cooking/cleaning
Gifting
Providing for the family
Care for children and elderly
Sexual performance
Fidelity
Intimacy
Social respect

Of these things, which ones are really important to you?
Can you tell me about a time when you were angry at
　　your spouse about one of these things?

7. How has your marriage changed since you have had children? (Note: alter question if no children.)

Purpose: To elicit information about changes in marital relationships that occur with parenthood, especially with regard to gender dynamics and role of love/emotion in relationship.

Probes:
　　Ask about:
　　Time together
　　Do you try to spend time together without the children?
　　Husband vs. wife involvement in childcare
　　Effects on sex
　　Relationship stronger/weaker—and in what ways
　　Resources/financial demands
　　What do you think it would be like if you did not have children?

8. How do you manage money in your family?

Purpose: To look at money management as an aspect of gender, individuality, and marital power dynamics.

Probes:
　　Do you have your own money?
　　What do you spend it on?
　　Does your spouse have his/her own money?
　　What does he/she spend it on?
　　Do you have joint/shared money?
　　What do you spend joint/shared money on?
　　What was the last major purchase in your household?
　　Who decided?
　　How did you decide?
　　Tell me about a time when you disagreed about a purchase; what happened?

9. I am interested in learning more about how you decide what is best for your children.

Purpose: To elicit information about the ways in which household decisions are made and how this reflects and/or produces certain gender dynamics and feelings/meanings with regard to the marriage relationship.

Probes:
　　Ask about:
　　Schooling

School fees
Child illness episodes
Discipline
Get specific examples:
What did your spouse want?
What did you want?
How did you resolve it?

10. Tell me about the last time you had an argument with your spouse.

Purpose: To understand how arguments/disputes reflect gender and relationship
dynamics.
Probes:
What was the argument about?
What did you want to do?
What did your spouse want to do?
Did anyone intervene or help in resolving the conflicts?
How did it end up?
Who had the most influence on the outcome?
Did the woman go back to her natal home (go back to her place)?
Did the argument get violent?

11. Has there ever been violence in your relationship?

Purpose: To understand how violence reflects and affects gendered power dynamics.
Probes:
Has your spouse ever hit you?
Have you ever hit your spouse?

12. How involved is your family in the affairs of your marriage?

Purpose: To situate marriage within a wider framework of kinship and community, and to
elicit information about the extent to which marriage is an individual/dyadic project
vs. a collective one. It is important to learn about both how this plays out and how
couples feel about it—e.g., do they resent or take for granted in-law interference, and
along what dimensions?
Probes:
Examples of family involvement: visits, fights, arguments
Help in the form of money, moral support, in-kind support, labor
Advice about children
Advice about roles of husband/wife or mother/father
How does respondent feel about all these things?

13. How involved is your spouse's family in the affairs of your marriage?

Purpose: To situate marriage within wider framework of kinship and community and to elicit information about extent to which marriage is individual/dyadic project vs. a collective one. It is important to learn about both how this plays out and how couples feel about it—e.g., do they resent or take for granted in-law interference, and along what dimensions?

Probes:
>Examples of family involvement: visits, fights, arguments
>Help: money, moral support, in-kind support, labor
>Advice about children
>Advice about roles of husband/wife or mother/father
>How does respondent feel about all these things?

Interview 3

Part I: Marital Ideals and Intimacy

1. How would you say your marriage differs from your parents'?

Purpose: To elicit information about changes in the social organization of gender in marriage over generations/time.

Probes:
>**Ask about:**
>Your courtship
>Whose permission did your parents need to get married compared to you?
>Sleeping/residence arrangements
>How much time do you spend together?
>What do you do together?
>What are the things you want to do to be a good parent?
>How are the things that you do in this marriage different
>>than what your mother/father did?
>How are the things that your partner does different than what his/her father/mother
>>did? (Probes: the way you talk to each other, the things you talk about.)

2. How would you like your children's marriages to differ from yours?

Purpose: To assess respondent's satisfaction with his/her own marriage [by learning about his or her] advice to children; to explore changing marital ideals.

Probes:
>**Ask about:**
>What would you tell them to look for in a spouse?
>Their courtship
>Whose permission will they need to get married compared to you?

Sleeping/residence arrangements
How much time will they spend together?
What will they do together?
The things they will do to be good parents
How are the things they will do in marriage different than what you did?
The way they will talk to each other
The things they will talk about

3. What are the best things about your marriage?

4. What are the aspects of your marriage that have been disappointing?

I know this is very private, but I'd like to ask you some questions about sex. I want to remind you that you don't have to answer any questions if you don't want to.

Purpose: To understand the role of sex in marriage, especially the extent to which sexual relations are paramount (or not) in the construction of the marriage relationship.

5. First, tell me what you knew about sex before you got married.

Purpose: To provide an innocuous introduction to the topic.
Probes:
How did you learn these things? (Examples: school, newspapers, peers, magazines, movies, boyfriends/girlfriends.)

6. Tell me about the first time you and your spouse were physically intimate.

(not necessarily sex—the first kiss, holding hands, whatever makes sense locally)

7. What about the first time you had sex?

8. Tell me about your sex life with your spouse now.

9. What is/are the reason(s) you have sex with your spouse?

10. How frequently do you have sex now?

11. Do you talk to your spouse about sex? If yes, in what way?
Probes:
Can you tell your spouse what feels good or doesn't feel good?
Do you joke about sex?

12. Who initiates sex in your marriage?

13. Tell me about what usually happens when you and your partner are going to have sex.

Probes:

How do you express to your partner that you want to have sex?

What do you and your partner do to get ready (warm up) for sex?

Do you and your partner touch each other for very long before intercourse?

14. Do you enjoy sex with your spouse?

Probes:

Do you enjoy it more, less, or the same as when you first began your relationship?

What are the other ways in which your intimacy has

changed over the course of the marriage?

15. How important is pleasurable sex with your spouse/in your marriage?

16. What would happen in your marriage if your partner were not happy with the sexual relationship?

Probes:

What would happen if you weren't happy?

17. Do couples here have sex if the woman is menstruating?

Probes:

How about other times?

What if one partner does not want to have sex, can she/he say no?

How?

18. Did your partner ever ask you to engage in a particular kind of sex that you didn't want to engage in?

Probes:

Ask about:

Using a condom

Having oral/anal sex, etc.

19. Have you and/or your partner ever done anything to plan the number of children you have?

Purpose: To elicit information about spousal communication about contraception and to look at contraceptive decision-making as an indicator of the kinds of relationships people have.

Probes:
Do you ever talk about it with your partner?
Have you ever used contraception in your marriage? Why?
What kind(s) have you used?
How did you and/or your partner decide on those ways of regulating fertility?

Part II: Extramarital Opportunity Structures, the Social Organization of Extramarital Sex, and HIV

I realize these are incredibly private matters (renew promise of confidentiality), but I want to ask you some questions about extramarital sexual relationships.

20. Some people in (community) have sex outside marriage, for various reasons. What are some of the circumstances in which this happens?

Probes:
What are some of the reasons why it happens?
Note: In asking this question, remember to introduce the topic gently and in a way that suggests that good people might also be tempted.

21. Have you ever had a sexual relationship outside your marriage?

Purpose: To obtain information about actual experiences of extramarital sex and their context/meaning.

Probes:
If yes, tell me about the most recent time this happened.
How did you meet this person?
Tell me about this person.
During what stage of your marriage did this take place?
How long did the relationship last?
[If it ended:] How did it end?
Who knew about the relationship?
How did you feel about it then?
How do you feel about it now?

22. What were the circumstances and reasons that led to this?

Purpose: To explore the opportunity structures of extramarital relationships.
Probes:
> **Possible circumstances:**
> Where were you when this happened?
> Where you were living at this time?
> Were you living with your spouse?
> Did you have sex because you needed money?
> Did you have sex because you had money?
> Were you encouraged or expected by others to have an extramarital relationship?
> What was your relationship with your spouse like?
> How were you feeling at the time (lonely, angry, horny, entitled, lusty, in love)?

23. Tell me about what your relationship with this person was like.

Probes:
> How would you characterize this relationship (was your
>   partner a sex worker, love interest, etc.)?
> **Ask about:**
> Autonomy and independence
> Communication
> Work
> Affect
> Role expectations
> Money
> Arguments and violence
> The involvement of others
> Best and most disappointing aspects
> Risks and benefits
> How different from marriage

24. Tell me about the sexual relationship with this person.

Probes:
> **Ask about:**
> Reasons
> Frequency
> Talking
> Initiation
> Describe an episode of sex
> Pleasure
> Experimentation
> How was the sex different than the sex with your spouse?

25. Did you/your partner want a pregnancy in this relationship?

Purpose: To elicit information on contraceptive use in extramarital relations.
Probes:
  Did you or your partner think about the risk of pregnancy?
  Did you or your partner do anything to reduce the risk of pregnancy?
  Did you talk about contraception with your partner?
  If you used it, how did you negotiate contraception?
  What types of contraceptives did you use?
  Who obtained them?

26. Did you ever think about the risk of HIV in this relationship? [Ask about STDs, if relevant to field site.]

Purpose: To elicit respondent's HIV risk management practices.

27. If yes, did you do anything about it?

Probes:
  Ask about:
  Discussions with partner
  Partner choice
  Condom use
  Other sexual practices related to risk or risk reduction—e.g., oral sex, anal sex

28. If you've had several extramarital relationships, how have they been different?

29. *If no sexual relationship outside marriage:* Have you ever wanted to have sex with someone other than your spouse?

Purpose: To help explore gender differences in penalties of extramarital sex.
Probes:
  If so, how often?

30. Did you ever suspect or find out that your spouse has ever had sex outside your marriage? What can you tell me about it? [Remind them that you don't have access to information from the other interview and that you will not share this information with anyone.]

31. Have you ever talked with your spouse about extramarital relations? If yes, describe.

32. Have you ever talked with your spouse about HIV? If yes, describe.

33. Have you ever talked with your spouse about ways to reduce the risk of HIV transmission in your relationship?

Purpose: To elicit HIV risk management practices.
Probes:
    What are the things that you've talked about?
    What are the things that you've actually done to reduce risk, if anything?
    Ask about:
    Discussions with partner
    Condom use
    Other sexual practices related to risk or risk reduction—e.g., oral sex, anal sex

34. Have you ever thought about HIV?

Probes:
    What did you do about it?
    Have you ever talked to anybody about HIV?

35. We are interested in learning about things that put married people at risk of HIV infection. What do you think are the things that put married people at risk?

Probes:
    What do you think would make married men less likely to become infected with HIV?
    Married women?

36. Do you have any questions for me?

After the interview, provide respondent with basic information on HIV and AIDS. The nature of this information will be determined at each field site, but might include HIV transmission routes, risk reduction techniques, nearby counseling and testing centers, and local HIV agencies and support organizations.

Appendix III. Detailed Listing of Plans for Participant Observation, High-Priority Locations

As suggested by the title, this instrument presents the high-priority areas for participant observation, representing the team's consensus about the spaces in which we were most likely to observe phenomena relevant to answering our shared questions. The set of instruments we developed also included a list of lower-priority sites for participant observation, which is not reproduced here. Each of us used these instruments as guides in determining where to spend time and what to look for over the course of our fieldwork.

SOCIAL SPACES

TThings to look for specifically	Vital questions to answer

Patterns of socializing

Gender, social networks, and prestige hierarchies

    How do men socialize with other men?

    How do women socialize with other women?

    To what extent do men's social networks and activities shape extramarital relationships?

    How are men's patterns of socializing related to economic factors?

Staging of extramarital sex

    What are the social spaces in which men and women spend time together outside of the home, and how does the organization of these spaces shape nonmarital heterosexual relationships?

    Where does commercial sex happen? (bars, houses, out of town)

    Who controls these spaces? (state, police, commercial interests)

Vital questions to answer: What is the social geography of extramarital sex?

What is the difference here between men's
"heterosexual" and "homosexual"
relationships (using these categories as
general placeholders)?

Are there any regulations about condom use
in different commercial sex venues?

Are these regulations enforced? By whom?

The lived experience of marriage and family life in public

Marital communication and socializing—tone and content

How do couples act together in public?

Do they even ever appear in public as
couples? If so, where?

Are these spaces for heterosociality new?
Public? Commercial? How are they
shaped by social class?

Gender and life-course differences in physical autonomy

What are the local single-sex social spaces?

In what circumstances do women go out by
themselves?

Where do men go by themselves?

What is perceived to be safe for women?

What is perceived to be safe for men?

How does the public face of couples
help us learn about the diversity
of marital practices in terms of:

Affect?

Work?

Power: Individual autonomy/
control over one's spouse?

Decision-making (as both
an affective process and
a manifestation of power
differences)?

How children fit into family-
building?

How sex fits into family-building?

Social constructions of sexuality

Sexual identities

What are the local categories through which
people understand sexual identity?

What are people's attitudes toward various
sexual identities?

What is the moral landscape of object choice
(sex of partner)?

Presentation of sexual self (issues of
sexuality and gendered prestige/status
and stigma)—the strategic creation of a
sexual self for public consumption; dress,

What can we learn from the
media, coming-of-age rituals, and
other cultural forms about:

The nature and purpose of marital
sexuality?

Symbolic aspects of extramarital sex?

Local organization of sexual identities?

comportment, where they go, and who
they go with (can women say hello to
other people on the street? do they need
to be accompanied?)
Private sexual selves—how do issues of
self play out in the formation of sexual
relationships?
Beliefs/attitudes toward extramarital relations

Cultural ideals and extramarital sex

How do men and women react to stories about
different kinds of extramarital relationships?

Are some kinds seen differently than
others (e.g., another man's wife versus
a commercial sex worker or unmarried
woman, either within or outside of the
community)?

Are there different reasons for different kinds
of relationships?

Are there different risks for different kinds of
relationships?

Patterns of sexual joking and gossip,
especially about extramarital sex

Are there gender differences in how people
joke and talk about extramarital sex?

Are there generational differences in styles,
content, audiences?

What about relevant policies (i.e., public
policy/public health/legal regulation of
extramarital and nonmarital sex)?

What is the public discourse
about infidelity?

Marketplaces as social and sexual spaces

A space where we might be able to observe
gendered interactions between men and
women (like a U.S. shopping mall)

How do people flirt in the market?

Do married people shop together?

What is going on in marketplaces in
terms of self-presentation and sexual
advertisements?

What is the gendered division
of interaction and presentation
in places of commerce?

HOUSEHOLDS

Things to look for specifically	Vital questions to answer

Symbolic and material aspects of wedding rituals and household formation

Premarital relationships that do not lead to marriage (same- and opposite-sex)

Watch the unmarried adolescent children in families—how are they courting?

What do their premarital relationships involve?

Why do they sometimes not lead to marriage?

How do families intervene to try to control these relationships (or not)?

Gather stories of how families organize their children's weddings

Who marries them?

Who is involved in ritual and celebratory aspects—religious regulation of marriage, marriage rituals, pre-wedding counseling (formal and informal, including premarital counseling regarding HIV and other STDs)?

Marriage and social networks: How is the wedding celebrated? Who is invited?

Marriages and consumption: What do they wear? What do they receive as gifts? Who pays for what?

Look at where couples live immediately after marriage

What is involved in terms of setting up a household?

Where do the resources come from to establish these new households?

If residence is not neolocal, how long and under what circumstances do couples live with husband's (or wife's) kin?

How people marry is an important way of getting at what marriage is. For the participant observation on these topics, we are interested in learning about how these things work *in general* and how they are perceived to be changing over time. It is sometimes easier for people to tell the story of their courtship than to articulate their affective goals for a union, but courtship stories can reveal a lot about those affective goals.

Questions:

What can we learn about the social constructions of marriage from seeing how unions are formed?

Specifically: What is marriage for? What is sex in marriage for? What are the marital implications of extramarital sex?

How does the process of union formation differ across lines of:

Generation?

Social class?

Ethnic group?

Other significant local sources of diversity?

What is the relationship of these changes or sources of ideological/actual diversity to economic and cultural change (à la Collier, Yan, or Hirsch)?

Talk with people about the purpose of marriage
  Why do men marry?
  Why do women marry?
  What do they expect from marriage?
  What are the reasons for considering a
     marriage a success or failure?

**The lived experience of marriage and family
life—how do couples act at home?**
*Marital communication—tone and content—
how do couples talk to each other?*
  Fighting: What are some reasons for
     fighting? How do couples make up?
     How do couples use violence to resolve
     disputes?
  Joking: Do couples joke about sex? What are
     the jokes like? What else do couples joke
     about?
  What do couples talk about (money,
     children, sex, gossip, feelings, etc.)?
  Are there gender and life-course differences
     in physical autonomy?
  Control over one's own physical mobility:
     Who asks whose permission before going
     out? For an overnight journey? Do people
     sometimes not know where a spouse is or
     when he/she will return?
  Decisions about what to wear: Do you ever
     hear comments about things women can
     or cannot wear?
Affect
  Verbal expressions
  Physical expressions
  Telling secrets to a spouse
  Through gifts
  Affective disappointments
Socializing
  When are people not working?
  What are people doing when they are not
     working?
  Does it even make sense in your location to

Focus on six aspects of marriage,
in mapping out the diversity
of marital practices:
  Affect
  Work
  Power: Individual autonomy/control
     over one's spouse
  Decision-making (as both an affective
     process and a manifestation of power
     differences)
  How children fit into family-building
  How sex fits into family-building

How does relationship-level gender
inequality affect women's control of
men's behavior outside the house?

In other words, how much control
do women have of men?

How much control do men
have of women?

think of this division between work time
and social time? If not, how is socializing
organized?

Do couples spend "leisure time" together?

Do couples ever deliberately spend time
together without their children?

*Exchanges between the couple—are
there items in the house that men and
women have given each other?*

Ritual gift-giving

"Modern" gift-giving—Valentine's Day,
Mother's Day, etc.

*Patterns of eating—how do patterns
of eating demonstrate underlying
concepts about social hierarchy?*

Who serves whom during meals?

Do couples eat together?

Do parents and children eat together?

What about family and guests?

Who eats first and best?

Who gets seconds?

How are things different when guests are
present?

*Men's and women's contributions to
social reproduction—what is each
person's job in marriage?*

Food preparation

Childcare

Housework

Gardening

Animal husbandry

Helping children with schoolwork

Other tasks

MATERIAL CULTURE

Things to look for specifically	Vital questions to answer
Relationships/symbolic and material aspects of wedding rituals and household formation *The range of courtship practices/ how couples are created*	What can we learn about the social constructions of marriage from seeing the things that people buy when they set up how unions are formed?

What kinds of material exchanges take place during courtship? What kinds of gifts are sold as things that courting couples might exchange?

Are there special holidays for lovers? (Valentine's Day but also local holidays)

Paths to marriage

What do they wear?

What do they receive as gifts?

Who pays for what?

Where couples live immediately after marriage

What is involved in terms of setting up a household? (See Collier 1997 on this—what kinds of things do newlyweds "need"?)

Purpose of marriage

Why do men marry?

Why do women marry?

What do they expect from marriage?

What are the reasons for considering a marriage a success or failure?

What are the things that people buy to build relationships?

How does the way people engage with material culture differ across lines of:

Generation?

Social class?

Ethnic group?

Other significant local sources of diversity?

What is the relationship of these material goods to economic and cultural change?

Exchanges between the couple

Ritual gift-giving

"Modern" gift-giving—Valentine's Day, Mother's Day, etc.

Use this as a means to explore affective goals in marriage (and the commercialization of affect).

Sexual and intimate commodities

Lingerie

Sex toys (if they exist) and paraphernalia

Sexual media (magazines, romance novels)

Makeup

This is part of learning about the meanings of sexuality: Are certain goods used more for premarital sex, marital sex, or extramarital sex?

Domestic architecture

Who furnishes the houses?

What do houses "need" to have?

What sorts of furniture are available in furniture stores? (Do furniture stores even exist?)

How are houses decorated? (See Hirsch 2003, chapter 2, on domestic altars.)

Look at domestic architecture to get a sense of how family ideologies intersect with the material world.

What is the diversity in physical organization
of households across generational or
economic lines?

**Regulation of reproduction/contraceptive use/
disease prevention**

What kinds of contraceptive methods are
available without a prescription?

How popular are these?

To which kinds of women (or men) are they
targeted? (Ask vendors/pharmacists, look
at packaging)

How available are condoms?

For commercial sex, is condom use regulated
in any way?

How do condom or contraceptive campaigns
deal with extramarital sex, if at all?

Can people buy antibiotics for STDs over the
counter?

RELIGIOUS INSTITUTIONS

Things to look for specifically	Vital questions to answer
Religion and marital ideologies Religious regulation of marriage, divorce, and sexual behavior Religious ideologies about gender and family organization, including conflicts with the State	What are religious influences on these marital ideologies?
Relationships/symbolic and material aspects of wedding rituals and household formation *Religious messages about* Premarital sex/virginity Ideal partners Courtship practices *Paths to marriage* Who marries them? Religious regulation of marriage	What can we learn about the social constructions of marriage from seeing how unions are formed? Specifically: What is marriage for? What is sex in marriage for? What are the marital implications of extramarital sex?

Marriage rituals

Pre-wedding counseling (formal and
   informal), including premarital
   counseling regarding HIV and other
   STDs)

Purpose of marriage

Why do men marry?

Why do women marry?

What do religious ideologies tell them to
   expect from marriage?

HEALTH CLINICS/ORGANIZATION OF HEALTH SERVICES

Things to look for specifically   Vital questions to answer

Regulation of reproduction

Contraceptive use   What is the role of nonreproductive

   Access to services   sex in marriage?

   Preferred methods and why

   Interactions around contraceptive use   What is the role of children
      (couple, other family members,   in family-building?
      practitioners)

   Pamphlets or health education materials
      promoting specific methods

   Pamphlets or health education materials
      promoting fertility limitation

Local meanings of condoms

   How available are condoms?

   For commercial sex, is condom use regulated
      in any way?

   How do condom or contraceptive campaigns
      deal with extramarital sex, if at all?

Notes

Introduction
Epigraph: From *Suzette veut me lâcher*. Quoted in Thurman 1999: 112.
1. The writing in this chapter reflects the collective efforts of our group. Jennifer S. Hirsch first drafted this introduction in the summer of 2007, and Daniel Jordan Smith drafted a major revision in June 2008, but it has gone through dozens of rounds of editing since 2007, with significant additions contributed, excisions performed, and interventions made by each of the co-authors.
2. During the early years of the HIV epidemic in the United States, relatively little attention was paid to women. The disease was first diagnosed primarily among men, and the Centers for Disease Control's initial definitions of AIDS did not even include the specific AIDS-related causes of death most common among women. The invisibility of women is suggested by the fact that during those early years, women on the brink of death were ineligible to receive the Social Security disability payments for which men dying of Kaposi's sarcoma qualified, because the opportunistic infections from which women suffered did not qualify them for AIDS diagnoses (Anastos and Marte 1989; Amaro 1995).
3. Among the most important articles responding to this call for research on how social and cultural aspects of gender shape women's risk of HIV infection were Debruyn 1992; Farmer, Lindenbaum, and Good 1993; Heise and Elias 1995; Amaro 1995; de Zoysa, Sweat, and Denison 1996; and Zierler and Krieger 1997.
4. This attention to men in public health has been paralleled by a growing interest among social demographers in exploring "couple-level" factors that influence contraceptive use, reflecting a desire to apply a feminist optic to these issues. The reproductive health focus on men has also sprung from an acknowledgment that (despite the family planning field's traditional focus on women) men play an important role in reproduction and that it is not possible to analyze the interpersonal dynamics of fertility without understanding that it takes (at least) two to tango.
5. Pleck, Sonenstein, and Ku's frequently cited 1993 article, for example, analyzing data from a nationally representative sample of adolescent men, found that "males who hold traditional attitudes toward masculinity indicate having more sexual partners in the last year, a less intimate relationship at last intercourse with the current partner, and greater belief that relationships between women and men are adversarial—characteristics suggesting less intimacy in their heterosexual relationships. . . . Traditional masculinity ideology is thus associated with characteristics suggesting limitations in the quality of adolescent males' close heterosexual relationships, and increased risk of unintended pregnancy and sexually transmitted diseases, including AIDS." For more examples of research that focuses on how men's ideas about masculinity shape their sexual practices, see Go et al. 2003; Verma et al. 2004; Barker 2005; Barker and Ricardo 2005; Missildine, Parsons, and Knight 2006; O'Sullivan et al. 2006; Pulerwitz et al. 2006; Verma, Pulerwitz, and Mahendra 2006; and Pulerwitz and Barker 2007.
6. An element of gender inequality that we do not address centrally in this book is gender

violence, though we greatly appreciate how it both reflects and reinforces inequalities between men and women in intimate relationships. The contrast between men's sexual opportunity structures and women's experiences of coercion and violence highlights the way the social organization of sexuality reflects gendered inequalities. Certainly each of us know of instances when the latent violence of gendered inequalities in domestic power was expressed through more direct interpersonal violence—and violence was a particularly frequent means of dispute resolution in the Papua New Guinea field site. We did not, however, set out to study how gender violence figures in marriage or the organization of HIV risk, and so direct the reader to the ample literature on gender, violence, and HIV that does more justice to the complexity of the topic than we can do here (Merry 2009; Heise, Ellsberg, and Gottmoeller 2002; Esther 2002; Wojcicki 2008; van der Straten et al. 1995; Goldstein and Manlowe 1997).

7. Social scientists (e.g., Simmons 1979, Skolnik 1991) have used the term "companionate marriage" to describe relationships characterized by "intense psychological companionship, or friendship between husband and wife." By the end of the twentieth century, the idea that emotional intimacy and companionship are at the core of the marital bond in low-fertility, largely neolocal western societies had become widely accepted (Giddens 1992; Gillis, Tilly, and Levin 1992; Schneider and Schneider 1996; Collier 1997). A similar phenomenon had been identified by Caldwell in sub-Saharan Africa in 1968, when he noted that in Nigeria "a surprising proportion of women longed for a non-traditional marriage, one with much more spousal companionship and one where this companionship was reflected in sexual matters" (quoted in Orubuloye, Caldwell, and Caldwell 1997: 1201). Later, he referred to this as "the emotional nucleation" of the family (Caldwell 1976). Over the past forty years, this "emotional nucleation" has captured people's imaginations throughout the developing world (see Inhorn 1996; Hollos and Larsen 1997; Ahearn 2001; Yan 2003; Smith 2000, 2001; Reddy 2005; Wardlow 2006; Parikh 2004; Hirsch and Wardlow 2006; Hirsch 2003a; Padilla et al. 2007; Cole and Thomas 2009).

8. Prior to Sobo's work, Kline, Kline, and Oken (1992) and Worth (1989) also helped lay the foundation for these questions about love and risk by connecting women's condom use practices to broader issues of culture, inequality, and agency among minority women.

9. A third body of work on love and intimacy has explored changing forms of same-sex relations in diverse contexts. Some of this work within anthropology (e.g., Weston 1997, Reddy 2005) emphasizes how ties of affect create bonds of kinship and closely mirrors the work on love and the social production of heterosexuality. Other recent work (Sinnot 2004, Boellstorff 2005) has focused on the ways in which both nationalist discourses and globalization have shaped same-sex identities. Still other work (Wekker 2006) has examined the postcolonial and diasporic transformations of same-sex relationships in a context of dramatic economic decline.

10. The words "homosocial" and "heterosocial" denote forms of socializing that are primarily organized around, respectively, single-sex or mixed-sex social relationships. Here we primarily use the term "homosocial" to describe circumstances in which men spend leisure time with each other. Women are frequently present but, as others have also argued, the heterosexual activities that take place in these have become intertwined in important ways with how men use these settings to develop and strengthen their social relations with one another (Sedgwick 1985; Allison 1994; Bird 1996; Grazian 2007).

11. See, for example, Choi, Catania, and Dolcini 1994; Laumann 1994; Wiederman 1997; Atkins, Baucom, and Jacobson 2001; Allen et al. 2005; Blow and Hartnett 2005; Schensul et al. 2006; Burdette et al. 2007; Dollahite and Lambert 2007; Whisman, Gordon, and Chatav 2007; Allen et al. 2008; Atkins and Kessel 2008; Traeen and Martinussen 2008.

12. Examples of this genre of research on infidelity include Glassmann 2003; Ward 2004;

Allen and Atkins 2005; Gordon, Baucom, and Snyder 2005; Lusterman 2005; Martell and Prince 2005; McCarthy 2005; Orzeck and Lung 2005; Snyder and Doss 2005; Whisman and Wagers 2005; Dupree et al. 2007; Bagarozzi 2008; Butler, Seedall, and Harper 2008; Platt et al. 2008; Young 2008.

13. We think here of works such as Bamford 2007 or Carsten 2000 that articulate how the bonds of kinship are seen to be constituted not by the transmission of biological substance, but rather through relations of nurturing and care.

14. We present the ethnographic material in this book primarily in the present tense, shifting to the past tense when we describe historical aspects of each field site and to the past perfect for more abstract analyses. Our use of the present tense does not indicate that the conditions we describe in each field site are timeless and unchanging—indeed, throughout this volume, we go to great lengths to situate what people do within particular political and economic conditions. Rather, we use the present tense to achieve a more vivid and lively depiction of our fieldwork experiences and to bring readers into the everyday lives of people we encountered.

15. "Doi Moi" (Renovation) refers to a series of new economic reforms initiated in 1986 by the Vietnamese government. It marks a shift from a centrally planned economy to a market economy with a socialist direction.

Chapter 1

1. Holly Wardlow took the lead in writing the first half of this chapter, which frames our understanding of critical comparative anthropology and discusses it in relation to the history and politics of the comparative method in anthropology. Jennifer S. Hirsch drafted the first version of the chapter's second half, which describes our research methods—although portions of it draw heavily on the initial NIH grant proposal, which was such a collaborative effort that it is impossible to identify any one of us as a "lead author." Shanti Parikh, Harriet M. Phinney, Daniel Jordan Smith, and Constance A. Nathanson each made significant contributions to this chapter.

2. The notion of "thick description," in other words, refers to description that includes both the externally observable elements of a behavior as well as the contextually determined meanings of that behavior. It was first presented by Gilbert Ryle (1971) but was further developed in (and made famous by) Clifford Geertz's classic *The Interpretation of Cultures* (1973).

3. Richard G. Fox similarly asserts that "the comparative method and cross-cultural comparison too often sacrificed history and historical process in the pursuit of trite, superficial general laws" (2002: 167). However, invoking such scholars as Fred Eggan, Eric Wolf, and Sidney Mintz, he argues that in American anthropology there has always existed a "subaltern" comparative method (although it was not known as such) that examined "divergent outcomes of similar historical processes" (ibid.; see also Silverman 2005).

4. Reflexivity denotes research from a post-positivist standpoint, in which the researcher considers how the assumptions and social position he or she brings to the work shapes the findings. The term "experience-near," as developed by Geertz, refers to the categories and terms for experiences that are used by people in everyday life to talk about those experiences, in contrast to the more abstract terms used by experts. Geertz writes about the importance of working in experience-near terms as a strategy "to figure out what the devil [people] think they are up to" (1974: 29).

5. We designed the ethnographic field guide with the goal of developing trust by asking general questions about courtship, marriage, and family during the earlier interviews, and then asking questions related to sexuality and extramarital sex in the last interview after a rapport and trust had been established. Marital case study participants were interviewed in two or three sessions, allowing for more time and renewed personal contact, as well

as for more consideration on our parts of how their perceptions of us, and the particular relationship developed with each informant, might shape the stories they told us.

Chapter 2

1. The fieldwork on which this chapter draws was conducted as a collective enterprise. Sergio Meneses Navarro and Brenda Thompson contributed both to the data collection and to conversations throughout the course of the fieldwork about the meanings of what we were learning. My friends Estela Mata Rivera and Alan Lujambio García were keen observers of Degollado society and provided invaluable help by introducing us to many of the marital case study participants.

2. Because of space constraints, and this volume's overall focus on men's extramarital sexual relations, we leave those stories for another time.

3. Instituto Nacional de Estadística y Geografía (INEGI), "Working population by county, sex and primary occupation," *www.inegi.org.mx*; INEGI, *VII Censo general de población, 1960, Estado de Michoacán* (Mexico City: Estados Unidos Mexicanos, 1960); "El frijol prodedente de EU y Canada inunda el mercado Mexicano, a pesar de que aún no se autorizan cupos de importacion," *Mural* (March 15, 2004); " 'Impactan reglas de EU a productos nacionales': Hubo un incremento de importaciones de maíz, trigo, frijoles, y carne de cerdo y ave," *Mural* (May 10, 2004); "La preferencia por frutas y hortalizas de USA y Chile en México esta afectando a los productores mexicanos," *Mural* (June 14, 2004).

4. INEGI, "Total population by county, sex and five year age groups," *www.inegi.org.mx.*

5. The town lacks the rich indigenous crafts traditions found in other Mexican states such as Oaxaca and Michoacan, but an enterprising local figure began a stone-carving initiative, working the soft pink sandstone known as *cantera* into fountains, sculpture, and colonial-style architecture details. The industry now provides employment for hundreds of local men (and a few women), and exports its products to North America, as well as (reportedly) Europe and the Middle East. For more on economic development in the face of the pressures of globalization, see "La secretaría de turismo promueve al estado con tazas que llevan la leyenda: 'Jalisco es México,' pero las tazas son hechas en China," *Mural* (March 27, 2004); "Los productos Chinos desplazan a los productores nacionales de Mexico," *Mural* (April 21, 2004); "Falsifican en China talavera de Puebla," *Mural* (May 24, 2004); "Recomiendan a las empresas Mexicanas reorientar su mercado exportador hacia EU para competir con los productos Chinos," *Mural* (June 7, 2004). For reference to the planting of agave, see "La falta de integración de las cadenas productivas agroalimentarias engarzan desempleo," *Mural* (March 1, 2004).

6. Unmarried young women and men do sometimes go together for casual dinners of *tacos* or *sopes* at *cenadurías*, which are usually located in the front bedrooms of private homes. One of these was reported to have a secret room where lovers could tryst; whether or not this was true, the insistent local gossip about goings-on in the back room highlights the unseemliness of unmarried people slipping away from the town's watchful eye.

7. The only circumstances under which young women break out of this transnational circle of surveillance is when they have already stepped over the moral line. Young women who have shamed their families through premarital pregnancies frequently strike out as *madres solteras* (single mothers) away from the prying eyes of neighbors, having already failed their natal families.

8. A *compadre* is the godfather of one's child (the feminine is *comadre*). In Mexico, *compadrazgo* (literally, "being *compadres* or *comadres* with someone"; no equivalent term exists in English) is an important kinship form, through which relations of affect and obligation are formalized and strengthened.

9. I was initially confused by the notion that men who had spent an evening with women doing lap-dances would then seek out male sex workers, but over time it came to make sense in the broader context of men's flexibility regarding object choice.

10. I could never confirm the rumor that married men from Degollado had been sighted there, because every time Estela and I would make a plan to go together, her husband (who was always worried about my bad influence) would invent a crisis (such as pretending his mother was dying) to interrupt our plans.

11. The United States is perceived to be a place where, as I was told by one young woman, "women go through men like Kleenex" and by another that "se casan y descasan con la misma facilidad" (there they marry and divorce with the same ease)—a land of easy women and loose morals.

12. As people say, "Dime con quien andas y te dire quien eres" (tell me who you run with and I will tell you who you are). An element of this is that people choose who they run with as part of the process of constructing who they are.

13. The phrase "small towns have big gossip" is the local version of the name of a recent telenovela, *Pueblo chico, infierno grande* (Small Town, Big Hell), which apparently focused on the scandals and suffering simmering just below the surface in small-town Mexico.

14. If a woman forgoes this ritual establishment of sexual innocence and then ends up getting pregnant before marriage, she runs the risk that her partner will deny that the child is his and insist that she is trying to trap him. After marriage, having firmly established herself as sexually virtuous allows a woman the freedom to develop a wider repertoire of marital sexual acts without fearing recrimination or humiliation.

15. Although the other chapters in this book provide ample evidence that the Catholic Church is hardly the only institution propagating ideologies that base a woman's moral standing on her sexual behavior—and although, to his credit, the Señor Cura in Degollado no longer posts the marriage announcements of virgins and non-virgins in different colors, as was the practice of his predecessor—it is clear that this division of women into *muchachas decentes o putas* (virgins and whores) has been heavily influenced by the Church.

16. Even as the material world out of which couples build sexual intimacy is transformed by consumer products and images that were not available in rural Mexico a generation ago, the Church continues to assert its authority to make distinctions between permitted and prohibited sexuality. Through the Christian Family Movement, whose local leaders teach the marriage preparation classes young couples are required to attend before they marry in the Church, modern Catholicism disseminates the notion of "la sexualidad al servicio de amor" (sex in the service of love) in which mutual sexual pleasure, caring, shared religious faith, a commitment to reproduction, and physical intimacy intertwine to elevate mere "genitality" into a moment of physical and spiritual communion that profoundly strengthens the family (for example, see Tomás Melendo Granados, "La sexualidad al servicio de amor y la unión conyugal," *es.catholic.net*, July 16, 2008).

17. In the spring of 2004, we attended a First Communion party at a social hall in La Piedad, a mid-sized city twenty kilometers from Degollado, which was notable for the fact that the parents of the child were a lesbian couple. Some of the men we met that night were married (to women, not to each other), but they were there with their male lovers or with friends, gathering in a hidden social parallel universe. These nascent networks of individuals forming families of choice could be read either as evidence of the fragility of Mexican heteronormativity (since all these individuals, men and women, were gathering in a community organized around same-sex desire) or as evidence of its intractability (there was a great deal of secrecy surrounding the location and nature of this event, and those with whom we spoke had no intention of assuming a public homosexual or lesbian identity—particularly not those from small towns such as Degollado).

18. Of course, many times, the gesture actually does lead to the deep and passionate kiss.

Chapter 3

1. Stephanie Nolen, "Focus," *Globe and Mail* (Toronto), October 18, 2003; Sharon LaFraniere, "AIDS now compels Africa to challenge widows' 'cleansing,'" *New York Times*, May 11, 2005.

2. The rise of modern Nigerian marriage is certainly not the equivalent of or reducible to some sort of women's movement or feminist revolution. It would be inaccurate to present women as the advocates of modern marriage and men as its opponents. The story is much more complex and nuanced.

3. "Pepper-soup joints" are restaurants that specialize in various dishes spiced with hot pepper. These establishments commonly serve beer and are regularly patronized by men looking for a spot to entertain their lovers.

4. The arrival of cell phone service in Nigeria around 2001 has added an interesting twist to the separation of social spaces. These days, it is quite common for married men to provide cell phones to their unmarried lovers; yet, phone calls can easily transgress the normal spatial boundaries. Wives often call men when they are out with their girlfriends, and I have watched countless men lie and quickly end these calls. Men shared with me a number of strategies to preserve the boundaries between marriage and family and extramarital sex. First, most men found it necessary to provide their wives with phones if they did not already have one, so that a woman would have no reason to answer or use her husband's phone. Second, when men entered their girlfriends' numbers into their cell phones' address books, they used fake names (usually male names) in case their wives ever snooped at the records of recent ingoing and outgoing calls. Finally, some men simply maintained several phones, using different lines for different purposes and keeping the lines used with girlfriends at work or in their cars rather than bringing them into their marital homes. But even with the challenges posed by cell phones, most married men's lovers are careful about trying to obey cultural rules regarding the boundaries between relationships of marriage and infidelity.

5. It was impossible to get the married women I interviewed to talk about their own participation in extramarital sex. All denied they had been unfaithful themselves, though they could tell stories of other women who had engaged in extramarital sex. I am quite sure some of the women have had extramarital sex, but because it is much more socially risky for them than for men, I also think it is reasonable to assume that fewer married women than married men are unfaithful to their spouses. Whereas I am arguing that men's extramarital sex happens *because* of a whole range of socially organized opportunity structures, to the extent that women have extramarital sex, it happens *despite* all the social impediments designed to prevent it.

6. For additional literature on gender and sexual negotiations in the context of the AIDS epidemic, see Susser 2001; Susser and Stein 2000.

Chapter 4

1. Anh Binh (Older Brother Binh) is a pseudonym, as are all of the names of other informants and case study participants. Individuals such as Tran Thi Van Anh, a sociologist who was interviewed as someone who had studied these issues, are identified by their actual names. In keeping with Vietnamese convention, the full names of Vietnamese scholars are listed when their works are cited, both out of respect and in order to avoid confusion. The data for this chapter comes from ethnographic fieldwork conducted among the majority ethnic group in Hanoi, the Kinh, from February through July 2004. The research was carried out by Harriet M. Phinney in collaboration with Nguyen Huu Minh, vice director of the Institute of Sociology (IOS) at the Vietnamese Academy of Social Sciences (VASS) in Hanoi and Vietnamese researchers from VASS.

2. Tran Thi Van Anh (Institute for Family and Gender Studies, Hanoi), personal communication, 2004.

3. For examples of social science research on sexuality in Vietnam, see Dang Nguyen Anh and Le Bach Duong n.d.; Blanc 2004; Colby, Nghia Huu Cao, and Doussantousse 2004; Le Bach Duong 2001; Ghuman et al. 2006; Go et al. 2003; Go et al. 2002; Tran Duc Hoa et al. 2007; Khuat Thu Hong 1998; Khuat Thu Oanh 2004; Nguyen Minh Thang, Vu Thu Huong, and Blanc 2002; Nguyen Thi Than Thuy, Lindan, Nguyen Xuan Hoan, Barclay, and Ha Ba Kiem 2000; Trung Nam Tran et al. 2004.

4. According to a Family Health International report, "Married male respondents estimated that based on personal experience, 70–90 percent of men they know had sex outside of marriage" (Tran Duc Hoa et al. 2007: 15).

5. For articles that do discuss the intersection between HIV infection and Doi Moi policies, see Tran Duc Hoa et al. 2007; Micollier 2004a, 2004c; Nguyen-Vo Thu-Huong 2002.

6. The market also targets women, but in a different way: whereas the market provides men with sexual services, it provides women with products geared toward their sexual and maternal selves, such as clothing, jewelry, lingerie, makeup, cribs, and strollers. Cribs and strollers symbolize a modern Western lifestyle.

7. Walters 2004 provides qualitative and quantitative evidence to demonstrate the value of prostitution to the Vietnamese economy at many levels.

8. During the early 1990s, karaoke bars were principally places where friends could go to sing. Some karaoke bars became known as *karaoke om* (hugging karaoke), where waitresses would keep the male singers company. Men used to tease each other by asking whether they had "karaoke arm" at the end of the evening. Gradually some businesses, big and small, began to provide private rooms for their male clients to sing with pretty girls. Some *bia hoi* (fresh beer) establishments became *bia om* (hugging beer) places, but these are public and not as popular as the *karaoke om*. At the same time, not all karaoke bars cater to men who are looking for women.

9. For a detailed description of the different kinds of sex workers in Hanoi, the kind of establishments they work in, and the range in cost, see Trung Nam Tran et al. 2004.

10. The "Happy Family" is notably different from the State's 1980s efforts to enact "The New Culture Family" campaign. The goal of that campaign had been to build a "new family" based on unity, equality, and mutual affection. The campaign promoted stable families, tried to reduce husbands' resistance to wives participating in social lives and employment opportunities outside the home, encouraged husbands to contribute to household labor, and advised parents on the necessity of educating their children (Pham Van Bich 1999). The "Happy Family" campaign represents a shift from a focus on building the nation to the economic success of the family, its withdrawal of support for women to work outside the home, and its lack of emphasis on the affective nature of marital relations.

11. Prior to Doi Moi, political standing had been considered an important factor for many individuals when choosing a spouse (Phinney 2008a).

12. Women's sexual needs are recognized but far less talked about. We talked to one woman whose husband, quite a bit older than she, was no longer able to satisfy her sexual needs. She said she secretly found sexual satisfaction elsewhere, but without telling her husband.

13. When we began this project, research on older women's sexual desires was scant. Our interviews with older women gave us the impression that many had not enjoyed or did not have the opportunity to enjoy sexual intercourse. One older woman said she had only ever had sex with her clothes on and in the dark. There was no privacy or space to experiment sexually with her husband. One woman did not enjoy sexual intercourse because she found it painful.

14. In this case, our informant did not acquiesce; she eventually divorced her husband, left

town, and moved to Hanoi, where she found another man to marry. Such accounts, however, are uncommon.

15. Tran Thi Van Anh, personal communication, 2004.

16. "The introduction of the market economy meant the loss of tens of thousands of state jobs. The evidence to date is that more women have been laid off from state-sector jobs than men" (Werner 2002: 34). This has led many women to turn to the informal sector and to home-based work, keeping women closer to home than their husbands.

17. This is ironic, because it reinforces the visible commodification of women's sexuality and bodies that allows the sex industry and sexualized leisure to flourish.

18. For an elaboration on the subject of the "eroticized" wife, see Nguyen-Vo Thu-Huong 2002.

19. I heard this joke frequently from married men (in their mid-twenties to late thirties) when I was living in Hanoi in the early 1990s and again in 2004. According to the folklorist Tran Quoc Vuong, whom I interviewed in 1996, it is thought to be a new joke that emerged after the advent of Doi Moi.

20. Migration studies indicate that 75 percent of the migrants are between the ages of thirteen and nineteen, and 48 percent are between the ages of twenty-four and thirty-three. Men migrate in slightly larger numbers than women. Hanoi currently has a population of 2.5 million, plus additional immigrants (300,000) from other provinces. As the population of Hanoi has grown, so has its urban land area. In 1960, the land area was fifty-eight square kilometers, and by 1998 it had grown to ninety-one square kilometers and is expected to grow to one hundred twenty-one square kilometers by 2010 (DiGregorio, Rambo, and Yanagisawa 2003). For further discussion on urban changes, see Douglas et al. 2002. For an in-depth study of female migrants, see Ha Thi Phuong Tien and Ha Quang Ngoc 2001.

21. For an examination of the way in which the changing mode of governing contributed to the increase in the sex industry, see Nguyen-Vo Thu-Huong 1998.

22. This ease of mobility can be compared to the situation during the early 1990s, when bicycling was the dominant mode of transport and there were very few cell phones.

23. Although we did not conduct any research among men who had migrated into the city, small-scale behavioral studies indicate that such men do seek the services of sex workers in Vietnam. See Nguyen Minh Thang, Vu Thu Huong, and Blanc 2002. On the relationship between migration and HIV in other countries, see Campbell 1997 and Hirsch et al. 2002.

24. Prior to Doi Moi, the government dictated what kinds of clothing people could buy, making such decisions as what kind of bathing suits were appropriate for women. For a discussion on changes in consumer goods, see Drummond 2006.

25. While I was in Hanoi in 2004, I was invited to a neighborhood Women's Union meeting. A university professor who teaches linguistics gave the women gathered together on a Thursday night a lecture on how to speak in a "cultured" manner. He advised them not to speak loudly or with harsh voices, but to speak softly. This was one route to becoming a civilized and refined individual.

26. If men used condoms with these extramarital sexual partners, there would be no inherent relation between these patterns of extramarital sexual intercourse and married women's HIV risk. Men we interviewed who engage in extramarital sexual intercourse typically said they used condoms with sex workers. However, behavioral studies of sex workers and their clients in Hanoi have indicated that condom use is low (Nguyen Minh Thang et al. 2002). In addition, the extremely high abortion rate in Vietnam indicates that many men are not using condoms to protect against pregnancy or sexually transmitted diseases (Henshaw, Singh, and Haas 1999). One divorced man said that there is no need to use a condom with high-class sex workers because they are clean. None of the men we interviewed felt it was necessary to use a condom with girlfriends or wives. Should one do so, both would be suspicious.

Chapter 5

1. Huli people tend to live in dispersed households rather than in centralized villages, and each family property is encircled by moat-like trenches, some eight or nine feet deep. Although often muddy and slippery, they can provide a high degree of privacy.

2. Many thanks to my field assistants: Ken Angobe, Luke Magala, Thomas Mindibi, and Michael Parali. They conducted almost all of the interviews with married men, and they were helpfully blunt about interview questions that didn't work. Moreover, they were all wonderfully and sometimes poignantly candid about the research process and about the uncomfortable things they were learning about their peers. I could not have asked for a better research team.

3. In 2002, some Huli—angry that they were not receiving more benefits from PJV—toppled many of the pylons, closing the mine for more than two months and causing PJV to lose millions of dollars. In order to prevent any similar recurrence, PJV opened a community liaison office in Tari, employed a number of Huli men as community liaison officers, and undertook a variety of development projects, such as building schools, maintaining roads, and paying "youth groups" (often ad hoc groups of unemployed young men) to carry out infrastructure repairs (such as cutting the grass on the Tari airstrip).

4. The causes of this rapid downward spiral into chaos during the early 2000s are complex, but many analysts blame provincial government corruption; the unequal distribution of royalties and other benefits from the gold, oil, and natural gas projects in the province; and longstanding ethnic conflict, particularly between the Huli and the Mendi (Haley and May 2007).

5. The Papua New Guinea National AIDS Council Secretariat and Partners (2008) estimated a 2009 HIV prevalence of 2.56 percent, with a projected increase to a more than 5 percent prevalence by 2012. The available epidemiological data indicate that unprotected heterosexual intercourse is the predominant mode of transmission, that almost equal numbers of men and women are HIV-positive, and that women are being infected at younger ages than men. Moreover, Papua New Guinea has a high prevalence of untreated sexually transmitted infections, which is likely contributing to the rapid spread of the HIV epidemic (Passey 1998; Malau and Crockett 2000). Tari District Hospital began testing for HIV in 1996, and by mid-2004 had documented seventy-two cases. The head nurse was familiar with all seventy-two documented AIDS cases, and her description of each case indicated that at least nineteen of the thirty-one women who were HIV-positive or who had died of AIDS-related illnesses were cases of husband-to-wife transmission. The remaining women had been infected either before marriage (when a woman was a student, for example) or through sex work.

6. This did not automatically preclude polygamy. Sometimes it was agreed that the second wife would live in her own house and that the husband would visit her but live in his first wife's house. Alternatively, if the first wife was much older than the second and had indicated that she was no longer interested in sex, then the husband would live with the second wife and visit the first. In point of fact, polygamy is increasingly rare among the Huli, primarily because few men can afford bridewealth for additional wives, but also because of condemnation of the practice by all area churches, many women's resistance to it, and perhaps an uneasy sense that people from other areas of Papua New Guinea who have never been polygamous or who have given it up think of the Huli as backwards in part because of their polygamy.

7. When I returned to Tari in 2006, a few very low-cost "guest houses" had sprung up, primarily to service laborers associated with PJV—for example, long-distance truckers delivering materials for the building of schools. A few women I knew sold sex at these guest houses.

8. From 1970 to 1995, a demographic database was maintained by the Tari Research Unit,

a branch of the Papua New Guinea Institute of Medical Research, through a system in which Huli men were hired to keep track of 500–1,000 people on their own clan territories and report all demographic events monthly.

9. Because Huli society is changing so rapidly, some people—especially in the younger generation—are ambivalent about or even openly rejecting of this construction of marital sexuality.

Chapter 6

1. This chapter would not have been possible without the generous support of Iganga residents, and particularly the men and women who entrusted me and my research team with sometimes culturally embarrassing answers to our even more culturally inappropriate questions about intimacy and sex. It is not intended to expose "exotic" sex practices of the "other" (for infidelity exists everywhere); rather, it attempts to address residents' deep concerns about the inhumane effects that HIV and fear of it have had on their communities, families, and intimate relationships. It is with this in mind that I respectfully write this chapter. All names in this article are pseudonyms. All identifiable characteristics of our informants have been removed to protect their confidentiality.

2. Like many of the middle-class and wealthy men in our study, Charles asked that I conduct his interview. Given the overlapping networks of Lusoga-speakers and public interest in behaviors of elite men, it may be that these men thought their secrets would be safest if not revealed directly to someone from within. One of our participants offered a different interpretation: he suggested that he wanted me to get the story right about being a man in Uganda.

3. In scholarship on Africa, the term "middle-class" refers to a socioeconomic group of educated Africans that began to emerge during the colonial period as part of an attempt to create a group of Africans who would serve as intermediaries between laborers (whether on farms, in industries, or in mines) and European rulers. For an extended discussion on class formation in Africa and the emergence of the African middle class see, for example, Mamdani 1976 on Uganda, and West 2002 on Zimbabwe. Anthropologist James Ferguson (1999) uses the terms "cosmopolitans" and "localists" to discuss two different social groups in Zambia whose orientation is either global or more local, respectively.

4. *Basoga* (plural) are the people; *Musoga* (singular) refers to one person; *Lusoga* is the language. *Basoga* also refers to customs or things belonging to this group, such as Basoga proverbs or marital practices. Before Idi Amin expelled East Indians from Uganda in 1972, Iganga had had a large number of Asian businesses. Since the late 1980s, Indians slowly have migrated back to Iganga Town. Initially, many of them opened fabric shops along Main Street. In the last decade or so, their presence has dramatically increased and they have branched out into a variety of other commercial businesses, including grocery and retail stores, electronics stores, and restaurants.

5. For scholarly articles that detail Uganda's early HIV prevention strategy, see Lyons 1997; Parkhurst 2001; Putzel 2004.

6. In Africa, the prevalence of HIV in selected antenatal (or prenatal) clinics is the most important source of data for HIV surveillance or monitoring. In countries with a generalized epidemic, these "HIV surveillance" (or sentinel) sites provide most of the official information about a country's HIV prevalence rate in the adult population as well as new infections, or incidence. At prenatal sentinel sites, anonymous blood samples from pregnant women are randomly selected to be tested for HIV. The percentage rate of infection among this sample is thought to represent prevalence in the wider population of adults between the ages of 15 and 49.

7. Social historians have produced a rich body of literature on gender and colonialism in sub-Saharan Africa. This literature examines how various colonial projects implemented

by the colonial administration, Christian missionaries, and European corporations tended to reinforce gender inequality through legal systems, economic policies, and Christian civilizing and domesticity efforts. These works also emphasize various ways in which ordinary women sought to utilize colonial structures or circumvent them to gain some agency. See Allman and Tashjian 2000; Cooper 1997; Jeater 1993; Musisi 1991; Schmidt 1992; and Summers 2000.

8. The Marriage and Divorce Acts of 1904 were intended to regulate secular marriages, the 1904 Marriages of Africans Act concerned non-Christian marriages, and the 1906 Marriage and Divorce of Mohammedans Act related to Muslims.

9. For useful reviews of the influence and significance of the Pentecostal movement around sub-Saharan Africa, see Gifford 1998 and Meyer 2004.

10. According to historical cultural convention, the process of betrothal was initiated by an agreement between the prospective groom and the father (or guardian, usually a man) of the bride. Betrothal was solemnized by the groom making a formal visit to the father of the bride (called "an introduction"), during which he presented a "letter" with money. The union was official after a ceremony between the groom's and bride's families established the bridewealth, which solidified the bond between the two families.

11. Major sugar plantations exist near Iganga; however, this does not seem to be a common type of work for men in the area. Rather, the manual labor force at the sugar companies is dominated by Nilotic groups from northern Uganda.

12. Connell (1995) and others use the term to refer to masculine practices of men who are marginalized from capitalist or other power structures. This seems particularly relevant here, because as men express fear and anxiety over the gender equality movement in Uganda, their own marginal status vis-à-vis global capital and politics becomes evident. For an excellent discussion of protest masculinity, see Wardlow, this volume.

13. Historically, *nakyewombekeire* referred to divorced or widowed women who went back to their fathers' lands or elsewhere and lived alone. Today, it also refers to single young women who are not attached to fathers or husbands and do not live with men.

14. Luganda is the most widely spoken African language in Uganda. It is spoken by the Baganda, who are the predominant ethnic group in the capital. Luganda is closely related to Lusoga, the indigenous language of Iganga. Everyone I met in Iganga understood Luganda, and in fact, people can often write Luganda better than Lusoga, given the elite position of the Baganda during colonial times, and because the Lusoga orthography was not standardized until recently.

15. I heard several women point out the irony in the final scene: Sophie exposes the mistress by pulling off her wig, yet Sophie herself is wearing a wig. As one woman remarked, "Who is the fake one?"

16. In the song, "helper" is a derogatory word used to refer to the mistress who acts as a surrogate in taking care of the man's sexual or emotional needs when the wife does not want to or is too tired to.

17. H. Abdallah, "Wives can divorce cheating husbands," *The Monitor* (Kampala, Uganda), March 11, 2004.

18. Women commonly expressed appreciation to the interviewer that someone cared enough about such mundane occurrences as infidelity and the marital problems it caused. More than a few women ended their three-part interview sessions by thanking the interviewer for listening to their grievances without passing judgment. Many women even commented on the need for marital counseling centers.

Conclusion

1. The first draft of the sections on extramarital opportunity structures and social risk was written by Constance A. Nathanson, and the sections on sexuality theory and policy

were drafted by Jennifer S. Hirsch. All of this book's authors, however, contributed in substantial ways to the chapter and to the underlying analysis that is represented here.

2. The table could be further complicated by adding the dimensions of social class and historical time (i.e., social change). We would argue, however, that each of these two variables operates through its impact on the relative availability of partners, space, and time.

3. These spaces are also, of course, an incentive. We defer discussion of the incentive dimension of opportunity structures to the next section.

4. Mary Douglas defines "risk" as "the probability of an event combined with the magnitude of the gains and losses that will entail." However, as she observes (and in her own usage), "From a complex attempt to reduce uncertainty, [risk] has become a decorative flourish on the word 'danger' " (2002: 40). "Risk," as it has come to be used by the public and by almost everyone else as well, means "unacceptable danger."

5. For an example of public shaming, see Kate Zernike and Abby Goodnough, "Lawmaker quits over e-mail sent to teenage pages," *New York Times*, September 30, 2006.

6. For more on the history of needle exchange policies in the United States, see Nathanson 2007.

7. The pledge requirement meant that organizations conducting any form of HIV prevention with commercial sex workers were in practice prohibited from working to enhance their access to medical care or to help protect them from police brutality, much less to work for decriminalization of sex work. The requirement did not go unopposed, and indeed the government of Brazil publicly refused to take any further money from the US government under those conditions, despite the considerable size of that country's epidemic and its corresponding need for prevention funding. See Steinglass 2005 and Masenior and Beyrer 2007.

8. For perspectives that differ from Epstein's, see Campbell 2003; Pisani 2008; Stillwagon 2006; and Thornton 2008.

9. Uganda's famous 1990s slogan on posters and billboards was "Love Carefully: Zero grazing is the answer." Zero grazing, a practice of having cattle stay in one place to eat, implied sticking to one partner.

10. In all fairness, there is a politics to this as well, as it represents our collective commitment to the progressive notion that governments can and should create the conditions that promote health.

11. *www.hekhshertzedek.org.*

12. While it may be inconceivable, not to mention inappropriate, to suggest internationally funded interventions that would have the goal of doing away with these homosocial spaces as a strategy for HIV prevention, it is hardly inconceivable that indigenous feminist movements might at some point call into question the legitimacy of these physical spaces and social institutions. In the United States, for example, the role of all-male clubs has been sharply reduced over the past several decades, so that a male politician aspiring to higher office would now be as unlikely to join an all-male club as he would be to join a club that did not admit blacks or Jews.

13. The widely replicated Men as Partners (MAP) programs, for example, seek to promote gender equality and reduce the risk of HIV transmission and domestic violence through encouraging men to critique particular attitudes and beliefs about masculinity; see *www.engenderhealth.org.*

14. This quote comes from the title of a post dated May 10, 2007, on the blog Kusala (*kusala1.blogspot.com/2007/05/men-are-in-fact-dogs.html*).

Bibliography

Abu-Lughod, L. (1991). Writing against culture. In *Recapturing Anthropology: Working in the Present*, ed. R. G. Fox, 137–62. Santa Fe: School of America Research Press.

Adams, V., and S. L. Pigg, eds. (2005). *Sex in Development: Science, Sexuality, and Morality in Global Perspective*. Durham: Duke University Press.

Ahearn, L. M. (2001). *Invitations to Love: Literacy, Love Letters, and Social Change in Nepal*. Ann Arbor: University of Michigan Press.

Allen, B. (1995). At your own risk: Studying Huli residency. In *Papuan Borderlands: Huli, Duna, and Ipili Perspectives on the Papua New Guinea Highlands*, ed. A. Biersack, 141–72. Ann Arbor: University of Michigan Press.

———. (2007). The setting: Land, economics and development in the Southern Highlands. In Haley and May 2007, 35–36.

Allen, E. S., and D. C. Atkins. (2005). The multidimensional and developmental nature of infidelity: Practical applications. *Journal of Clinical Psychology* 61 (11): 1371–82.

Allen, E. S., D. C. Atkins, D. H. Baucom, D. K. Snyder, K. C. Gordon, and S. P. Glass. (2005). Intrapersonal, interpersonal, and contextual factors in engaging in and responding to extramarital involvement. *Clinical Psychology* 12 (2): 101–30.

Allen, E. S., G. K. Rhoades, S. M. Stanley, H. J. Markman, T. Williams, J. Melton, et al. (2008). Premarital precursors of marital infidelity. *Family Process* 47 (2): 243–59.

Allison, A. (1994). *Nightwork: Sexuality, Pleasure, and Corporate Masculinity in a Tokyo Hostess Club*. Chicago: University of Chicago Press.

Allman, J., and V. Tashjian. (2000). *I Will Not Eat Stone: A Women's History of Colonial Asante, 1900–1925*. Portsmouth, NH: Heinemann.

Amaro, H. (1995). Love, sex, and power: Considering women's realities in HIV prevention. *American Psychologist* 50.

Anarfi, J. K. (1993). Sexuality, migration and AIDS in Ghana: A socio-behavioural study. *Health Transition Review* 3 (Supplement): 45–67.

Anastos, K., and C. Marte. (1989). Women—the missing persons in the AIDS epidemic. *Health/PAC Bulletin*. Winter: 6–15.

Appadurai, A. (1988). Putting hierarchy in its place. *Cultural Anthropology* 3 (1): 36–49.

———. (1996). *Modernity at Large: Cultural Dimensions of Globalization*. Minneapolis: University of Minnesota Press.

Atkins, D. C., D. H. Baucom, and N. S. Jacobson. (2001). Understanding infidelity: Correlates in a national random sample. *Journal of Family Psychology* 15 (4): 735–49.

Atkins, D. C., and D. E. Kessel. (2008). Religiousness and infidelity: Attendance, but not faith and prayer, predict marital fidelity. *Journal of Marriage and the Family* 70 (2): 407–18.

Avieli, N. (2007). Dog meat, music, song birds and orchids: The politics of Vietnamese masculinity. Paper presented at "Modernities and Dynamics of Tradition in Vietnam: Anthropological Approaches," Binh Chau Resort, Vietnam, December 15–18.

Bagarozzi, D. A. (2008). Understanding and treating marital infidelity: A multidimensional model. *American Journal of Family Therapy* 36 (1): 1–17.

Ballard, C. (1994). The centre cannot hold: Trade networks and sacred geography in the Papua New Guinea highlands. *Archaeology in Oceania* 29 (3): 130–48.

———. (2002). A history of Huli society and settlement in the Tari Region. *Papua New Guinea Medical Journal* 45 (1–2): 8–14.

Bamford, S. C. (2007). *Biology Unmoored: Melanesian Reflections on Life and Biotechnology.* Berkeley: University of California Press.

Barker, G. (2005). *Dying to Be Men: Youth, Masculinities, and Social Exclusion.* London: Routledge.

Barker, G., and C. Ricardo. (2005). Young men and the construction of masculinity in sub-Saharan Africa: Implications for HIV/AIDS, conflict, and violence. In *Social Development Papers, Conflict Prevention and Reconstruction.* Washington, DC: World Bank.

Barss, P. G. (1991). Health impact of injuries in the highlands of Papua New Guinea: A verbal autopsy study. PhD diss., Johns Hopkins University.

Barth, F. (1987). *Cosmologies in the Making: A Generative Approach to Cultural Variation in Inner New Guinea.* Cambridge, UK: Cambridge University Press.

———. (1999). Comparative methodologies in the analysis of anthropological data. In Bowen and Petersen 1999, 78–89.

———. (2005). Britain and the commonwealth. In Barth et al. 2005.

Barth, F., A. Gingrich, R. Parkin, and S. Silverman, eds. (2005). *One Discipline, Four Ways: British, German, French, and American Anthropology.* Chicago: University of Chicago Press.

Bernstein, E. (2007). Buying and selling the "girlfriend experience": The social and subjective contours of market intimacy. In Padilla et al. 2007, 186–202.

Beyrer, C. (2008). Hidden yet happening: The epidemics of sexually transmitted infections and HIV among men who have sex with men in developing countries. *Sexually Transmitted Infections* 84 (6): 410–12.

Bird, S. R. 1996. Welcome to the men's club: Homosociality and the maintenance of hegemonic masculinity. *Gender and Society* 10 (2): 120–32.

Blanc, M.-E. (2004). Sex education for Vietnamese adolescents in the context of the HIV/AIDS epidemic: The NGOs, the school, the family and the civil society. In Micollier 2004b, 241–62.

Blankenship, K. M., S. R. Friedman, S. Dworkin, and J. E. Mantell. (2006). Structural interventions: Concepts, challenges and opportunities for research. *Journal of Urban Health* 83 (1): 59–72.

Blau, P. M. (1994). *Structural Contexts of Opportunities.* Chicago: University of Chicago Press.

Bledsoe, C. H. (1990). Transformations in sub-Saharan African marriage and fertility. *Annals of the American Academy of Political and Social Science* 510:115–25.

Bledsoe, C. H., and G. Pison, eds. (1994). *Nuptiality in Sub-Saharan Africa: Contemporary Anthropological and Demographic Perspectives.* Oxford: Clarendon Press.

Blow, A. J., and K. Hartnett. (2005). Infidelity in committed relationships II: A substantive review. *Journal of Marital and Family Therapy* 31 (2): 217–33.

Blundo, G., and J.-P. Olivier de Sardan. (2006). *Everyday Corruption and the State: Citizens and Public Officials in Africa.* London: Zed Books.

Boas, F. (1940 [1896]). *Race, Language and Culture.* New York: Macmillan.

Boellstorff, T. (2005). *The Gay Archipelago: Sexuality and Nation in Indonesia.* Princeton: Princeton University Press.

Boholm, A. (2003). The cultural nature of risk: Can there be an anthropology of uncertainty? *Ethnos* 68 (2): 159–78.

Bourdieu, P. (1990). *The Logic of Practice.* Stanford: Stanford University Press.

Bourgois, P. (1996). In search of masculinity: Violence, respect and sexuality among Puerto Rican crack dealers in East Harlem. *British Journal of Criminology* 36 (3): 412–27.

Bowen, J. R., and R. Petersen. (1999). Introduction: Critical comparisons. In Bowen and Petersen 1999, 1–20.

———, eds. (1999). *Critical Comparisons in Politics and Culture*. Cambridge, UK: Cambridge University Press.

Brennan, D. (2004). *What's Love Got To Do with It? Transnational Desires and Sex Tourism in the Dominican Republic*. Durham: Duke University Press.

———. (2007). Love work in a tourist town: Dominican sex workers and resort workers perform at love. In Padilla et al. 2007, 203–25.

Briggs, C. (2003). *Stories in the Time of Cholera: Racial Profiling during a Medical Nightmare*. Berkeley: University of California Press.

Bryant, R. (2002). The purity of spirit and the power of blood: A comparative perspective on nation, gender and kinship in Cyprus. *Journal of the Royal Anthropological Institute* 8 (3): 509–30.

Burdette, A. M., C. G. Ellison, D. E. Sherkat, and K. A. Gore. (2007). Are there religious variations in marital infidelity? *Journal of Family Issues* 28 (12): 1553–81.

Butler, M. H., R. B. Seedall, and J. M. Harper. (2008). Facilitated disclosure versus clinical accommodation of infidelity secrets: An early pivot point in couple therapy; Part 2: Therapy ethics, pragmatics, and protocol. *American Journal of Family Therapy* 36 (4): 265–83.

Caldwell, J. C. (1976). Toward a restatement of demographic transition theory. *Population and Development Review* 2:321–66.

Caldwell, J. C., P. Caldwell, and P. Quiggin. (1989). The social context of AIDS in sub-Saharan Africa. *Population and Development Review* 19 (1): 185–233.

Campbell, C. (1997). Migrancy, masculine identities and AIDS: The psychosocial context of HIV transmission on the South African gold mines. *Social Science and Medicine* 45: 273–81.

———. (2003). *Letting Them Die: Why HIV/AIDS Intervention Programmes Fail*. Bloomington: Indiana University Press.

Carrier, J. (1985). Mexican male bisexuality. *Journal of Homosexuality* 11 (1–2): 75–85.

———. (1989). Sexual behavior and spread of AIDS in Mexico. *Medical Anthropology* 10 (2–3): 129–42.

———. (1994). Review of *Bisexuality and HIV/AIDS: A Global Perspective*, by R. Tielman, M. Carballo, and A. Hendriks. *Journal of Homosexuality* 26 (4): 178–81.

———. (1995). *De Los Otros: Intimacy and Homosexuality Among Mexican Men*. New York: Columbia University Press.

Carrillo, H. (2001). *The Night Is Young: Sexuality in Mexico in the Time of AIDS*. Chicago: University of Chicago Press.

———. (2004). Sexual migration, cross-cultural sexual encounters, and sexual health. *Sexuality Research and Social Policy* 1 (3): 58–70.

Carsten, J. (2000). *Cultures of Relatedness: New Approaches to the Study of Kinship*. Cambridge, UK: Cambridge University Press.

Cerrutti, M., and D. S. Massey. (2001). On the auspices of female migration from Mexico to the United States. *Demography* 38 (2): 187–200.

Cerwonka, A., and L. Malkki. (2007). *Improvising Theory: Process and Temporality in Ethnographic Fieldwork*. Chicago: University of Chicago Press.

Charsley, K., and A. Shaw. (2006). South Asian transnational marriages in comparative perspective. *Global Networks Affairs* 6 (4): 331–33.

Chen, A. (1999). Lives at the center of the periphery, lives at the periphery of the center: Chinese American masculinities and bargaining with hegemony. *Gender and Society* 13 (5): 584–607.

Cheng, S. (2007). Romancing the club: Love dynamics between Filipina entertainers and GIs in US military camp towns in South Korea. In Padilla 2007, 226–51.

Choi, K. H., J. A. Catania, and M. M. Dolcini. (1994). Extramarital sex and HIV risk behavior among US adults: Results from the National AIDS Behavioral Survey. *American Journal of Public Health* 84 (12): 2003–7.

Chukwuezi, B. (2001). Through thick and thin: Igbo rural-urban circularity, identity, and investment. *Journal of Contemporary African Studies* 19 (1): 55–66.

Clark, J. (1997). State of desire: Transformations in Huli sexuality. In *Sites of Desire/Economies of Pleasure: Sexualities in Asia and the Pacific*, ed. L. Manderson and M. Jolly, 191–211. Chicago: University of Chicago Press.

Clifford, J. (1988). *The Predicament of Culture: Twentieth-Century Ethnography, Literature, and Art*. Cambridge, MA: Harvard University Press.

Colby, D., Nghia Huu Cao, and S. Doussantousse. (2004). Men who have sex with men and HIV in Vietnam: A review. *AIDS Education and Prevention* 16:45–54.

Cole, J., and L. M. Thomas, eds. (2009). *Love in Africa*. Chicago: University of Chicago Press.

Cole, J., and E. Wolf. (1974). *The Hidden Frontier: Ecology and Ethnicity in an Alpine Valley*. New York: Academic Press.

Cole, S. C. (1991). *Women of the Praia: Work and Lives in a Portuguese Coastal Community*. Princeton: Princeton University Press.

Collier, J. F. (1997). *From Duty to Desire: Remaking Families in a Spanish Village*. Princeton: Princeton University Press.

Comaroff, J., and J. Comaroff. (1986). Christianity and colonialism in South Africa. *American Ethnologist* 13 (1): 1–22.

———. (1992). *Ethnography and the Historical Imagination*. Boulder: Westview Press.

———. Connell, R. (1987). *Gender and Power: Society, the Person, and Sexual Politics*. Stanford: Stanford University Press.

———. (1995). *Masculinities*. St. Leonards, Australia: Allen and Unwin.

———. (2003). Masculinities, change, and conflict in global society: Thinking about the future of men's studies. *Journal of Men's Studies* 11 (3): 249–67.

Connell, R., and G. W. Dowsett. (1999). "The unclean motion of the generative parts": Frameworks in Western thought on sexuality. In Parker and Aggleton 1999, 179–96.

Cooper, B. M. (1997). *Marriage in Maradi*. Portsmouth, NH: Heinemann.

Cornwall, A. (2002). Spending power: Love, money, and the reconfiguration of gender relations in Ada-Odo, Southwestern Nigeria. *American Ethnologist* 29 (4): 963–80.

Counts, D. (1993). The fist, the stick and the bottle of bleach: Wife bashing and suicide in a Papua New Guinea society. In *Contemporary Pacific Societies: Studies in Development and Change*, ed. V. S. Lockwood, T. Harding, and B. Wallace, 249–55. Englewood Cliffs, NJ: Prentice-Hall.

Craig, D. (2002). *Familiar Medicine: Everyday Health Knowledge and Practice in Today's Vietnam*. Honolulu: University of Hawai'i Press.

D'Emilio, J. (1997). *Intimate Matters: A History of Sexuality in America*. Chicago: University of Chicago Press.

———. (1998). *Sexual Politics, Sexual Communities: The Making of a Homosexual Minority in the United States, 1940–1970*. Chicago: University of Chicago Press.

Dang Nguyen Anh, and Le Bach Duong. (n.d.). *Issues of Sexuality and Gender in Vietnam: Myths and Realities of Penile Implants and Sexual Stimulants*. Hanoi: Institute of Sociology.

Das, V. (1995). National honor and practical kinship: Unwanted women and children. In *Conceiving the New World Order: The Global Politics of Reproduction*, ed. F. D. Ginsburg and R. Rapp, 212–33. Berkeley: University of California Press.

de Munck, V. (2000). Introduction: Units for describing and analyzing culture and society. *Ethnology* 39 (4): 279–92.

———. (2002). Contemporary issues and challenges for comparativists: An appraisal. *Anthropological Theory* 2 (1): 5–19.

de Zalduondo, B., and J. M. Bernard. (1995). Meanings and consequences of sexual-economic exchange: Gender, poverty, and sexual risk behavior in urban Haiti. In Parker and Gagnon 1995, 155–80.

de Zoysa, I., M. D. Sweat, and J. A. Denison. (1996). Faithful but fearful: Reducing HIV transmission in stable relationships. *AIDS* 10 (Supplement): S197–S204.

Debruyn, M. (1992). Women and AIDS in developing countries. *Social Science and Medicine* 34 (3): 249–62.

DiGregorio, M., A. T. Rambo, and M. Yanagisawa. (2003). Clean, green, and beautiful: Environment and development under the Renovation economy. In Hy Van Luong 2003.

Dinan, C. (1983). Sugar daddies and gold-diggers: White collar single women in Accra. In *Female and Male in West Africa*, ed. C. Oppong, 31–48. London: Allen, and Unwin.

Dollahite, D. C., and N. M. Lambert. (2007). Forsaking all others: How religious involvement promotes marital fidelity in Christian, Jewish, and Muslim couples. *Review of Religious Research* 48 (3): 290–307.

Donham, D. (2001). Thinking temporally or modernizing anthropology. *American Anthropologist* 103 (1): 134–49.

Douglas, M. (2002). *Risk and Blame: Essays in Cultural Theory*. New York: Routledge.

Douglass, M., M. DiGregorio, V. Pichaya, P. Boonchuen, M. Brunner, W. Bunjamin, et al. (2002). *The Urban Transition in Vietnam*. Vietnam: United Nations Development Programme.

Drummond, L. B. W. (2000). Street scenes: Practices of public and private space in urban Vietnam. *Urban Studies* 37 (12): 2377–91.

———. (2006). Gender in post–Doi Moi Vietnam: Women, desire, and change. *Gender, Place and Culture* 13 (3): 247–50.

Du, S. (2002). *"Chopsticks Only Work in Pairs": Gender Unity and Gender Equality among the Lahu of Southwest China*. New York: Columbia University Press.

Dupree, W. J., M. B. White, C. S. Olsen, and C. T. Lafleur. (2007). Infidelity treatment patterns: A practice-based evidence approach. *American Journal of Family Therapy* 35 (4): 327–41.

Dvorak, G. (2008). "The Martial Islands": Making Marshallese masculinities between American and Japanese militarism. *Contemporary Pacific* 20 (1): 55–86.

Dworkin, S. L., and A. A. Ehrhardt. (2007). Going beyond "ABC" to include "GEM": Critical reflections on progress in the HIV/AIDS epidemic. *American Journal of Public Health* 97 (1): 13–18.

Earl, C. (2003). Leisure and social mobility in Ho Chi Minh City. In *Social Inequality in Vietnam and the Challenges to Reform*, ed. P. Taylor. Singapore: Institute of Southeast Asian Studies.

Eggan, F. (1950). *Social Organization of the Western Pueblos*. Chicago: University of Chicago Press.

———. (1954). Social anthropology and the method of controlled comparison. *American Anthropologist* 56 (5): 743–63.

———. (1966). *The American Indian: Perspectives for the Study of Social Change*. Chicago: Aldine Publishing.

Ember, C., and M. Ember. (2001). Father absence and male aggression: A re-examination of the comparative evidence. *Ethos* 29 (3): 296–314.

Epprecht, M. (2008). *Heterosexual Africa? The History of an Idea from the Age of Exploration to the Age of AIDS*. Athens: Ohio University Press.

Epstein, H. (2005). God and the fight against AIDS. *New York Review of Books* 52 (7), April 28.
———. (2007). *The Invisible Cure: Why We Are Losing the Fight Against AIDS in Africa*. New York: Picador.
Esther, E. M. (2002). Gender, violence, and HIV: Women's survival in the streets. *Culture, Medicine, and Psychiatry* 26 (1): 33–54.
Fallers, L. (1957). Some determinants of marriage stability in Basoga: A reformulation of Gluckman's hypothesis. *Africa* 27:106–23.
———. (1969). *Law without Precedent: Legal Ideas in Action in the Courts of Colonial Busoga*. Chicago: University of Chicago Press.
Family Health International. (2007). *Behind the Pleasure: Sexual Decision Making Among High-Risk Men in Urban Vietnam*. Hanoi: FHI.
Fardon, R. (1990). *Localizing Strategies*. Washington, DC: Smithsonian Institution Press.
Farmer, P. (1999). *Infections and Inequalities: The Modern Plagues*. Berkeley: University of California Press.
Farmer, P., M. Connors, and J. Simmons, eds. (1996). *Women, Poverty, and AIDS: Sex, Drugs, and Structural Violence*. Monroe, ME: Common Courage Press.
Farmer, P., S. Lindenbaum, and M. J. D. V. Good. (1993). Women, poverty and AIDS: An introduction. *Culture, Medicine, and Psychiatry* 17 (4): 387–97.
Feldman-Savelsburg, P. (1994). Plundered kitchens and empty wombs: Fear of infertility in the Cameroonian grassfields. *Social Science and Medicine* 39 (4): 463–74.
Ferguson, J. (1999). *Expectations of Modernity: Myths and Meanings of Urban Life on the Zambian Copperbelt*. Berkeley: University of California Press.
Fortes, M. (1978). Parenthood, marriage, and fertility in West Africa. *Journal of Development Studies* 14 (4): 121–48.
Foucault, M. (1985). *The History of Sexuality*. New York: Pantheon.
———. (1991). Governmentality. In *The Foucault Effect: Studies in Governmentality*, ed. G. Burchell, C. Gordon, and P. Miller, 167–68. Chicago: University of Chicago Press.
Fox, A. M. (2009). Poverty or inequality as an underlying cause of HIV in Africa? The HIV-poverty thesis re-examined. PhD diss., Columbia University.
Fox, R. G. (2002). The study of historical transformation in American anthropology. In Gingrich and Fox 2002, 167–84.
Fox, R. G., and A. Gingrich. (2002). Introduction to Gingrich and Fox 2002, 1–24.
Frankel, S. (1980). "I am dying of man": The pathology of pollution. *Culture, Medicine, and Psychiatry* 4:95–117.
———. (1986). *The Huli Response to Illness*. Cambridge, UK: Cambridge University Press.
Friedman, S. R., and K. O'Reilly. (1997). Sociocultural interventions at the community level. *AIDS* 11:S201–S208.
Friedman, S. R., and G. Reid. (2002). The need for dialectical models as shown in the response to HIV/AIDS epidemic. *International Journal of Sociology and Social Policy* 22 (4/5/6): 177–200.
Fullilove, M. T., R. E. Fullilove, K. Haynes, and S. Gross. (1990). Black women and AIDS prevention: A view towards understanding the gender rules. *Journal of Sex Research* 27 (1): 47–64.
Gammeltoft, T. (1999). *Women's Bodies, Women's Worries: Health and Family Planning in a Vietnamese Rural Commune*. London: Routledge.
Geertz, C. (1973). Thick description: Toward an interpretive theory of culture. In *The Interpretation of Cultures: Selected Essays*. New York: Basic Books, 3–30.
———. (1974). "From the native's point of view": On the nature of anthropological understanding. *Bulletin of the American Academy of Arts and Sciences* 28 (1): 26–45.
Ghuman, S., M. L. Vu, T. H. Vu, and J. E. Knodel. (2006). Continuity and change in premarital sex in Vietnam. *International Studies in Family Planning* 32:166–74.

Giddens, A. (1992). *The Transformation of Intimacy: Sexuality, Love and Eroticism in Modern Societies.* Berkeley: University of California Press.

Giebel, C. (2001). Museum-Shrine: Revolution and its tutelary spirit in the village of My Hoa Hung. In *The Country of Memory: Remaking the Past in Late Socialist Vietnam,* ed. Hue-Tam Ho Tai. Berkeley: University of California Press.

Gifford, P. (1998). *African Christianity: Its Public Role.* London: Hurst.

Gillis, J. R., L. A. Tilly, and D. Levine. (1992). *The European Experience of Declining Fertility, 1850–1970: The Quiet Revolution.* Cambridge, MA: Blackwell.

Gingrich, A., and R. G. Fox. (2002). *Anthropology, by Comparison.* New York: Routledge.

Glasse, R. M. (1968). *Huli of Papua: A Cognatic Descent System.* Paris: Mouton.

———. (1974). Le masque de la volupté: Symbolisme et antagonisme sexuels sur les hauts plateaux de Nouvelle-Guinée. *L'Homme* 14:79–86.

Glassmann, M. (2003). Patterns of infidelity and their treatment, 2nd edition. *American Journal of Family Therapy* 31 (3): 229–31.

Global HIV Prevention Working Group. (2007). *Bringing HIV Prevention to Scale: An Urgent Global Priority. www.globalhivprevention.org.*

Gluckman, M. (1958). *Analysis of a Social Situation in Modern Zululand.* Manchester: Manchester University Press.

Glynn, J. R., M. Caraël, B. Auvert, M. Kahindo, J. Chege, R. Musonda, et al. (2001). Why do young women have a much higher prevalence of HIV than young men? A study in Kisumu, Kenya and Ndola, Zambia. *AIDS* 15 (Supplement 4): S51–S60.

Glynn, J. R., M. Caraël, A. Buvé, R. M. Musonda, and M. Kahindo. (2003). HIV risk in relation to marriage in areas with high prevalence of HIV infection. *Journal of Acquired Immune Deficiency Syndromes* 33:526–35.

Go, V. F., V. M. Quan, A. Chung, et al. (2002). Gender gaps, gender traps: Sexual identity and vulnerability to sexually transmitted diseases among women in Vietnam. *Social Science and Medicine* 55:467–81.

Go, V. F., C. J. Sethulakshmi, M. E. Bentley, S. Sivaram, A. K. Srikrishnan, S. Solomon, et al. (2003). When HIV-prevention messages and gender norms clash: The impact of domestic violence on women's HIV risk in slums of Chennai, India. *AIDS and Behavior* 7 (3): 263–72.

Godelier, M., and M. Strathern. (1991). *Big Men and Great Men: Personifications of Power in Melanesia.* Cambridge, UK: Cambridge University Press.

Goldman, L. (1983). *Talk Never Dies: The Language of Huli Disputes.* London: Tavistock.

Goldring, L. (1996a). Blurring borders: Constructing transnational community in the process of US-Mexico migration. *Research in Community Sociology* 6:69–104.

———. (1996b). Gendered memory: Constructions of rurality among Mexican transnational migrants. In *Creating the Countryside: The Politics of Rural and Environmental Discourse,* ed. M. DuPuis and P. Vandergeest, 303–29. Philadelphia: Temple University Press.

Goldstein, D. M. (2003). *Laughter Out of Place: Race, Class, Violence, and Sexuality in a Rio Shantytown.* Berkeley: University of California Press.

Goldstein, N., and J. L. Manlowe. (1997). *The Gender Politics of HIV/AIDS in Women: Perspectives on the Pandemic in the United States.* New York: New York University Press.

González, L. (1974). *San José de Gracia: Mexican Village in Transition.* Austin: University of Texas Press.

Gordon, K. C., D. H. Baucom, and D. K. Snyder. (2005). Treating couples recovering from infidelity: An integrative approach. *Journal of Clinical Psychology* 61 (11): 1393–1405.

Gray, R. H., D. Serwadda, G. Kigozi, F. Nalugoda, and M. Wawer. (2006). Uganda's HIV prevention success: The role of sexual behavior change and the national response. Commentary on Green, Halperin, Nantulya, and Hogle 2006. In *AIDS and Behavior* (10) 4: 347–50.

Grazian, D. (2007). The girl hunt: Urban nightlife and the performance of masculinity as collective activity. *Symbolic Interaction* 30 (2): 221–43.

Green, E. C. (2003). *Rethinking AIDS Prevention: Learning from Successes in Developing Countries*. Westport, CT: Praeger Publishers.

Green, E. C., D. T. Halperin, V. Nantulya, and J. A. Hogle. (2006). Uganda's HIV prevention success: The role of sexual behavior change and the national response. *AIDS and Behavior* 10 (4): 335–46.

Green, E. C., and K. Witte. (2006). Can fear arousal in public health campaigns contribute to the decline of HIV prevalence? *Journal of Health Communication* 11 (3): 245–59.

Greene, M. (2006). *SysteMALEtizing: Resources for Engaging Men in Sexual and Reproductive Health.* Washington, DC: Interagency Gender Working Group.

Gregor, T., and D. Tuzin. (2001). Comparing gender in Amazonia and Melanesia: A theoretical orientation. In *Gender in Amazonia and Melanesia: An Exploration of the Comparative Method*, ed. T. A. Gregor and D. Tuzin, 1–16. Berkeley: University of California Press.

Gugler, J. (2002). The son of a hawk does not remain abroad: The urban-rural connection in Africa. *African Studies Review* 45 (1): 21–41.

Gupta, G. R., D. Whelan, and K. Allendorf. (2003). Integrating gender into HIV/AIDS programmes: A review paper. Geneva: World Health Organization.

Gutiérrez, R. A. (1991). *When Jesus Came, the Corn Mother Went Away: Marriage, Sexuality, and Power in New Mexico, 1500–1846.* Stanford: Stanford University Press.

Gutmann, M. C. (1996). *The Meanings of Macho: Being a Man in Mexico City.* Berkeley: University of California Press.

———. (2003). *Changing Men and Masculinities in Latin America.* Durham: Duke University Press.

Guyer, J. (1994). Lineal identities and lateral networks: The logics of polyandrous motherhood. In Bledsoe and Pison 1994, 231–52.

Ha Thi Phuong Tien, and Ha Quang Ngoc. (2001). *Female Labour Migration: Rural-Urban.* Hanoi: Women's Publishing House.

Ha Vu. (2002). *The Harmony of Family and the Silence of Women: Sexual Behavior Among Married Women in Two Northern Rural Areas in Vietnam.* New York: Columbia University Research Track.

Haley, N. (2007). Cosmology, morality and resource development: Southern Highlands Province election outcomes and moves to establish a separate Hela Province. In Haley and May 2007, 57–68.

Haley, N., and R. J. May, eds. (2007). *Conflict and Resource Development in the Southern Highlands of Papua New Guinea.* Canberra: Australian National University E Press. *epress.anu.edu.au.*

Halperin, D., and H. Epstein. (2004). Concurrent sexual partnerships help to explain Africa's high HIV prevalence: Implications for prevention. *Lancet* 364 (9428): 4–6.

Halperin, D. T., M. J. Steiner, M. Cassell, E. Green, N. Hearst, and D. Kirby. (2004). The time has come for common ground on preventing sexual transmission of HIV. *Lancet* 364 (9449): 1913–15.

Hammar, L. (1992). Sexual transactions on Daru: With some observations on the ethnographic enterprise. *Research in Melanesia* 16:21–54.

———. (1996). Bad canoes and *bafalo*: The political economy of sex on Daru Island, Western Province, Papua New Guinea. *Genders* 23:212–43.

Hannerz, U. (1996). *Transnational Connections: Culture, People and Places.* London: Routledge.

Hardon, A. P., D. Akurut, C. Comoro, C. Ekezie, H. F. Irunde, T. Gerrits, et al. (2007). Hunger, waiting time and transport costs: Time to confront challenges to ART adherence in Africa. *AIDS Care* 19 (5): 658–65.

Harris, G. T. (1972). Labor supply and economic development in the Southern Highlands. *Oceania* 43:123–39.

Heise, L., and C. Elias. (1995). Transforming AIDS prevention to meet women's needs: A focus on developing countries. *Social Science and Medicine* 40 (7): 931–43.

Heise, L., M. Ellsberg, and M. Gottmoeller. (2002). A global overview of gender-based violence. *International Journal of Gynecology and Obstetrics* 78 (Supplement 1): S5–S14.

Henderson, R. (1972). *The King in Every Man: Evolutionary Trends in Onitsha Ibo Society and Culture*. New Haven: Yale University Press.

Henshaw, S. K., S. Singh, and T. Haas. (1999). The incidence of abortion worldwide. *International Family Planning Perspectives* 25:S30–S38.

Herdt, G. H. (1981). *Guardians of the Flutes: Idioms of Masculinity*. New York: McGraw-Hill.

———, ed. (1984). *Ritualized Homosexuality in Melanesia*. Berkeley: University of California Press.

———. (1987). *The Sambia: Ritual and Gender in New Guinea*. Fort Worth: Harcourt Brace Jovanovich.

Hirsch, J. S. (1990). Between the missionaries' position and the missionary position: Mexican dirty jokes and the public (sub)version of sexuality. *Critical Matrix* 5:1–27.

———. (2003a). *A Courtship after Marriage: Sexuality and Love in Mexican Transnational Families*. Berkeley: University of California Press.

———. (2003b). Anthropologists, migrants, and health research: Confronting cultural appropriateness. In *American Arrivals: Anthropology Engages the New Immigration*, ed. N. Foner, 229–57. Santa Fe: School of American Research Press.

———. (2004). "Un noviazgo despues de Ser Casados": Companionate marriage, sexual intimacy and fertility regulation in modern Mexico. In *Qualitative Demography: Categories and Contexts in Population Studies*, ed. S. Szreter, A. Dharmalingam, and H. Sholkamy, 249–75. Oxford: Oxford University Press.

———. (2008). Catholics using contraceptives: Religion, family planning, and interpretive agency in rural Mexico. *Studies in Family Planning* 39 (2): 93–104.

Hirsch, J. S., J. Higgins, M. Bentley, and C. Nathanson. (2002). The social constructions of sexuality: Marital infidelity and sexually transmitted disease—HIV risk in a Mexican migrant community. *American Journal of Public Health* 92:1227–37.

Hirsch, J. S., and S. Meneses Navarro. (2009). "Que gusto estar de vuelta en mi tierra": The sexual geography of transnational migration. In Thomas, Haour-Knipe, and Aggleton 2009.

Hirsch, J. S., S. Meneses Navarro, B. Thompson, M. Negroni, B. Pelcastre, and C. del Rio. (2007). The inevitability of infidelity: Sexual reputation, social geographies, and marital HIV risk in rural Mexico. *American Journal of Public Health* 97 (6): 986–96.

Hirsch, J. S., M. Muñoz-Laboy, C. M. Nyhus, K. M. Yount, and J. A. Bauermeister. (2009). They "miss more than anything their normal life back home": Masculinity and extramarital sex among Mexican migrant men in Atlanta. *Perspectives in Sexual and Reproductive Health* 41 (1): 23–32.

Hirsch, J. S., and C. A. Nathanson. (1998). Demografía informal: Cómo utilizar las redes sociales para construir una muestra etnografica sistematica de mujeres mexicanas en ambos lados de la frontera. *Estudios Demograficos y de Desarolio Urbano, México, DF; El Colegio de Mexico* 12 (1 and 2): 177–99.

———. (2001). Some traditional methods are more modern than others: Rhythm, withdrawal and the changing meanings of gender and sexual intimacy in the Mexican companionate marriage. *Culture, Health and Sexuality* 3 (4): 413–28.

Hirsch, J. S., and H. Wardlow, eds. (2006). *Modern Loves: The Anthropology of Romantic Love and Companionate Marriage*. Ann Arbor: University of Michigan Press.

Hochschild, A. R. (2003). *The Commercialization of Intimate Life: Notes from Home and Work*. Berkeley: University of California Press.

Hodgson, D. L. (2000). My daughter belongs to the government now. In *"Wicked" Women and the Reconfiguration of Gender in Africa*, ed. D. L. Hodgson and S. A. McCurdy, 149–67. Portsmouth, NH: Heinemann.

Holland, J., C. Ramazanoglu, S. Scott, S. Sharpe, and R. Thompson. (1990). Sex, gender and power: Young women's sexuality in the shadow of AIDS. *Sociology of Health and Illness* 12 (3): 336–50.

Hollos, M., and U. Larsen. (1997). From lineage to conjugality: The social context of fertility decisions among the Pare of Northern Tanzania. *Social Science and Medicine* 45 (3): 361–72.

Holy, L., ed. (1987a). *Comparative Anthropology*. Oxford: Basil Blackwell.

———. (1987b). Description, generalization and comparison: Two paradigms. Introduction to Holy 1987a.

Hue-Tam Ho Tai. (1992). *Radicalism and the Origins of the Vietnamese Revolution*. Cambridge, MA: Harvard University Press.

Hunt, N. R. (1991). Noise over camouflaged polygamy, colonial morality taxation, and a woman-naming crisis in Belgian Africa. *Journal of African History* 32 (3): 471–94.

Hunter, M. (2002). The materiality of everyday sex: Thinking beyond "prostitution." *African Studies* 61 (1): 99–120.

———. (2005). Cultural politics and masculinities: Multiple partners in historical perspective in KwaZulu-Natal. *Culture, Health and Sexuality* 7 (4): 389–403.

Hy Van Luong, ed. (2003). *Postwar Vietnam: Dynamics of a Transforming Society*. Lanham, MD: Rowman and Littlefield.

Iganga Municipality Profile. (2004). *www.amicaall.org/publications*.

Illouz, E. (1997). *Consuming the Romantic Utopia: Love and the Cultural Contradictions of Capitalism*. Berkeley: University of California Press.

Inhorn, M. C. (1996). *Infertility and Patriarchy: The Cultural Politics of Gender and Family Life in Egypt*. Philadelphia: University of Pennsylvania Press.

Interagency Coalition on AIDS and Development. (2005). Annotated bibliography: Gender, HIV/AIDS, and development. Ottawa: ICAD. *www.icad-cisd.com*.

Jacka, J. K. (n.d.). Land tenure, migration, and socioenvironmental changes in relation to gold mining at Porgera, Papua New Guinea. Manuscript under review.

Jeater, D. (1993). *Marriage, Perversion, and Power: The Construction of Moral Discourse in Southern Rhodesia, 1894–1930*. Oxford: Oxford University Press.

Jochelson, K., M. Mothibeli, and J. P. Leger. (1991). Human immunodeficiency virus and migrant labor in South Africa. *International Journal of Health Services* 21 (1): 157–73.

Kalema Commission. (1965). Report of the Commission on Marriage, Divorce and the Status of Women. Entebbe, Uganda: Government Printer.

Kaler, A. (2004). The moral lens of population control: Condoms and controversies in Southern Malawi. *Studies in Family Planning* 35 (2): 105–15.

Karanja, W. W. (1987). "Outside wives" and "inside wives" in Nigeria: A study of changing perceptions in marriage. In Parkin and Nyamwaya, 247–61.

Kelly, P. (2008). *Lydia's Open Door: Inside Mexico's Most Modern Brothel*. Berkeley: University of California Press.

Khuat Thu Hong. (1998). Study on sexuality in Vietnam: The known and unknown issues. Regional working paper, Population Council South and East Asia.

Khuat Thu Oanh. (2004). *How Do Vietnamese Youth Learn About Sexuality in the Family?* Hanoi: Institute for Social Development Studies.

Kimmel, M. S. (1987). *Changing Men: New Directions in Research on Masculinity*. Newbury Park, CA: Sage.

Kitschelt, H. (1986). Political opportunity structures and political protest: Anti-nuclear movements in four democracies. *British Journal of Political Science* 16:57–85.

Kline, A., E. Kline, and E. Oken. (1992). Minority women and sexual choice in the age of AIDS. *Social Science and Medicine* 34 (4): 447–57.

Knauft, B. M. (2002). *Critically Modern: Alternatives, Alterities, Anthropologies*. Bloomington: Indiana University Press.

Kuper, A. (2002). Comparison and contextualization: Reflections on South Africa. In Gingrich and Fox 2002, 143–66.

Kwiatkowski, L. (2008). Political economy and the health and vulnerability of battered women in Northern Vietnam. In *The Economics of Health and Wellness: Anthropological Perspectives*, ed. D. C. Wood, 199–226. Oxford: Elsevier.

Lamphere, L., and M. Z. Rosaldo, eds. (1974). *Women, Culture, and Society*. Stanford: Stanford University Press.

Lancaster, R. N. (1992). *Life Is Hard: Machismo, Danger, and the Intimacy of Power in Nicaragua*. Berkeley: University of California Press.

Laumann, E. (1994). *The Social Organization of Sexuality: Sexual Practices in the United States*. Chicago: University of Chicago Press.

Lavu, K. (2007). Porgera Joint Venture's presence in the Southern Highlands Province. In Haley and May 2007, 129–34.

Le Bach Duong. (2001). *Sexuality Research in Vietnam: A Review of the Literature*. Hanoi: Ford Foundation.

Le Minh Giang. (2007). Laboring in the space between state and family: Young men, migration, and HIV vulnerability in late socialist Vietnam. Paper presented at "Modernities and Dynamics of Tradition in Vietnam: Anthropological Approaches," Binh Chau Resort, Vietnam, December 15–18.

Le Thi. (1999). Social policies to prevent and contain prostitution in Vietnam. In *Ten Years of Progress: Vietnamese Women from 1985 to 1995*, ed. Le Thi and Do Thi Binh. Hanoi: Hanoi Women's Publishing House.

Lehmann, D. (2002). Demography and causes of death among the Huli in the Tari Basin. *Papua New Guinea Medical Journal* 45:51–62.

Lehmann, D., J. Vail, P. Vail, J. Crocker, H. Pickering, M. Alpers, and the Tari Demographic Surveillance Team. (1997). *Demographic Surveillance in Tari, Southern Highlands Province, Papua New Guinea: Methodology and Trends in Fertility and Mortality between 1979 and 1993*. Goroka: Papua New Guinea Institute of Medical Research.

Lemke, T. (2001). "The birth of bio-politics": Michel Foucault's lecture at the College de France on neo-liberal governmentality. *Economy and Society* 30:190–207.

Levine, R. (2001). The schooling of women: Maternal behavior and child environments. *Ethos* 29 (3): 259–70.

Levinson, B. A. U. (2005). Citizenship, identity, democracy: Engaging the political in the anthropology of education. *Anthropology and Education Quarterly* 36 (4): 329–40.

Lichter, D. T., F. B. LeClerc, and D. K. McLaughlin. (1991). Local marriage markets and the marital behavior of black and white women. *American Sociological Review* 96 (January): 843–67.

Luke, N. (2005). Confronting the "sugar daddy" stereotype: Age and economic asymmetries and risky sexual behavior in urban Kenya. *International Family Planning Perspectives* 31 (1): 6–14.

Lurie, M., B. Williams, K. Zuma, D. Mkaya-Mwamburi, G. P. Garnett, M. D. Sweat, et al. (2003). Who infects whom? HIV-1 concordance and discordance among migrant and non-migrant couples in South Africa. *AIDS* 17 (5): 2245–52.

Lusterman, D. D. (2005). Helping children and adults cope with parental infidelity. *Journal of Clinical Psychology* 61 (11): 1439–51.

Lyons, M. (1997). The point of view: Perspectives on AIDS in Uganda. In *AIDS in Africa and the Caribbean*, ed. G. Bond, J. Kreniske, I. Susser, and J. Vincent, 131–48. Boulder: Westview Press.

———. (2004). Mobile populations and HIV/AIDS in East Africa. In *HIV and AIDS in Africa: Beyond Epidemiology*, ed. E. Kalipeni, S. Craddock, J. R. Oppong, and J. Gosh, 175–90. Oxford: Blackwell.

MacIntyre, M. (2008). Police and thieves, gunmen and drunks: Problems with men and problems with society in Papua New Guinea. *Australian Journal of Anthropology* 19 (2): 179–93.

Mahoney, R. (1995). *Kidding Ourselves: Babies, Breadwinning, and Bargaining Power*. New York: Basic Books.

Mai Thi Tu, and Le Thi Nham Tuyet. (1978). *Women in Vietnam*. Hanoi: Foreign Languages Publishing House.

Malau, C., and S. Crockett. (2000). HIV and development the Papua New Guinea way. *Development Bulletin* 52:58–60.

Malungo, J. R. S. (2001). Sexual cleansing (kusalazya) and levirate marriage (kunkilila mung'anda) in the era of AIDS: Changes in perceptions and practices in Zambia. *Social Science and Medicine* 53 (3): 371–82.

Mamdani, M. (1976). *Politics and Class Formation in Uganda*. New York: Monthly Review Press.

Mann, K. (1994). The historical roots and cultural logic of outside marriage in colonial Lagos. In Bledsoe and Pison 1994, 167–93.

Mann, S. (2000). The male bond in Chinese history and culture. *American Historical Review* 105 (5): 1600–1614.

Marcus, G., and M. Fischer. (1986). *Anthropology as Cultural Critique: An Experimental Moment in Human Sciences*. Chicago: University of Chicago Press.

Marcus, G. E. (1995). Ethnography in/of the world-system: The emergence of multi-sited ethnography. *Annual Review of Anthropology* 24:95–117.

Marr, D. (1981). *Vietnamese Tradition on Trial 1920–1940*. Berkeley: University of California Press.

———. (2003). A passion for modernity: Intellectuals and the media. In Hy Van Luong 2003.

Martell, C. R., and S. E. Prince. (2005). Treating infidelity in same-sex couples. *Journal of Clinical Psychology* 61 (11): 1429–38.

Masenior, N. F., and C. Beyrer. (2007). The US anti-prostitution pledge: First Amendment challenges and public health priorities. *Plos Medicine* 4 (7): 1158–61.

Mason, K. O. (1994). HIV transmission and the balance of power between women and men: A global view. *Health Transit Review* 4 (Supplement): 217–40.

Mbulaiteye, S., C. Mahe, J. Whitworth, A. Ruberantwari, J. Nakiyingi, A. Ojwiya, et al. (2002). Declining HIV-1 incidence and associated prevalence over 10 years in a rural population in south-west Uganda: A cohort study. *Lancet* 360:41–46.

McCarthy, B. W. (2005). Treating infidelity: Therapeutic dilemmas and effective strategies. *Journal of Sex and Marital Therapy* 31 (1): 81–82.

McGrath J. W., C. B. Rwabukwali, D. A. Schumann, J. Pearson-Marks, S. Nakayima, B. Namande, et al. (1993). Anthropology and AIDS: The cultural context of sexual risk behaviour among urban Baganda women in Kampala, Uganda. *Social Science and Medicine* 36 (4): 429–39.

McNally, S. (2007). Constructing HIV in Vietnam. Paper presented at "Modernities and Dynamics of Tradition in Vietnam: Anthropological Approaches," Binh Chau Resort, Vietnam, December 15–18.

Meel, B. L. (2003). The myth of child rape as a cure for HIV/AIDS in Transeki: A case report. *Medicine, Science, and the Law* 43 (1): 85–88.

Merry, S. E. (2006). *Human Rights and Gender Violence: Translating International Law into Local Justice*. Berkeley: University of California Press.

———. (2009). *Gender Violence: A Cultural Perspective*. Oxford: Wiley-Blackwell.

Meyer, B. (2004). Christianity in Africa: From African independent to Pentecostal-charismatic churches. *Annual Review of Anthropology* 33: 447–74.

Meyer, D. S., and S. Staggenborg. (1996). Movements, countermovements, and the structure of political opportunity. *American Journal of Sociology* 101 (May): 1628–60.

Mgalla, Z., and R. Pool. (1997). Sexual relationships, condom use and risk perception among female bar workers in north-west Tanzania. *AIDS Care* 9 (4): 407–16.

Micollier, E. (2004a). Introduction. In Micollier 2004b.

———, ed. (2004b). *Sexual Cultures in East Asia: The Social Construction of Sexuality and Sexual Risk in a Time of AIDS*. London: Routledge.

———. (2004c). Social significance of commercial sex work: Implicitly shaping a sexual culture? In Micollier 2004c, 3–22.

Mill, J. E., and J. K. Anarfi. (2002). HIV risk environment for Ghanaian women: Challenges to prevention. *Social Science and Medicine* 54 (3): 325–37.

Ministry of Health and ORC Macro. (2006). *Uganda HIV/AIDS Sero-behavioural Survey 2004–2005*. Calverton, MD: Ministry of Health and ORC Macro.

Missildine, W., J. T. Parsons, and K. Knight. (2006). Split ends: Masculinity, sexuality and emotional intimacy among HIV-positive heterosexual men. *Men and Masculinities* 8 (3): 309–20.

Morris, H. F. (1967). Marriage law in Uganda: Sixty years of attempted reform. In *Family Law in Asia and Africa*, ed. J. N. D. Anderson. New York: Praeger.

Muñoz-Laboy, M., J. S. Hirsch, and M. A. Quispe-Lazaro. (2009). Loneliness as a sexual risk factor for male Mexican migrant workers. *American Journal of Public Health* 99 (5).

Munroe, R. L. (2001). Father absence, social structure, and attention allocation in children: A four-culture comparison. *Ethos* 29 (3): 315–28.

Murray, L., L. Moreno, S. Rosario, J. Ellen, M. Sweat, and D. Kerrigan. (2007). The role of relationship intimacy in consistent condom use among female sex workers and their regular paying partners in the Dominican Republic. *AIDS and Behavior* 11 (3): 463–70.

Musisi, N. B. (1991). Women, "elite polygyny," and Buganda state formation. *Signs* 16 (4): 757–86.

Nadel, S. F. (1952). Witchcraft in four African societies: An essay in comparison. *American Anthropologist* 54 (1): 18–29.

Nader, L. (1994). Comparative consciousness. In *Assessing Cultural Anthropology*, ed. R. Borofsky, 84–94. New York: McGraw-Hill.

Nathanson, C. A. (2007). *Disease Prevention as Social Change: The State, Society, and Public Health in the United States, France, Great Britain, and Canada*. New York: Russell Sage Foundation.

Nathanson, C. A., and R. Schoen. (1993). A bargaining theory of sexual behavior in women's adolescence. In *Proceedings of the IUSSP International Population Conference, Montreal*, 1:285–97. Liège, Belgium: International Union for the Scientific Study of Population.

Newmann, S., P. Sarin, N. Kumarasamy, E. Amalraj, M. Rogers, P. Madhivanan, et al. (2004). Marriage, monogamy and HIV: A profile of HIV-infected women in South India. *International Journal of STD and AIDS* 11:250–53.

Ngo Thi Ngan Binh. (2007). Imagination of a new political subjectivity: The social logics of "diplomatic" drinking in Ho Chi Minh City. Paper presented at "Modernities and Dynamics of Tradition in Vietnam: Anthropological Approaches," Binh Chau Resort, Vietnam, December 15–18.

Nguyen Huu Minh (1998). Tradition and change in Vietnamese marriage patterns in the Red River Delta. PhD diss., University of Washington.

Nguyen Minh Thang, Vu Thu Huong, and M.-E. Blanc. (2002). Sexual behavior related to HIV/AIDS: Commercial sex and condom use in Hanoi, Vietnam. *Asia-Pacific Population Journal* 17:41–52.

Nguyen Thi Than Thuy, C. P. Lindan, Nguyen Xuan Hoan, J. Barclay, and Ha Ba Kiem. (2000). Sexual risk behavior of women in entertainment services, Vietnam. *AIDS and Behavior* 4:93–101.

Nguyen-Vo Thu-Huong. (1998). Governing the social: Prostitution and liberal governance in Vietnam during marketization. PhD diss., University of California.

———. (2002). Governing sex: Medicine and governmental intervention. In *Gender, Household, State: Doi Moi in Vietnam*, ed. J. Werner and D. Belanger. Ithaca: Cornell University Southeast Asia Program Publications.

Nichter, M. (2002). The social relations of therapy management. In *New Horizons in Medical Anthropology: Essays in Honour of Charles Leslie*, ed. M. Nichter and M. Lock, 81–110. New York: Routledge.

O'Leary, A. (2000). Women at risk for HIV from a primary partner: Balancing intimacy. *Annual Review of Sex Research* 11:191–234.

O'Sullivan, L. F., A. Harrison, R. Morrell, A. Monroe-Wise, and M. Kubeka. (2006). Gender dynamics in the primary sexual relationships of young rural South African women and men. *Culture, Health and Sexuality* 8 (2): 99–113.

Oanh, K. T. H. (2004). *How Do Vietnamese Youth Learn About Sexuality in the Family?* Hanoi: Institute for Social Development Studies.

Obbo, C. (1987). The old and the new in East African elite marriages. In Parkin and Nyamwaya 1987, 263–80.

Orubuloye, I. O., J. Caldwell, and P. Caldwell. (1997). Perceived male sexual needs and male sexual behavior in Southwest Nigeria. *Social Science and Medicine* 44 (8): 1195–1207.

Orzeck, T., and E. Lung. (2005). Big-five personality differences of cheaters and non-cheaters. *Current Psychology* 24 (4): 274–86.

Ottenburg, S. (1959). Ibo receptivity to change. In *Continuity and Change in African Cultures*, ed. W. Bascom and R. Herskovits. Chicago: University of Chicago Press.

Padilla, M. (2007). *Caribbean Pleasure Industry: Tourism, Sexuality, and AIDS in the Dominican Republic*. Chicago: University of Chicago Press.

Padilla, M., J. S. Hirsch, M. Muñoz-Laboy, R. E. Sember, and R. G. Parker, eds. (2007). *Love and Globalization: Transformations of Intimacy in the Contemporary World*. Nashville: Vanderbilt University Press.

Pan American Health Organization. (2008). Fact sheet: Gender and HIV/AIDS. New York: World Health Organization. *www.paho.org*.

Papua New Guinea National AIDS Council Secretariat and Partners. (2008). *UNGASS 2008 Country Progress Report: Papua New Guinea*. Port Moresby: PNGNAC.

Parikh, S. (2001). Desire, romance, and regulation: Youth sexuality in Uganda's time of AIDS. PhD diss., Yale University.

———. (2005). From auntie to disco: The bifurcation of risk and pleasure in sex education in Uganda. In *Sex in Development: Science, Sexuality, and Morality in Global Perspective*, ed. V. Adams and S. L. Pigg, 125–57. Durham: Duke University Press.

———. (2007). The political economy of marriage and HIV: The ABC approach, "safe infidelity," and managing moral risk in Uganda. *American Journal of Public Health* 97 (7): 1198–1208.

Parker, R. (1985). "Masculinity, femininity, and homosexuality: On the anthropological interpretation of sexual meanings in Brazil. *Journal of Homosexuality* 11 (3–4): 155–63.

———. (1991). *Bodies, Pleasures, and Passions*. Boston: Beacon.

———. (2001). Sexuality, culture, and power in HIV/AIDS research. *Annual Review of Anthropology* 30:163.

Parker, R., and P. Aggleton, eds. (1999). *Culture, Society and Sexuality: A Reader*. New York: Routledge.

———. (2003). HIV and AIDS-related stigma and discrimination: A conceptual framework and implications for action. *Social Science and Medicine* 57 (1): 13–24.

Parker, R., and C. Caceres. (1999). Alternative sexualities and changing sexual cultures among Latin American men. *Culture, Health and Sexuality* 1 (3): 201–6.

Parker, R., and D. Easton. (1998). Sexuality, culture, and political economy: Recent developments in anthropological and cross-cultural sex research. *Annual Review of Sex Research* 9:1.

Parker, R., D. Easton, and C. H. Klein. (2000). Structural barriers and facilitators in HIV prevention: A review of international research. *AIDS* 14:S22–S32.

Parker, R., and J. H. Gagnon, eds. (1995). *Conceiving Sexuality: Approaches to Sex Research in a Postmodern World*. New York: Routledge.

Parker, R., R. Petchesky, and R. Sember, eds. (2007). *Sex Politics: Reports from the Frontlines*. New York: Sexuality Policy Watch. *www.sxpolitics.org*.

Parkhurst, J. (2001). The crisis of AIDS and the politics of response: The case of Uganda. *International Relations* 15:69–87.

———. (2002). The Ugandan success story? Evidence and claims of HIV-1 prevention. *Lancet* 360 (9326): 78–80.

Parkin, D., and D. Nyamwaya, eds. (1987). *Transformations of African Marriage*. Manchester: Manchester University Press.

Pashigian, M. J. (2002). Conceiving the happy family: Infertility and marital politics in Northern Vietnam. In *Infertility Around the Globe: New Thinking on Childlessness, Gender, and Reproductive Technologies*, ed. M. Inhorn and F. Van Balen, 134–51. Berkeley: University of California Press.

Passey, M., C. Mgone, S. Lupiwa, N. Suve, S. Tiwara, T. Lupiwa, et al. (1998). Community-based study of sexually transmitted diseases in rural women in the highlands of Papua New Guinea: Prevalence and risk factors. *Sexually Transmitted Infections* 74:120–27.

Peacock, J. (2002). Action comparison: Efforts towards a global and comparative yet local and active anthropology. In Gingrich and Fox 2002, 44–69.

Peel, J. D. Y. (1987). History, culture and the comparative method: A West African puzzle. In Holy 1987a, 88–118.

Pelzer, K. (1993). Socio-cultural dimensions of Renovation in Vietnam: Doi Moi as dialogue and transformation in gender relations. In *Reinventing Vietnamese Socialism*, ed. W. S. Turley and M. Selden. Toronto: York University.

Petchesky, R., and K. Judd, eds. (1998). *Negotiating Reproductive Rights: Women's Perspectives Across Countries and Cultures*. London: Zed Books.

Pettus, A. (2003). *Between Sacrifice and Desire: National Identity and the Governing of Femininity in Vietnam*. New York: Routledge.

Pham Van Bich. (1999). *The Vietnamese Family in Change: The Case of the Red River Delta*. Surrey: Curzon Press.

Phan Thi Thu Hien. (n.d.). Sexual coercion within marriage: A qualitative study in a rural area of Quanh Tri, Vietnam. MA thesis, University of Amsterdam.

Phinney, H. M. (2002). Asking for the essential child: Revolutionary transformations in reproductive space in northern Vietnam. PhD diss., University of Washington.

———. (2005). Asking for a child: The refashioning of reproductive space in post-war northern Vietnam. *Asia Pacific Journal of Anthropology* 6 (3): 215–30.

———. (2008a). Objects of affection: Vietnamese discourses on love and emancipation. *Positions: East Asia Cultures Critique* 16 (2): 329–58.

———. (2008b). "Rice is essential but tiresome; you should get some noodles": Doi Moi and the political economy of men's extramarital sexual relations and marital HIV risk in Hanoi, Vietnam. *American Journal of Public Health* 98 (4): 650–60.

Pickering, H., M. Okongo, B. Nnalusiba, K. Bwanika, and J. Whitworth. (1997). Sexual networks in Uganda: Casual and commercial sex in a trading town. *AIDS Care* 9 (2): 199–208.

Pigg, S. L. (1997). Authority in translation: finding, knowing, naming and training "traditional birth attendants" in Nepal. In *Childbirth and Authoritative Knowledge: Cross-Cultural Perspectives*, ed. R. E. Davis-Floyd and C. F. Sargent, 233–62. Berkeley: University of California Press.

Pilkington, C. J., W. Kern, and D. Indest. (1994). Is safer sex necessary with a "safe" partner? Condom use and romantic feelings. *Journal of Sex Research* 31 (3): 203–10.

Pisani, E. (2008). *The Wisdom of Whores: Bureaucrats, Brothels and the Business of AIDS*. New York: Norton.

Platt, R. A., D. P. Nalbone, G. Casanova, and J. Wetchler. (2008). Parental conflict and infidelity as predictors of adult children's attachment style and infidelity. *American Journal of Family Therapy* 36 (2): 149–61.

Pleck, J. H., F. L. Sonenstein, and L. C. Ku. (1993). Masculinity ideology: Its impact on adolescent males' heterosexual relationships. *Journal of Social Issues* 49 (3): 11–29.

Preston-Whyte, E. (1999). Reproductive health and the condom dilemma: Identifying situation barriers to condom use in South Africa. In *Resistances to Behavioral Change to Reduce HIV/AIDS Infection in Predominantly Heterosexual Epidemics in Third World Countries*, ed. J. Caldwell, P. Caldwell, J. Anarfiet, K. Awusabo-Asare, J. Ntozi, I. O. Orubuloye, et al. Canberra: Australian National University.

Pulerwitz, J., H. Amaro, W. De Jong, S. L. Gortmaker, and R. Rudds. (2002). Relationship power, condom use and HIV risk among women in the USA. *AIDS Care* 14 (6): 789–800.

Pulerwitz, J., and G. Barker. (2007). Measuring attitudes toward gender norms among young men in Brazil: Development and psychometric evaluation of the GEM Scale. *Men and Masculinities* 10:322.

Pulerwitz, J., G. Barker, M. Segundo, and M. Nascimento. (2006). *Promoting More Gender-Equitable Norms and Behaviors Among Young Men as an HIV/AIDS Prevention Strategy*. Washington, DC: Population Council.

Putzel, J. (2004). The politics of action on AIDS: A case study of Uganda. *Public Administration and Development* 24:19–30.

Radcliffe-Brown, A. R. (1950). Introduction. In Radcliffe-Brown and Forde 1950, 1–85.

Radcliffe-Brown, A. R., and D. Forde, eds. (1950). *African Systems of Kinship and Marriage*. London: Oxford University Press.

Razack, S. (2002). "Outwhiting the white guys": Men of colour and peacekeeping violence. *UNKC Law Review* 71 (2): 331–54.

Rebhun, L. A. (1999). *The Heart Is an Unknown Country: Love in the Changing Economy of Northeast Brazil*. Stanford: Stanford University Press.

Reddy, G. (2005). *With Respect to Sex: Negotiating Hijra Identity in South India*. Chicago: University of Chicago Press.

Reiter, R. R. (1975a). Introduction. In Reiter 1975b.

———, ed. (1975b). *Toward an Anthropology of Women*. New York: Monthly Review Press.

Rich, A. (1980). Compulsory heterosexuality and lesbian existence. *Signs* 5 (4): 631–60.

Romero-Daza, N., and D. Himmelgreen. (1998). More than money for your labor: Migration and the political economy of AIDS in Lesotho. In *The Political Economy of AIDS*, by M. Singer, 185–204. Amityville, NY: Baywood Publishers.

Rouse, R. (1991). Mexican migration and the social space of postmodernism. *Diaspora* 1 (1): 8–23.

Rubin, G. (1975). The traffic in women: Notes on the political economy of sex. In Reiter 1975b, 157–210.

Rydstrom, H. (2006). Sexual desires and "social evils": Young women in rural Vietnam. *Gender, Place and Culture* 13: 283–301.

Ryle, G. (1971). *Collected Papers.* Vol. 2. London: Hutchinson.

Sahlins, M. (1993). Goodbye to *Tristes Tropes*: Ethnography in the context of modern world history. *Journal of Modern History* 65:1–25.

Sanday, P. R. (2002). *Women at the Center: Life in a Modern Matriarchy.* Ithaca: Cornell University Press.

Sanday, P. R., and R. G. Goodenough, eds. (1990). *Beyond the Second Sex: New Directions in the Anthropology of Gender.* Philadelphia: University of Pennsylvania Press.

Sanders, E. J., S. M. Graham, H. S. Okuku, et al. (2007). HIV-1 infection in high risk men who have sex with men in Mombasa, Kenya. *AIDS* 21 (18): 2513–20.

Sandfort, T. G. M., J. Nel, E. Rich, et al. (2008). HIV testing and self-reported HIV status in South African men who have sex with men: Results from a community-based survey. *Sexually Transmitted Infections* 84 (6): 425–29.

Schensul, S. L., A. Mekki-Berrada, B. K. Nastasi, R. Singh, J. A. Burleson, et al. (2006). Men's extramarital sex, marital relationships and sexual risk in urban poor communities in India. *Journal of Urban Health* 83 (4): 614–24.

Scheper-Hughes, N. (1992). *Death without Weeping: The Violence of Everyday Life in Brazil.* Berkeley: University of California Press.

Schmidt, E. (1992). *Peasants, Traders, and Wives.* Portsmouth, NH: Heinemann.

Schneider, J., and P. Schneider. (1996). *Festival of the Poor: Fertility Decline and the Ideology of Class in Sicily, 1860–1980.* Tucson: University of Arizona Press.

———. (2002). The Mafia and al-Qaeda: Violent and secretive organizations in comparative and historical perspective. *American Anthropologist* 104 (3): 776–82.

Schoepf, B. G. (1988). Women, AIDS, and economic crisis in central Africa. *Canadian Journal of African Studies* 22 (3): 625–44.

———. (1997). AIDS, gender, and sexuality during Africa's economic crisis. In *African Feminism: The Politics of Survival in Sub-Saharan Africa*, ed. G. Mikell, 310–32. Philadelphia: University of Pennsylvania Press.

———. (2001). International AIDS research in anthropology: Taking a critical perspective on the crisis. *Annual Review of Anthropology* 30:335–61.

Schwandt, M., C. Morris, A. Ferguson, E. Ngugi, and S. Moses. (2006). Anal and dry sex in commercial sex work, and relation to risk for sexually transmitted infections and HIV in Meru, Kenya. *Sexually Transmitted Infections* 82:392–96.

Sedgwick, E. K. (1985). *Between Men: English Literature and Male Homosocial Desire.* New York: Columbia University Press.

Setel, P. (1995). AIDS as a paradox of manhood and development in Kilimanjaro, Tanzania. *Social Science and Medicine* 43 (8): 1169–78.

———. (1999). *A Plague of Paradoxes: AIDS, Culture, and Demography in Northern Tanzania.* Chicago: University of Chicago Press.

Sharma, A., E. Buklisi, P. Gorbach, et al. (2008). Sexual identity and risk of HIV/STI among men who have sex with men in Nairobi. *Sexually Transmitted Diseases* 35 (4): 352–54.

Shelton, J., D. Halperin, V. Nantulya, M. Potts, and H. Gayle. (2004). Partner reduction is crucial for balanced "ABC" approach to HIV prevention. *British Medical Journal* 328:891–93.

Sherrif, R. (2000). Exposing silence as cultural censorship: A Brazilian case. *American Anthropologist* 102 (1): 114–32.

Silverman, S. (2005). The United States. In Barth et al. 2005.

Simmons, C. (1979). Companionate marriage and the lesbian threat. *Frontiers* 4 (3): 54–59.

Sinnot, M. (2004). *Toms and Dees: Transgender Identity and Female Same-Sex Relationships in Thailand*. Honolulu: University of Hawai'i Press.

Skolnik, A. (1991). *Embattled Paradise: The American Family in an Age of Uncertainty*. New York: Basic Books.

Smith, D. J. (2000). "These girls today na war-o": Premarital sexuality and modern identity in southeastern Nigeria. *Africa Today* 47 (3–4): 98–120.

———. (2001). Romance, parenthood, and gender in a modern African society. *Ethnology* 40 (2): 129–51.

———. (2002). "Man no be wood": Gender and extramarital sex in contemporary Southeastern Nigeria. *Ahfad Journal* 19 (2): 4–23.

———. (2003). Imagining HIV/AIDS: Morality and perceptions of personal risk in Nigeria. *Medical Anthropology* 22 (4): 343–72.

———. (2006). Cell phones, social inequality, and contemporary culture in southeastern Nigeria. *Canadian Journal of African Studies* 40 (3): 496–523.

———. (2007). Modern marriage, extramarital sex, and HIV risk in southeastern Nigeria. *American Journal of Public Health* 97 (6): 997–1005.

———. (2008). *Intimacy, infidelity, and masculinity in southeastern Nigeria*. In *Intimacies*, ed. W. Jankowiak. New York: Columbia University Press.

Snyder, D. K., and B. D. Doss. (2005). Treating infidelity: Clinical and ethical directions. *Journal of Clinical Psychology* 61 (11): 1453–65.

Sobo, E. J. (1995a). *Choosing Unsafe Sex: AIDS-Risk Denial Among Disadvantaged Women*. Philadelphia: University of Pennsylvania Press.

———. (1995b). Finance, romance, social support, and condom use among impoverished inner-city women. *Human Organization* 54 (2): 115–28.

Solomon, H., K. M. Yount, and M. T. Mbizvo. (2007). "A shot of his own": The acceptability of a male hormonal contraceptive in Indonesia. *Culture, Health and Sexuality* 9 (1): 1–14.

South, S. J., and K. M. Lloyd. 1995. "Spousal Alternatives and Marital Dissolution." *American Sociological Review* 60:21–35.

South, S. J., K. Trent, and Y. Shen. (2001). Changing partners: Toward a macrostructural-opportunity theory of marital dissolution. *Journal of Marriage and the Family* 63 (3): 743–54.

Steinglass, M. (2005). The question of rescue. *New York Times Magazine*, July 24.

Stewart, R. G. (1992). *Coffee: The Political Economy of an Export Industry in Papua New Guinea*. Boulder: Westview Press.

Stoneburner, R., and D. Low-Beer. (2004). Population-level HIV declines and behavioral risk avoidance in Uganda. *Science* 302:714–18.

Strathern, A., and M. Lambek. (1998). Embodying sociality: Africanist-Melanesianist comparisons. Introduction to *Bodies and Persons: Comparative Perspectives from Africa and Melanesia*, ed. M. Lambek and A. Strathern, 1–25. Cambridge, UK: Cambridge University Press.

Stuart, B. (2004). Declining HIV rates in Uganda: Due to cleaner needles, not abstinence or condoms. *International Journal of STD and AIDS* 15 (7): 440–41.

Summers, C. (2000). Whips and women: Forcing change in eastern Uganda during the 1920s. Paper presented in the "Development and Change in East Africa" seminar, University of Nairobi, Kenya. July.

Susser, I. (2001). Sexual negotiations in relation to political mobilization: The prevention of HIV in comparative context. *Journal of AIDS and Behavior* 5 (2): 163–72.

———. (2002). Health rights for women in the age of AIDS. *International Journal of Epidemiology* 31:45–48.

Susser, I., and Z. Stein. (2000). Culture, sexuality and women's agency in the prevention of HIV/AIDS in southern Africa. *American Journal of Public Health* 90 (7): 1042–49.

Tarrow, S. (1998). *Power in Movement: Social Movements and Contentious Politics*. New York: Cambridge University Press.

Taussig, M. T. (1999). *Defacement: Public Secrecy and the Labor of the Negative*. Stanford: Stanford University Press.

Thomas, F., M. Haour-Knipe, and P. Aggleton. (2009). *Mobility, Sexuality and AIDS*. London: Routledge.

Thompson, B. (2005). Protecting your image: An ethnographic look at courtship and sexuality from the perspective of muchachas in a Mexican migrant-sending town. MPH thesis, Emory University.

Thornton, R. J. (2008). *Unimagined Community: Sex, Networks, and AIDS in Uganda and South Africa*. Berkeley: University of California Press.

Thurman, J. (1999). *Secrets of the Flesh: A Life of Colette*. New York: Knopf.

Tien, H. T. P., and H. Q. Ngoc. (2001). *Female Labour Migration: Rural-Urban*. Hanoi: Women's Publishing House.

Tiwara, S., M. Passey, A. Clegg, C. Mgone, S. Lupiwa, N. Suve, et al. (1996). High prevalence of trichomonal vaginitis and chlamydial cervicitis among a rural population in the Highlands of Papua New Guinea. *Papua New Guinea Medical Journal* 39:234–38.

Toft, S. (1985). Domestic violence in Papua New Guinea. (Monograph No. 3.) Port Moresby: Law Reform Commission of Papua New Guinea.

Tomsen, S. (1997). "A top night": Social protest, masculinity and the culture of drinking violence. *British Journal of Criminology* 37 (1): 9102.

Traeen, B., and M. Martinussen. (2008). Extradyadic activity in a random sample of Norwegian couples. *Journal of Sex Research* 45 (4): 319–28.

Tran Duc Hoa, S. Cohen, Nguyen Quy Nghi, Le Thuy Duong, Nguyen Thi Van, Pham Minh Anh, et al. (2007). *Behind the Pleasure: Sexual Decision-Making Among High-Risk Men in Urban Vietnam*. Hanoi: Family Health International.

Truitt, A. (2008). On the back of a motorbike: Middle-class mobility in Ho Chi Minh City, Vietnam. *American Ethnologist* 35 (1): 3–19.

Trung Nam Tran, R. Detels, Nguyen Tran Hien, et al. (2004). Drug use, sexual behaviors and practices among female sex workers in Hanoi, Vietnam—a qualitative study. *International Journal of Drug Policy* 15:189–95.

Uchendu, V. C. (1965). *The Igbo of Southeast Nigeria*. Fort Worth: Holt, Rinehart and Winston.

UNAIDS. (2008). Report on the Global AIDS Epidemic. Geneva: Joint United Nations Programme on HIV/AIDS.

UNAIDS, UNFPA, and UNDP. (2004). *Women and HIV/AIDS: Confronting the Crisis*. New York: Joint United Nations Programme on HIV/AIDS, United Nations Fund for Population Activities, and United Nations Development Fund for Women.

UNAIDS/WHO. (2008). *Epidemiological Fact Sheets on HIV and AIDS: Uganda, 2008 Update*. Geneva: UNAIDS/WHO Working Group on Global HIV/AIDS and STI Surveillance. *www.who.int/hiv*.

UNESCAP. (2003). *Economic and Social Progress in Jeopardy: HIV/AIDS in the Asian and Pacific Region*. New York: United Nations Economic and Social Commission for Asia and the Pacific. *www.unaids.org.vn*.

United Nations. (2003). *World Urbanization Prospects: The 2003 Revision*. New York: United Nations Publications.

United Nations Children's Fund. (2002). *Young People and HIV/AIDS: Opportunity in Crisis*. New York: UNCF.

United Nations Development Fund for Women. (2001). Gender dimensions of HIV/AIDS in

India. In *Summaries of Community-Based Research on the Gender Dimensions of HIV/AIDS.* New York: UNDFW.

United Nations Human Development Report 2007/2008. (2008). *Fighting Climate Change: Human Solidarity in a Divided World.* New York: United Nations.

Vail, J. (2002). Social and economic conditions at Tari. *Papua New Guinea Medical Journal* 45:113–27.

———. (2007). Community-based development in Tari—present and prospects. In Haley and May 2007, 107–22.

van der Straten, A., R. King, O. Grinstead, A. Serufilira, and S. Allen. (1995). Couple communication, sexual coercion and HIV risk reduction in Kigali, Rwanda. *AIDS* 9 (8): 935–44

van Griensven, F. (2007). Men who have sex with men and their HIV epidemics in Africa. *AIDS* 21 (10): 1361–62.

van Griensven, F., and E. J. Sanders. (2008). Understanding HIV risks among men who have sex with men in Africa. *Sexually Transmitted Diseases* 35 (4): 355–56.

Vance, C. (1991). Anthropology rediscovers sexuality: A theoretical comment. *Social Science and Medicine* 33 (8): 875–84.

Verma, R. K., J. Pulerwitz, and V. Mahendra. (2006). Challenging and changing gender attitudes among young men in Mumbai, India. *Reproductive Health Matters* 14 (28): 135–43.

Verma, R. K., J. Pulerwitz, V. Mahendra, and J. van Dam. (2004). From research to action: Addressing masculinity and gender norms. *Indian Journal of Social Work* 65 (4): 634–54.

VNMOH (Vietnamese Ministry of Health). (2005). *HIV/AIDS Estimates and Projections 2005–2010.* www.unaids.org.vn.

Walker, G. W. (2006). Disciplining protest masculinity. *Men and Masculinities* 9 (1): 5–22.

Walters, I. (2004). Dutiful daughters and temporary wives: Economic dependency on commercial sex in Vietnam. In Micollier 2004b.

Ward, D. B. (2004). Treating infidelity: Therapeutic dilemmas and effective strategies. *Journal of Marital and Family Therapy* 30 (4).

Ward, R. G. (1990). Contract labor recruitment from the highlands of Papua New Guinea, 1950–1974. *International Migration Review* 24 (2): 273–96.

Wardlow, H. (2002a). Headless ghosts and roving women: Specters of modernity in Papua New Guinea. *American Ethnologist* 29 (1): 5–32.

———. (2002b). Giving birth to *Gonolia*: "Culture" and sexually transmitted disease among the Huli of Papua New Guinea. *Medical Anthropology Quarterly* 16 (2): 151–75.

———. (2002c). Passenger women: Changing gender relations in the Tari Basin. *Papua New Guinea Medical Journal* 45 (1–2): 142–46.

———. (2004). Anger, economy and female agency: Problematizing "prostitution" and "sex work" in Papua New Guinea. *Signs* 29:1017–40.

———. (2006a). All's fair when love is war: Romantic passion and companionate marriage among the Huli of Papua New Guinea. In Hirsch and Wardlow 2006, 51–77.

———. (2006b). *Wayward Women: Sexuality and Agency in a New Guinea Society.* Berkeley: University of California Press.

———. (2007). Men's extramarital sexuality in rural Papua New Guinea. *American Journal of Public Health* 97 (6): 1006–14.

———. (2008a). "She liked it best when she was on top": Intimacies and estrangements in Huli men's marital and extramarital relationships. In *Intimacies: Love and Sex across Cultures,* ed. W. Jankowiak, 194–223. New York: Columbia University Press.

———. (2008b). "You have to understand: some of us are glad AIDS has arrived": Christianity and condoms among the Huli of Papua New Guinea. In *Making Sense of AIDS: Culture,*

Sexuality and Power in Melanesia, ed. L. Butt and R. Eves, 187–205. Honolulu: University of Hawai'i Press.

———. (2009). Labour migration and HIV risk in Papua New Guinea. In Thomas, Haour-Knipe, and Aggleton 2009.

Wardlow, H., and J. S. Hirsch. (2006). Introduction. In Hirsch and Wardlow 2006.

Warr, D. J., and P. M. Pyett. (1999). Difficult relations: Sex work, love and intimacy. *Sociology of Health and Illness* 21 (3): 290–309.

Watney, S. (1999). Safer sex as community practice. In Parker and Aggleton 1999.

Wawer, M. J., R. Gray, D. Serwadda, Z. Namukwaya, F. Makumbi, N. Sewankambo, et al. (2005). Declines in HIV prevalence in Rakai, Uganda: Not as simple as ABC. Paper presented at the 12th Conference on Retroviruses and Opportunistic Infections, Boston.

Weeks, J. (1986). *Sexuality*. London: Tavistock Publications.

———. (1989). *Sex, Politics, and Society: The Regulation of Sexuality Since 1800*. New York: Longman.

Wekker, G. (2006). *The Politics of Passion: Women's Sexual Culture in the Afro-Surinamese Diaspora*. New York: Columbia University Press.

Werner, J. (2002). Gender, household, state: Renovation (Doi Moi) as a social process in Vietnam. In *Gender, Household, State: Doi Moi in Vietnam*, ed. J. Werner and D. Belanger, 29–48. Ithaca: SEAP Publications.

West, M. O. (2002). *The Rise of an African Middle Class: Colonial Zimbabwe, 1898–1965*. Bloomington: Indiana University Press.

Whisman, M. A., K. C. Gordon, and Y. Y. Chatav. (2007). Predicting sexual infidelity in a population-based sample of married individuals. *Journal of Family Psychology* 21 (2): 320–24.

Whisman, M. A., and T. P. Wagers. (2005). Assessing relationship betrayals. *Journal of Clinical Psychology* 61 (11): 1383–91.

Whiting, B., and J. Whiting. (1975). *Children of Six Cultures*. Cambridge, MA: Harvard University Press.

Wiederman, M. W. (1997). Extramarital sex: Prevalence and correlates in a national survey. *Journal of Sex Research* 34 (2): 167–74.

Wingood, G. M., and R. J. DiClemente. (2000). Application of the theory of gender and power to examine HIV-related exposures, risk factors, and effective interventions for women. *Health Education and Behavior* 27 (5): 539–65.

Wojcicki, J. M. (2008). "She drank his money": Survival sex and the problem of violence in taverns in Gauteng Province, South Africa. *Medical Anthropology Quarterly* 16 (3): 268–93.

Wolf, E. (1999). *Envisioning Power: Ideologies of Dominance and Crisis*. Berkeley: University of California Press.

———. (2001). *Pathways of Power: Building an Anthropology of the Modern World*. Berkeley: University of California Press.

Wong, M. L., I. Lubek, B. C. Dy, S. Pen, S. Kros, and M. Chhi. (2003). Social and behavioural factors associated with condom use among direct sex workers in Siem Reap, Cambodia. *Sexually Transmitted Infections* 79 (2): 163–65.

Worth, D. (1989). Sexual decision-making and AIDS: Why condom promotion among vulnerable women is likely to fail. *Studies in Family Planning* 20 (6): 297–307.

Yan, Y. (2003). *Private Life Under Socialism: Love, Intimacy, and Family Change in a Chinese Village, 1949–1999*. Stanford: Stanford University Press.

Young, K. S. (2008). Internet sex addiction: Risk factors, stages of development, and treatment. *American Behavioral Scientist* 52 (1): 21–37.

Young, R. M., and I. H. Meyer. (2005). The trouble with "MSM" and "WSW": Erasure of the sexual-minority person in public health discourse. *American Journal of Public Health* 95 (7): 1144–49.

Zaba, B. W., L. M. Carpenter, J. T. Boerma, S. Gregson, J. Nakiyingi, and M. Urassa. (2000). Adjusting ante-natal clinic data for improved estimates of HIV prevalence among women in sub-Saharan Africa. *AIDS*: 2741–50.

Zaloom, C. (2004). The productive life of risk. *Cultural Anthropology* 19 (3): 365–91.

Zierler, S., and N. Krieger. (1997). Reframing women's risk: Social inequalities and HIV infection. *Annual Review of Public Health* 18:401–36.

Zimmer-Tamakoshi, L. (1997). Wild pigs and dog men: Rape and domestic violence as women's issues in Papua New Guinea. In *Gender in Cross-Cultural Perspective*, ed. C. B. Brettell and C. F. Sargent, 538–53. Upper Saddle River, NJ: Prentice-Hall.

Index

Page numbers in bold indicate illustrations.

About the Authors

Jennifer S. Hirsch, Associate Professor of Sociomedical Sciences in the Mailman School of Public Health at Columbia University, is the author of *A Courtship after Marriage: Sexuality and Love in Mexican Transnational Families* and co-editor of two recent volumes on the comparative anthropology of love.

Holly Wardlow, Associate Professor of Anthropology at the University of Toronto, is the author of *Wayward Women: Sexuality and Agency in a New Guinea Society.*

Daniel Jordan Smith, Associate Professor of Anthropology and Associate Director of the Population Studies and Training Center at Brown University, is the author of *A Culture of Corruption: Everyday Deception and Popular Discontent in Nigeria.*

Harriet M. Phinney is a lecturer at Seattle University.

Shanti Parikh is Assistant Professor of Anthropology, Washington University in St. Louis.

Constance A. Nathanson, Professor of Clinical Sociomedical Sciences and Professor of Population and Family Health in the Mailman School of Public Health at Columbia University, is the author of *Disease Prevention as Social Change* and *Dangerous Passage: The Social Control of Sexuality in Women's Adolescence.*